AWAKENINGS

BY OLIVER SACKS

Migraine

Awakenings

A Leg to Stand On

The Man Who Mistook His Wife for a Hat

Seeing Voices

Oliver Sacks

AWAKENINGS

HarperPerennial
A Division of HarperCollinsPublishers

I am grateful to the following for quotations from copyright material: from Ernest Jones, *The Life and Work of Sigmund Freud,* to Mrs Katherine Jones, The Hogarth Press Ltd and Basic Books Inc.; from *The Complete Poems of D. H. Lawrence,* to Laurence Pollinger Ltd and the Estate of the late Mrs Frieda Lawrence, William Heinemann Ltd and The Viking Press Inc.; from Ludwig Wittgenstein, *Philosophical Investigations,* to the literary executors of Ludwig Wittgenstein, Basil Blackwell & Mott Ltd and The Macmillan Company, New York; from John Maynard Keynes, *Collected Writings,* to the Royal Economic Society, Macmillan, London and Basingstoke, Ltd and St Martin's Press Inc.; from T. S. Eliot, *Collected Poems 1909–1962,* to Faber & Faber Ltd and Harcourt Brace Jovanovich Inc.

First HarperPerennial edition

Designed by Helene Berinsky

Library of Congress Cataloging-in-Publication Data

Sacks, Oliver W.
  Awakenings / Oliver Sacks.
    p. cm.
  "First Perennial Library edition"—T.p. verso.
  Originally published: London : Duckworth, 1973.
  Includes bibliographical references and index.
  ISBN 0-06-097368-4 (pbk.)
    1. Parkinsonism, Postencephalitic—Case studies. 2. Encephalitis, Epidemic—Complications and sequelae—Case studies. 3. Dopa—Therapeutic use—Case studies. I. Title.
RC382.S23 1990
616.8'32—dc20   90-4914

90 91 92 93 94 CC/FG 10 9 8 7 6 5 4 3 2 1

To the memory of W. H. Auden
and A. R. Luria

. . . and now, a preternatural
birth in returning to life
from this sickness

—DONNE

CONTENTS

Acknowledgements xiii

Preface to the Original Edition xvii

Preface to the 1990 Edition xxi

Foreword to the 1990 Edition xxv

Prologue

PARKINSON'S DISEASE AND PARKINSONISM 3

THE SLEEPING-SICKNESS *(Encephalitis Lethargica)* 12

THE AFTERMATH OF THE SLEEPING-SICKNESS (1927–67) 20

LIFE AT MOUNT CARMEL 24

THE COMING OF L-DOPA 28

Awakenings

FRANCES D. 39

MAGDA B. 67

ROSE R. 74

ROBERT O. 88

HESTER Y. 95

ROLANDO P. 116

MIRIAM H. 128

LUCY K. 140

MARGARET A. 148

MIRON V.   161

GERTIE C.   165

MARTHA N.   170

IDA T.   176

FRANK G.   180

MARIA G.   183

RACHEL I.   188

AARON E.   190

GEORGE W.   198

CECIL M.   202

LEONARD L.   203

Perspectives

PERSPECTIVES   223

AWAKENING   235

TRIBULATION   243

ACCOMMODATION   265

Epilogue (1982)   277

Postscript (1990)   313

Appendices

A HISTORY OF THE SLEEPING-SICKNESS   319

'MIRACLE' DRUGS: FREUD, WILLIAM JAMES,
AND HAVELOCK ELLIS   323

THE ELECTRICAL BASIS OF AWAKENINGS   327

BEYOND L-DOPA   333

PARKINSONIAN SPACE AND TIME   339

CHAOS AND AWAKENINGS   351

AWAKENINGS ON STAGE AND SCREEN   367

Glossary 387

Bibliography 395

Index 402

Photo insert follows page 184

ACKNOWLEDGEMENTS

My first (and infinite) debt is to the remarkable patients at Mount Carmel Hospital, New York, whose stories I relate in this book, and to whom *Awakenings* was originally dedicated.

It is difficult now, looking back over a quarter of a century, to recall all of those at Mount Carmel who were concerned with our patients, and who directly or indirectly contributed to *Awakenings;* but I have warm memories of the nursing staff – Ellen Costello, Eleanor Gaynor, Janice Grey, and Melanie Epps; of the medical staff – Walter Schwartz, Charles Messeloff, Jack Sobel, and Flora Tabbador; of our speech therapist, and my closest helpmate in the crucial three years when our patients were being awakened, Margie Kohl Inglis; of our EEG technician, who was my collaborator on 'The Electrical Basis of Awakenings,' Chris Carolan; of our pharmacist, Bob Malta, who spent hours encapsulating L-DOPA, surrounded by clouds of dopaminergic dust; and of devoted occupational and physiotherapists. I have to single out our music therapists – Kitty Stiles in the early years of our patients' awakenings, and Connie Tomaino since – with whom I have had the closest relation, for music has been the profoundest non-chemical medication for our patients.

I owe a special debt to my English colleagues at the Highlands Hospital, for enabling me to keep in touch with an extraordinary group of patients, profoundly similar to, yet profoundly different from, ours at Mount Carmel. In particular, I must acknowledge the friendly assistance of Gerald Stern and Donald Calne, who helped 'awaken' these patients in 1969; James Sharkey and Rodwin Jackson, who between them have looked after these patients since 1945; Bernard Thompson, a nurse who was with the patients for many years; and, above all, James Purdon Martin, who had known these (and other) post-encephalitic patients for more than sixty years. He made a special visit to Mount Carmel in 1969, to see our patients in the first flush of their 'awakenings,' and was thereafter something of a father figure and a guide.

Innumerable other colleagues and friends have helped me, or *Awakenings,* along the way: D. P. dePaola, Roger Duvoisin, Stanley Fahn (and the Basal Ganglia Club), Ilan Golani, Elkhonon Goldberg, Mark Homonoff, William Langston, Andrew Lees, Margery Mark, Jonathan Mueller, H. Narabayashi, Isabelle Rapin, Robert Rodman, Israel Rosenfield, Sheldon Ross, Richard Shaw, Bob Wasserman. Among these I should especially mention Jonathan Miller, who preserved a copy of the 1969 manuscript, when I had destroyed the original, and conveyed this to Colin Haycraft, my first editor-publisher (and who, much later, was to make the remarkable BBC film portrait of Ivan Vaughan, *Ivan*); Eric Korn, who helped edit the 1976 edition; Lawrence Weschler, who knew many of the post-encephalitic patients at Mount Carmel, and has discussed aspects of *Awakenings* with me in every way, intensively, for ten years; and Ralph Siegel, who is now working with me on chaos theory and 'awakenings.'

A special place must be reserved for those colleagues who are themselves patients, and who know and can describe the world of the Parkinsonian with an incomparable authority, from the inside. Among these have been Ivan Vaughan, Sidney Dorros, and Cecil Todes (all of whom have written their own accounts of living with Parkinson's); and Ed Weinberger, who has provided powerful insights and images for me in innumerable ways. Many people with Tourette's syndrome have helped me to understand their own condition, a condition with many similarities to that of hyperkinetic encephalitis. Finally, my own post-encephalitic patient, Lillian Tighe, whom I have known now for over twenty years: Lillian was central in the documentary film of *Awakenings,* and was an inspiration during the making of the feature film of it too.

Many people have devoted their creative talents to writing, producing, or performing dramatic versions of *Awakenings:* first and foremost, Duncan Dallas, of Yorkshire Television, who made a beautiful documentary film of *Awakenings* in 1973 – this contains unforgettable images of the patients and events I write of in *Awakenings,* and I wish could be seen by everyone who reads it; Harold Pinter, who in 1982 sent me an extraordinary play *(A Kind of Alaska)* inspired by *Awakenings,* which was first performed in England at the National Theatre in October of that year; John Reeves, who produced a moving radio adaptation of *Awakenings* for the Canadian Broadcasting Corporation in 1987; Arnold Aprill of City Lit, who masterminded a remarkable stage version in Chicago in 1987; Carmel Ross, who produced an audio version of *Awakenings;* and now the cast and crew of the feature film of *Awakenings* – in particular, Walter Parkes and Larry Lasker, its producers; Steve Zaillian, its screenwriter; Penny Marshall, its director; and, of course, its great actors, Robert De Niro and Robin Williams.

Finally, I am grateful to my agent, Suzanne Gluck, and to the many editors of *Awakenings,* who have guided it through its many editions in the last seventeen years: Colin Haycraft, Ken McCormick, Julia Vellacott, Anne Freedgood, Mike Petty, Bill Whitehead, Jim Silberman, Rick Kot, and Kate Edgar. Though it is invidious to single out names, I must single out the first and the last of these: Colin Haycraft of Duckworth, whose faith in me, and *maieuticê technê,* allowed the original edition to be brought forth in 1973; and Kate Edgar, who has helped bring to birth this present, greatly enlarged edition.

In the second edition I made two very special acknowledgements – to W. H. Auden and A. R. Luria, who were mentors, friends, and 'awakeners' to me. I now omit these, but dedicate *Awakenings,* in gratitude and love, to the memory of these two men.

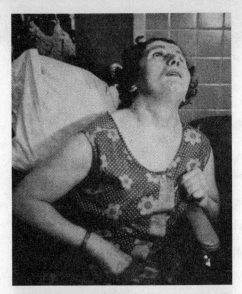

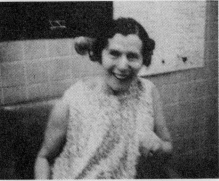

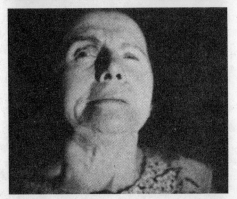

*Rose R.: entranced, awakened,
and blocked.*

PREFACE TO THE ORIGINAL EDITION

The theme of this book is the lives and reactions of certain patients in a unique situation – and the implications which these hold out for medicine and science. These patients are among the few survivors of the great sleeping-sickness epidemic *(encephalitis lethargica)* of fifty years ago, and their reactions are those brought about by a remarkable new 'awakening' drug (laevodihydroxy-phenylalanine, or L-DOPA). The lives and responses of these patients, which have no real precedent in the entire history of medicine, are presented in the form of extended case-histories or biographies: these form the major part of the book. Preceding these case-histories are introductory remarks on the nature of their illnesses, the sort of lives they have led since first being taken ill, and something about the drug which has transformed their lives. Such a subject might seem to be of very special or limited interest, but this, I believe, is by no means the case. In the latter part of the book, I have tried to indicate some of the far-reaching implications which arise from the subject – implications which extend to the most general questions of health, disease, suffering, care, and the human condition in general.

In a book such as this – about living people – a difficult, perhaps insuperable, problem arises: that of conveying detailed information without betraying professional and personal confidence. I have had to change the names of my patients, the name and location of the hospital where they live, and certain other circumstantial details. I have, however, tried to preserve what is important and essential – the real and full *presence* of the patients themselves, the 'feeling' of their lives, their characters, their illnesses, their responses – the essential qualities of their strange situation.

The general style of this book – with its alternation of narrative and reflection, its proliferation of images and metaphors, its remarks, repetitions, asides, and footnotes – is one which I have been impelled towards by the very nature of the subject-matter. My aim is not to make a system, or to see patients as systems, but to picture a world, a variety of worlds – the landscapes of being in which these patients reside. And the picturing of worlds requires not a static and systematic formulation, but an active exploration of images and views, a continual jumping-about and imaginative *movement*. The stylistic (and epistemological) problems encountered have been precisely those described by Wittgenstein in the Preface to *Philosophical Investigations* when he spoke of the necessity of depicting landscapes (thoughtscapes) by images and 'remarks':

> . . . This was, of course, connected with the very nature of the investigation. For this compels us to travel over a wide field of thought criss-cross in every direction. The . . . remarks in this book are, as it were, a number of sketches of landscapes which were made in the course of these long and involved journeyings. The same or almost the same points were always being approached from different directions, and new sketches made . . . Thus this book is really only an album.

Running throughout the book is a metaphysical theme – the notion that it is insufficient to consider disease in purely mechanical or chemical terms; that it must be considered equally in biological or metaphysical terms, i.e. in terms of organization and design. In my first book, *Migraine,* I suggested the necessity of such a *double* approach, and in the present work I develop this theme in much greater detail. Such a notion is far from new – it was understood very clearly in classical medicine. In present-day medicine, by contrast, there is an almost exclusively technical or mechanical emphasis, which has led to immense advances, but also to intellectual regression, and a lack of proper attention to the full needs and feelings of patients. This book represents an attempt to regain and restore this metaphysical attention.

I have found the writing unexpectedly difficult, although its ideas and intentions are simple and straightforward. But one cannot go straight forward unless the way is clear, and the way is *allowed*. One struggles to gain the right perspective, focus, and tone – and then, one loses it, all unawares. One must continually fight to regain it, to hold accurate awareness. I cannot better express the problems which have challenged me, and which my readers must challenge, than in the splendid words of Maynard Keynes in the Preface to his *General Theory:*

> The composition of this book has been for the author a long struggle of escape, and so must the reading of it be for most readers if the author's assault upon them is to be successful – a struggle of escape from habitual modes of thought and expression. The ideas which are here expressed so laboriously are extremely simple and should be obvious. The difficulty lies, not in the new ideas, but in escaping from the old ones, which ramify, for those brought up as most of us have been, into every corner of our minds.

Force of habit, and resistance to change – so great in all realms of thought – reaches its maximum in medicine, in the study of our most complex sufferings and disorders of being; for we are here compelled to scrutinize the deepest, darkest, and most fearful parts of ourselves, the parts we all strive to deny or not-see. The thoughts which are most difficult to grasp or express are those which touch on this forbidden region and re-awaken in us our strongest denials and our most profound intuitions.

O.W.S.

New York
February 1973

PREFACE TO THE
1990 EDITION

Awakenings has been through several editions and formats since its original appearance in 1973. There have been, over the years, all sorts of additions, subtractions, revisions, and other changes, which have sometimes been confusing to bibliographers and readers. The brief publishing history which follows may also help to trace the evolution of the present edition.

Awakenings was first published in 1973, by Duckworth, in England. The first U.S. edition was published by Doubleday in 1974. This included a little additional material: a dozen or so extra footnotes, and a short follow-up on Rolando P. (who had died when the U.K. edition was in press).

A paperback edition was brought out in 1976 by Penguin Books in England, and by Random House (Vintage Books) in the United States. This contained a huge additional mass of footnotes, some with the length and format of miniature essays, and amounting *in toto* to a third the length of the book. (These had been written during a period of enforced immobilization, in the autumn of 1974, when I was a patient myself – the period described in *A Leg to Stand On.*)

In the third edition, published in 1982 by Pan Books in England and in the United States the following year by Dutton, I added, in the form of an epilogue, detailed follow-ups on all the patients (by this time, I had seen nearly 200 patients with post-encephalitic syndromes, most of whom had been maintained on L-DOPA for eleven or twelve years), and a sort of meditation on the general nature of health, sickness, music, etc., as well as the specifics of L-DOPA and Parkinsonism. I also added an appendix on some new EEG observations I had been able to make with our patients. Still other observations and thoughts I put in (my favourite format of) footnotes – though I also acceded to a publisher's request that I remove all footnotes as such, incorporating them in the text wherever possible, and relegating what remained (often much shortened) to endnotes at the end of the book. Some 20,000 words of footnote material were entirely removed. (In 1987, in a new U.S. hardback published by Summit Books, I added a massive new foreword, otherwise keeping the book the same.) This 1982–3 edition was altogether neater, it was felt, than the 1976 one, but (to my mind, and many others) impoverished by the omission of so much material.

The need to correct this impoverishment, and restore the missing footnotes, coupled with the need to add a good deal more new material, has moved me to recast *Awakenings* once again, and rather radically, for this new 1990 edition. I have restored to its original form the most important part of the book – the *text* – relegating all additional and new material to footnotes and appendices. I have not, I should add, restored *all* the footnotes of the 1976 edition; some I felt constrained to shorten or remove. I cannot help feeling a sense of loss here, and a wondering whether (to paraphrase Gibbon) I may not have eradicated some choice flowers, some flowers of fancy, along with the weeds. I have also moved some of the longest 1976 footnotes (on the history of sleeping-sickness and on Parkinsonian space and time) to new appendices. I have not been able to resist adding a few further footnotes (but there are no more than a handful of these) and three newly-written appendices. The new material added has reference to the last surviving post-encephalitic patients (both in the United States and the United Kingdom); the remarkable advances in our understanding and treatment of Parkinsonism in the last six or seven years; some new theoretical formulations which have only emerged for me in the past few months; and finally, the striking dramatic and cinematic adaptations of *Awakenings* which have been created and shown in the last eight years, culminating in the feature film of *Awakenings* this year.

There are special difficulties in updating a book – at least a highly personal book composed largely of observation and reflection, of consciousness – for the subject is always evolving in one's mind. There may be formulations one no longer adheres to or believes in, formulations which are obsolete, in a way; and yet these formulations – some perhaps extravagant, some seemingly abortive, but others genuinely precursory and embryonic – have formed the path by which one arrived at one's present position. Therefore, although there are formulations in *Awakenings* I no longer agree with, I have left them, out of fidelity to the process by which such a book comes into being. And, by the same token, who knows what visions and revisions the 1990s have in store? I still see Parkinsonian patients with a sense of complete wonder, a sense that I have only touched the surface of an infinite condition, a sense that there may be wholly different ways of viewing it.

It is now 21 years since my patients' awakenings, and 17 years since this book was first published; yet, it seems to me, the subject is inexhaustible – medically, humanly, theoretically, dramatically. It is this which demands new additions and editions, and which keeps the subject for me – and, I trust, my readers – evergreen and alive.

O.W.S.

New York
March 1990

FOREWORD TO THE
1990 EDITION

Twenty-four years ago I entered the wards of Mount Carmel and
met the remarkable post-encephalitic patients who had been immured there since the great *encephalitis lethargica* (sleeping-sickness) epidemic just after the First World War. Von Economo,
who first described the *encephalitis lethargica* half a century before,
had spoken of the most affected patients as 'extinct volcanoes.' In
the spring of 1969, in a way which he could not have imagined,
which no one could have imagined or foreseen, these 'extinct
volcanoes' erupted into life. The placid atmosphere of Mount
Carmel was transformed – occurring before us was a cataclysm of
almost geological proportions, the explosive 'awakening,' the
'quickening,' of eighty or more patients who had long been
regarded, and regarded themselves, as effectively dead. I cannot
think back on this time without profound emotion – it was the
most significant and extraordinary in my life, no less than in the
lives of our patients. All of us at Mount Carmel were caught up
with the emotion, the excitement, and with something akin to
enchantment, even awe.

It was not a purely 'medical' excitement, any more than these
awakenings were a purely medical event. There was a tremendous *human* (even allegorical) excitement at seeing the 'dead'
awaken again – it was at this point that I conceived the title
Awakenings, taken from Ibsen's *When We Dead Awaken* – at seeing lives which one had thought irremediably blighted suddenly
bloom into a wonderful renewal, at seeing individuals in all their
vitality and richness emerge from the almost cadaveric state

where they had been frozen and hidden for decades. We had had inklings of the vivid personalities so long immured – but the full reality of these only emerged, indeed burst upon us, with our patients' awakenings.

I was exceedingly lucky to encounter such patients at such a time, in such working conditions. But they were not the only post-encephalitic patients in the world – there were, in the late '60s, still many thousands, some in large groups, in institutions all over the world. There was no major country *without* its complement of post-encephalitics. And yet *Awakenings* is the only existing account of such patients – their decades-long 'sleep' and, then, their dramatic 'awakening' in 1969.

I found this exceedingly peculiar at the time: why, I thought, were there not other accounts of what must be happening all over the world? Why, for example, was there not an 'Awakenings' from Philadelphia, where I knew of a group of patients not so dissimilar to my own? Why not from London, where the Highlands Hospital housed the largest post-encephalitic colony in England?[1] Or from Paris or Vienna, where the disease first struck?

There is no single answer to this; there were many things that mitigated against the sort of description, the 'biographic' approach, of *Awakenings.*

One factor that made *Awakenings* possible had to do with the nature of the *situation.* Mount Carmel is a chronic hospital, an asylum; and physicians in general avoid such hospitals, or visit them briefly, and leave as soon as they can. This was not always the case: in the last century, Charcot virtually lived in the Salpêtrière, and Hughlings-Jackson at the West Riding Asylum – the founders of neurology realised well that it was only in such hospitals that the depths and details of the profounder disorders could be explored and worked out. As a resident I myself had never been to a chronic hospital, and though I had seen a number of patients with post-encephalitic Parkinsonism and other problems in outpatient clinics, I had no idea how profound and

---

[1] There was a short, statistical paper by Calne et al. (1969), describing a six-week trial of L-DOPA in some of the Highlands patients, but there were no *biographical* accounts of 'awakenings' in these, or any other, patients.

strange the effects of post-encephalitic disease might be. I found coming to Mount Carmel, in 1966, a revelation. It was my first encounter with disease of a depth I had never seen, read of, or heard of, before. The medical literature on the sleeping-sickness had virtually come to a stop in 1935, so that the profounder forms of it, occurring later, had never been described. I would not have imagined it *possible* for such patients to exist; or, if they existed, to remain undescribed. For physicians do not go, and reports do not emerge, from the 'lower reaches,' these abysses of affliction, which are now (so to speak) beneath the notice of Medicine. Few doctors ever entered the halls and back wards of chronic hospitals and asylums, and few had the patience to listen and look, to penetrate the physiologies and predicaments of these increasingly inaccessible patients.

The 'other' side, the good side, of chronic hospitals is that what staff they have may work and live in them for decades, may become extraordinarily close to their charges, the patients, get to know and love them, recognize, respect them, *as people.* So when I came to Mount Carmel I did not just encounter 'eighty cases of post-encephalitic disease,' but eighty individuals, whose inner lives and total being was (to a considerable extent) known to the staff, known in the vivid, concrete knowing of relationship, not the pallid, abstract knowing of medical knowledge. Coming to this community – a community of patients, but also of patients and staff – I found myself encountering the patients as individuals, whom I could less and less reduce to statistics or lists of symptoms.

And, of course, this was a unique *time* for the patients, and for all of us. It had been established in the late 1950s that the Parkinsonian brain was lacking in the transmitter dopamine, and that it might therefore be 'normalised' if the level of dopamine could be raised. But attempts to do this, by giving L-DOPA (a precursor of dopamine) in milligram quantities, had failed persistently – until Dr George Cotzias, with great audacity, gave a group of patients L-DOPA in doses of a *thousand times* greater than had ever been used. With the publication of Cotzias's results in February 1967, the outlook for Parkinsonian patients was changed at a stroke: a sudden, unbelievable hope appeared – that patients hitherto able to look forward only to miserable and increasing disability might be (if not cured) transformed by the new drug. Life opened out once again, in imagination, for all our patients. For the first time in forty years they could believe in a future. The atmosphere from this time on was electric with excitement. One of the patients, Leonard L., when he heard of L-DOPA, rapped on his letterboard with mixed enthusiasm and irony, 'Dopamine is Resurrectamine. Cotzias is the Chemical Messiah.'

Yet it was not L-DOPA, or what it offered, which was so exciting for me when I first came as a young doctor, a year out of residency, to Mount Carmel. What excited me then was the spectacle of a disease that was never the same in two patients, a disease that could take any possible form – one rightly called a 'phantasmagoria' by those who first studied it. ('There is nothing in the literature of medicine,' wrote McKenzie in 1927, 'to compare with the phantasmagoria of disorder manifested in the course of this strange malady.') At this level of the fantastic, the phantasmagoric, the encephalitis was enthralling. Much more fundamentally, it was, by virtue of the enormous range of disturbances occurring at every level of the nervous system, a disorder that could show, far better than any other, how the nervous system was organised, how brain and behavior, at their more primitive levels, worked. The biologist, the naturalist, in me was enthralled by all this – and led me to start gathering data at this time for a book on primitive, subcortical behaviours and controls.

But then, over and above the disorder, and its direct effects, were all the responses of the patients to their sickness – so what confronted one, what one studied, was not just disease or physiology, but *people,* struggling to adapt and survive. This too was clearly realised by the early observers, above all Ivy McKenzie: 'The physician is concerned (unlike the naturalist) . . . with a single organism, the human subject, striving to preserve its identity in adverse circumstances.' In perceiving this, I became something more than a naturalist (without, however, ceasing to be one). There evolved a new concern, a new bond: that of commitment to the patients, the individuals under my care. Through them I would explore what it was like to be human, to *stay* human, in the face of unimaginable adversities and threats. Thus, while continually monitoring their organic nature – their complex, ever-changing pathophysiologies and biologies – my central study and concern became *identity* – their struggle to maintain identity – to observe this, to assist this, and, finally, to describe this. All this was at the junction of biology and biography.

This sense of the dynamics of illness and life, of the organism or subject striving to survive, sometimes under the strangest and darkest circumstances, was not a viewpoint which had been emphasised when I was a student or resident, nor was it one I found in the current medical literature. But when I saw these post-encephalitic patients, it was clearly and overwhelmingly true – indeed, it was the only way in which I *could* view them. Thus what had been dismissed disparagingly by most of my colleagues ('chronic hospitals – you'll never see anything interesting in *those* places') revealed itself as the complete opposite: an ideal situation in which to observe, to care, to explore. *Awakenings* would have been written, I think, even if there had not been any 'awakening': it would then have been *People of the Abyss* (or *Cinquante Ans de Sommeil,* as the French edition has it), a delineation of the stillness and darkness of these arrested and frozen lives, and of the courage and humour with which patients, nonetheless, faced life.

The intensity of feeling for these patients, and equally of intellectual interest and curiosity about them, bound us together as a community at Mount Carmel; and this intensity rose to a peak in 1969, the actual year of the patients' 'awakenings.' In the spring of that year, I moved to an apartment a hundred yards from the hospital and would sometimes spend twelve or fifteen hours a day with our patients. I was with the patients constantly – I grudged the hours of sleep – observing them, talking with them, getting them to keep notebooks, and keeping voluminous notes myself, thousands of words each day. And if I had a pen in one hand, I had a camera in the other: I was seeing such things as had never, perhaps, been seen before – and which, in all probability, would never be seen again; it was my duty, and my joy, to record and bear witness. Many others also dedicated themselves, spent countless hours in the hospital. All of us involved with the patients – nurses, social workers, therapists of every sort – were in constant communication: talking to each other excitedly in the passage, phoning each other on weekends and at night, constantly exchanging new experiences and ideas. The excitement, the enthusiasm, of that year was remarkable; *this,* it seems to me, was an essential part of the 'Awakenings' experience.

And yet, at the start, I scarcely knew what to expect. I had read the half-dozen reports on L-DOPA published in 1967 and '68, but felt my own patients to be very different. They did not have ordinary Parkinson's disease (like the other patients reported), but a post-encephalitic disorder of far greater complexity, severity, and strangeness. How would *these* patients, with their so-different disease, react? I felt I had to be cautious – almost exaggeratedly so. When, early in 1969, I embarked on the work which was later to become *Awakenings,* I conceived it in quite limited and narrowly 'scientific' terms – as a 90-day, double-blind trial of L-DOPA in a large group of patients who had become institutionalised after having encephalitis. L-DOPA was considered an experimental drug at this time, and I needed to get (from the Food and Drug Administration) a special investigator's licence to use it. It was a condition of such licences that one use 'orthodox' methods, including a double-blind trial, coupled with presentation of results in quantitative form.

But it became obvious within a month or less that the original format would have to be abandoned. The effects of L-DOPA in these patients was decisive – spectacular; while, as I could infer from the precise fifty percent failure rate, there was no significant placebo effect whatever. I could no longer, in good conscience, continue the placebo but had to try L-DOPA in every patient; and I could no longer think of giving it for 90 days and then stopping – this would have been like stopping the very air that they breathed. Thus what was originally conceived as a limited 90-day experiment was transformed instead into an historical experience: a story, in effect, of life for these patients as it had been before L-DOPA, and as it was changed, and as it was to become, after starting treatment with L-DOPA.

Thus I was impelled, willy-nilly, to a presentation of case-histories or biographies, for no 'orthodox' presentation, in terms of numbers, series, grading effects, etc., could have conveyed the historical reality of the experience. In August 1969, then, I wrote the first nine case-histories, or 'stories,' of *Awakenings*.

The same impulse, the same sense that one had to convey stories and phenomena – the drama of stories, the delight of phenomena – led me to write a number of letters to the editor, which I despatched to the *Lancet* and the *British Medical Journal* early the next year. I enjoyed writing these letters, and as far as I could gather, readers of these journals enjoyed reading them too. There was something about their format and style that allowed me to convey the wonder of the clinical experience, in a way that would have been quite impossible in a medical article.

I now decided to present my overall observations, and my general conclusions, while still adhering to an epistolary format. My earlier letters to the *Lancet* had been anecdotal (and everyone loves anecdotes); I had not yet attempted any general formulations. My first experiences, the patients' first responses, in the summer of '69, had been happy ones; there had been an astonishing, festive 'awakening,' at the time – but then all of my patients ran into trouble and tribulation. I observed, at this time, not only specific 'side-effects' of L-DOPA, but certain *general* patterns of trouble – sudden and unpredictable fluctuations of response, the rapid development of oscillations, the development of extreme sensitivity to L-DOPA, and, finally, the absolute impossibility of matching dose and effect – all of which I found dismaying in the extreme. I tried altering the dose of L-DOPA, but this no longer worked – the 'system' now seemed to have a dynamic of its own.

In the summer of 1970, then, in a letter to the *Journal of the American Medical Association,* I reported these findings, describing the total effects of L-DOPA in 60 patients whom I had maintained on it for a year. *All* of these, I noted, had done well at first; but all of them, sooner or later, had escaped from control, had entered complex, sometimes bizarre, and unpredictable states. These could not, I indicated, be seen as 'side-effects,' but had to be seen as integral parts of an evolving whole. Ordinary considerations and policies, I stressed, sooner or later ceased to work. There was a need for a deeper, more radical understanding.

My *JAMA* letter caused a furor among some of my colleagues. (See Sacks et al., 1970c and letters appearing in the December 1970 *JAMA.*) I was astonished and shocked by the storm that blew up; and, in particular, by the tone of some of the letters. Some colleagues insisted that such effects 'never' occurred; others that, even if they did, the matter should be kept quiet, lest it disturb 'the atmosphere of therapeutic optimism needed for the maximal efficiency of L-DOPA.' It was even thought, absurdly, that I was 'against' L-DOPA – but it was not L-DOPA but reductionism I was against. I invited my colleagues to come to Mount Carmel, to see for themselves the reality of what I had reported; none of them took up my invitation. I had not properly realised, until this time, the power of *wish* to distort and deny – and its prevalence in this complex situation, where the enthusiasm of doctors, and the distress of patients, might lie in unconscious collusion, equally concerned to wish away an unpalatable truth. The situation had similarities to what had occurred twenty years before, when cortisone was clothed with unlimited promise; and one could only hope that with the passage of time, and the accumulation of undeniable experience, a sense of reality would triumph over wish.

Was my letter too condensed – or simply confusing? Did I need to put things in the form of extended articles? With much labour (because it went against the grain, so to speak), I put everything I could in an orthodox or conventional format – papers full of statistics and figures and tables and graphs – and submitted these to various medical and neurological journals. To my amazement and chagrin, none was accepted – some of them, indeed, elicited vehemently censorious, even violent, rejections, as if there were something intolerable in what I had written. This confirmed my feeling that a deep nerve had been struck, that I had somehow elicited not just a medical, but a sort of epistemological, anxiety – and rage.[2]

---

[2] Five years later, it happened that one of the neurologists who had taken such exception to my letter in *JAMA* – he had said that my observations were beyond credibility – found himself chairing a meeting at which the documentary film of *Awakenings* was being shown. There is a particular point in the film at which various bizarre 'side-effects' and instabilities of drug reaction are shown in dizzying array, and I was fascinated to observe my colleague's reactions here. First, he stared amazed, and his mouth dropped open; it was as if he were seeing such things for the first time, and his reaction was one of innocent and almost childlike wonder. Then he flushed a dark and angry crimson – whether with embarrass-

I had not only cast doubt on what had appeared at first to be the extremely simple matter of giving a drug and being in control of its effects; I had cast doubt on predictability itself. I had (perhaps without fully realising it myself) hinted at something bizarre, a contradiction of ordinary ways of thinking, and of the ordinary, accepted picture of the world. A spectre of extreme oddness, of radical contingency, had come up – and all this was disquieting, confounding, in the extreme ('These things are so bizarre that I cannot bear to contemplate them' – Poincaré).

And so, by mid-1970 I was brought to a halt, at least so far as any publication was concerned. The work continued, full of excitement, unabated, and I accumulated (I dared to think) an absolute treasure of observations and of hypotheses and reflections associated with them, but I had no idea what to do with them. I knew that I had been given the rarest of opportunities; I knew that I had something valuable to say; but I saw no way of saying it, of being faithful to my experiences, without forfeiting medical 'publishability' or acceptance among my colleagues. This was a time of great bewilderment and frustration, considerable anger, and sometimes despair.

This impasse was broken in September of 1972, when the editor of *The Listener* invited me to write an article on my experiences. This was going to be my opportunity. Instead of the censorious rejections I was used to, I was actually being invited to write, being offered a chance to publish, fully and freely, what had been accumulating and building up, dammed up, for so long. I wrote 'The Great Awakening' at a single sitting – neither I nor the editor altered a single word – and it was published the following month. Here, with a sense of great liberation from the constraints of 'medicalising' and medical jargon, I described the wonderful panorama of phenomena I had seen in my patients. I

---

ment or mortification, I could not tell; these were the very things he had dismissed as 'beyond credibility,' and now he was being forced to see them for himself. Then he developed a curious *tic,* a convulsive movement of the head which kept turning it away from the screen he could no longer bear to see. Then, finally, with great abruptness and violence, and muttering to himself, he burst out of his seat, in mid-film, and rushed out of the room. I found this behaviour extraordinary and instructive, for it showed how profound, how utterly overwhelming, reactions to the 'incredible' and 'intolerable' might be.

described the raptures of their 'awakenings,' I described the torments that so often followed; but above all, it was *phenomena* which I was concerned to describe, with a neutral and phenomenological (rather than a therapeutic, or 'medical') eye.

But the picture, the theory, implied by the phenomena: this seemed to me to be of a revolutionary sort – 'a new neurophysiology,' as I wrote, 'of a quantum-relativistic sort.' These were bold words indeed; they excited me, and others – although I soon came to think that I had said too much, and too little. That there was *something,* assuredly, very strange going on – not quantality, not relativity, but something much commoner, yet stranger. I could not imagine what this was, in 1972, though it haunted me when I came to complete *Awakenings,* and rippled through it constantly, evasively, as half-tantalising metaphors.

The article in *The Listener* was followed (in contrast to the hateful *JAMA* experience of two years earlier) by a wave of interest, and a great number of letters, an exciting correspondence which lasted several weeks. This response put an end to my long years of frustration and obstruction and gave me a decisive encouragement and affirmation. I picked up my long discarded case-histories of 1969, added eleven more, and in two weeks completed *Awakenings.* The case-histories were the easiest to write; they wrote themselves, they stemmed straight from experience, and I have always regarded them with especial affection as the true and unassailable centre of *Awakenings.* The rest is disputable, the stories are so.

But the 1973 publication of *Awakenings,* while attracting much general attention, met the same cold reception from the profession as my articles had done earlier. There was not a single medical notice or review, only a disapproving or uncomprehending silence. There was one brave editor (of the *British Clinical Journal*) who spoke out on this, making *Awakenings* his 'editor's choice' for 1973, but commenting on 'the strange mutism' of the profession towards it.

I was devastated at this medical 'mutism,' but at the same time reassured and encouraged by the reaction of A. R. Luria. Luria himself, after a lifetime of minute neuropsychological observations, had himself published two extraordinary, almost novelistic case-histories – *The Mind of a Mnemonist* (in 1968) and *The Man with a Shattered World* (1972). To my intense pleasure, in the strange medical silence which attended the publication of *Awakenings,* I received a letter, two letters, from him; in the first, he spoke of his own 'biographic' books and approaches:

> Frankly said, I myself like very much the type of 'biographical' study, such as Sherashevsky [the Mnemonist] and Zazetski [the man with the 'shattered world'] . . . firstly because it is a kind of 'Romantic Science' which I wanted to introduce, partly because I am strongly *against* a formal statistical approach and *for* a qualitative study of personality, *for* every attempt to find *factors* underlying the structure of personality. [Letter of July 19, 1973, emphasis in original]

And in the second, he spoke of *Awakenings:*

> I received *Awakenings* and have read it at once with great delight. I was ever conscious and sure that a good clinical description of cases plays a leading role in medicine, especially in Neurology and Psychiatry. Unfortunately, the ability to describe which was so common to the great Neurologists and Psychiatrists of the 19th century [is] lost now, perhaps because of the basic mistake that mechanical and electrical devices can replace the study of personality . . . Your excellent book shows, that the important tradition of clinical case studies can be revived and with a great success. [Letter of July 25, 1973]

He then went on to ask me some specific questions, above all expressing his fascination that L-DOPA should be so various and unstable in effect.[3]

---

[3] He returned to this topic the following month, when he said that he had been fascinated by the case of Martha N., and the fact that she had responded to L-DOPA in six different ways: '*Why* was it different each time?' he asked, '*Why* could one not replay things again and again?' – questions I could not answer in 1973. It seemed to me typical of the genius of Luria that he had at once homed in on one of the central mysteries and challenges of *Awakenings* – the various and unrepeatable and unpredictable character of patients' responses – and been fascinated by this; whereas my neurological colleagues, by and large, had been

* * *

I had admired Luria infinitely since my medical school days, and before. When I heard him lecture in London in 1959, I was overwhelmed by his combination of intellectual power and human warmth – I had often encountered these separately, but I had not too often encountered them *together* – and it was exactly this combination which so pleased me in his work, and which made it such an antidote to certain trends in medical writing, which attempted to delete both subjectivity and reflection. Luria's early works had been, sometimes, a little stilted in character, but they grew in intellectual warmth, in wholeness, as he grew older, culminating in his two late works, *The Mind of a Mnemonist* and *The Man with a Shattered World.* I do not know how much either of these works influenced me, but they certainly emboldened me, and made it easier to write and publish *Awakenings.*

Luria often said that he had to write two sorts of books, wholly different but wholly complementary: 'classical,' analytic texts (like *Higher Cortical Functions in Man*) and 'romantic,' biographical books (like *The Mind of a Mnemonist* and *The Man with a Shattered World*). I was also conscious of this double need, and found there were always *two* books, potentially, demanded by every clinical experience: one more purely 'medical' or 'classical' – an objective description of disorders, mechanisms, syndromes; the other more existential and personal – an empathic entering into patients' experiences and worlds. Two such books dawned in me when I first saw our post-encephalitic patients: *Compulsion and Constraint* (a study of subcortical disorders and mechanisms) and *People of the Abyss* (a novelish, Jack Londonish book). They only came together, finally, in 1969 – to a book which tried to be *both* classical and romantic; to place itself at the intersection of biology and biography; to combine, as best it could, the modes of paradigm and art.

But *no* model, finally, seemed to suit my requirements – for what I was seeing, and what I needed to convey, was neither

---

frightened and dismayed by this, had tended to asseverate, 'It's not so, it's not so.'

purely classical nor purely romantic, but seemed to move into the profound realm of allegory or myth. Even my title, *Awakenings,* had a double meaning, partly literal, partly in the mode of metaphor or myth.

The elaborate case-history, the 'romantic' style, with its endeavour to present a whole life, the repercussions of a disease, in all its richness, had fallen very much out of favour by the middle of the century – and this, perhaps, was one reason for the 'strange mutism' of the profession when *Awakenings* was first published in 1973. But as the seventies progressed, this antipathy to case-history diminished – it even became possible (though difficult) to publish case-histories in the medical literature. With this thawing of atmosphere, there was a renewed sense that complex neural and psychic functions (and their disorders) *required* detailed and non-reductive narratives for their explication and understanding.[4]

At the same time, the unpredictable responses to L-DOPA I saw with my patients in 1969 – their sudden fluctuations and oscillations, their extraordinary 'sensitization' to L-DOPA, to *everything* – were now being seen, increasingly, by everyone. Post-encephalitic patients, it became clear, might show these bizarre reactions within weeks, sometimes days – whereas 'ordinary' Parkinsonian patients, with their more stable nervous systems, might not show them for several years. Yet, sooner or later, *all* patients maintained on L-DOPA started to show these strange, unstable states – and with the FDA approval of L-DOPA in 1970, their numbers mounted, finally to millions. And now, everybody found the same: the central promise of L-DOPA was confirmed, a million-fold – but so too was the central threat, the certainty of 'side-effects' or 'tribulations,' sooner or later.

Thus what had been surprising or intolerable when I first published *Awakenings* was – by the time the third edition was published in 1982 – confirmed for all my colleagues by their own,

---

[4] There has been a parallel movement in anthropology since 1970 – this had also been becoming meagre and mechanical – with a new, or renewed, insistence on what Clifford Geertz has dubbed 'thick' description.

undeniable experience. The optimistic and irrational mood of the early days of L-DOPA had changed to something more sober and realistic. This mood, well established by 1982, made the new edition of *Awakenings* acceptable, and even a classic, to my medical colleagues, where the original had been unacceptable nine years before.

It is the imagination of other people's worlds – worlds almost inconceivably strange, yet inhabited by people just like ourselves, people, indeed, who might *be* ourselves – that forms the centre of *Awakenings*. Other worlds, other lives, even though so different from our own, have the power of arousing the sympathetic imagination, of awakening an intense and often creative resonance in others. We may never have seen a Rose R., but once we have read of her we see the world differently – we can imagine her world, with a sort of awe, and with this our world is suddenly enlarged. A wonderful example of such a creative response was given by Harold Pinter in his play, *A Kind of Alaska;* this is Pinter's world, the landscape of his unique gifts and sensibility, but it is also Rose R.'s world, and the world of *Awakenings*. Pinter's play has been followed by several adaptations of *Awakenings* for stage and screen; each of these has drawn on different aspects of the book. Every reader will bring to *Awakenings* his own imagination and sensibilities, and will find, if he lets himself, his world strangely deepened, imbued with a new depth of tenderness and perhaps horror. For these patients, while seemingly so extraordinary, so 'special,' have in them something of the universal, and can call to everyone, awaken everyone, as they called to and awakened me.

I hesitated very greatly in regard to the original publication of our patients' 'story' and their lives. But they themselves encouraged me, and said to me from the first, 'Tell our story – or it will never be known.'

A few of the patients are still alive – we have known each other for twenty-four years now. But those who have died are in some sense not dead – their unclosed charts, their letters, still face me as I write. They still live, for me, in some very personal way. They were not only patients but teachers and friends, and the years I spent with them were the most significant of my life. I want something of their lives, their presence, to be preserved and live for others, as exemplars of human predicament and survival. This is the testimony, the only testimony, of a unique event – but one which may become an allegory for us all.

O.W.S.

New York
March 1990

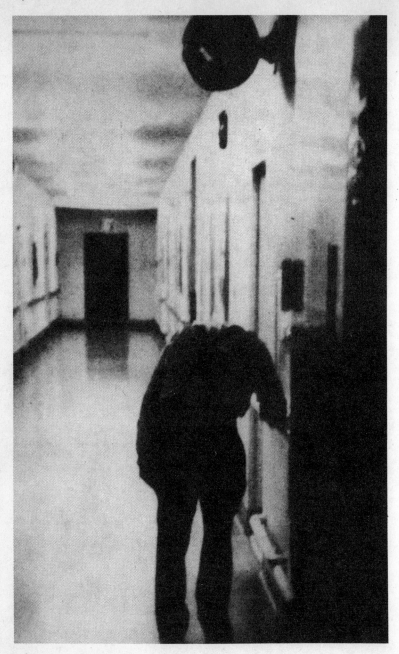

Seymour L. would often be frozen for hours like this in the corridor.

Prologue

PARKINSON'S DISEASE
AND PARKINSONISM

℺ In 1817, Dr James Parkinson – a London physician – published his famous *Essay on the Shaking Palsy,* in which he portrayed, with a vividness and insight that have never been surpassed, the common, important, and singular condition we now know as Parkinson's disease.

Isolated symptoms and features of Parkinson's disease – the characteristic shaking or tremor, and the characteristic hurrying or festination of gait and speech – had been described by physicians back to the time of Galen. Detailed descriptions had also appeared in the non-medical literature – as in Aubrey's description of Hobbes's 'Shaking Palsy.' But it was Parkinson who first saw every feature and aspect of the illness as a whole, and who presented it as a distinctive human condition or *form of behaviour.* [5]

---

[5] It is true, in a sense, that Parkinson had many 'predecessors' (Gaubius, Sauvages, de la Noë, and others) who had observed and classified various 'signs' of Parkinsonism. But there was a radical difference between Parkinson and these men – perhaps more radical than Parkinson himself allowed or admitted. Observers of Parkinsonism, before Parkinson himself, had been content to 'spot' various characteristics (in much the same way as one 'spots' trains or planes), and then to arrange these characteristics in classificatory schemes (somewhat as a butterfly-spotter, or would-be entomologist, might arrange his specimens according to colour and shape). Thus Parkinson's predecessors were entirely concerned with 'diagnosis' and 'nosology' – an arbitrary, pre-scientific diagnosis and nosology, based entirely on superficial characteristics and relationships: the Zodiacal charts of Sauvages and others represent a sort of pseudo-astronomy, first attempts to come to grips with the unknown. Parkinson's own initial observations were also made 'from the outside,' so to speak, from seeing Parkinsonians in the streets of London, inspecting their peculiarities of motion from a

Between 1860 and 1890, working amid the large population of chronically ill patients at the Salpêtrière in Paris, Charcot filled in the outline which Parkinson had drawn. In addition to his rich and detailed characterizations of the illness, Charcot perceived the important relations and affinities which existed between the symptoms of Parkinson's disease and those of depression, catatonia, and hysteria: indeed, it was partly in view of these striking relationships that Charcot called Parkinsonism 'a neurosis.'

In the nineteenth century, Parkinsonism was almost never seen before the age of fifty, and was usually considered to be a reflection of a degenerative process or defect of nutrition in certain 'weak' or vulnerable cells; since this degeneration could not actually be demonstrated at the time, and since its cause was unknown, Parkinson's disease was termed an idiosyncrasy or 'idiopathy.' In the first quarter of this century, with the advent of the great sleeping-sickness epidemic *(encephalitis lethargica),* a 'new'

---

distance. But his observations were deeper than those of his predecessors, deeper-rooted and more deeply related. Parkinson resembles a *genuine* astronomer, and London the field of his astronomical observations, and at this stage, through his eyes, we see Parkinsonians as bodies-in-transit, moving like comets or stars. Soon, moreover, he came to recognize that certain stars form a *constellation,* that many seemingly unrelated phenomena form a definite and constant 'assemblage of symptoms.' He was the first to recognize this 'assemblage' as such, this constellation or syndrome we now call 'Parkinsonism.'

This was a clinical achievement of the first magnitude, and Parkinsonism was one of the first neurological syndromes to be recognized and defined. But Parkinson was not merely talented – he was a man of genius. He perceived that the curious 'assemblage' he had noted was something more than a diagnostic syndrome – that it seemed to have a coherent inner logic and order of its own, that the constellation was a sort of *cosmos* . . . Sensing this, he now realized that inspection-at-a-distance, however acute, was insufficient if he wished to understand its nature; he realized it was necessary to meet actual patients, to engage them in clinical and dialogic encounter. With this he adopted an entirely different stance and concurrently with this a quite different language. He ceased to see Parkinsonians as remote objects in orbit, and saw them as patients and fellow human beings; he ceased to use diagnostic jargon, and used words indicative of *intention* and *action;* he ceased to see Parkinsonism as 'an assemblage of symptoms' and now thought of being-Parkinsonian as a strange form of *behaviour,* a peculiar and characteristic mode of Being-in-the-World. Thus Parkinson, compared to his predecessors, was a radical, a revolutionary, in two different ways: first in establishing a genuine empiricism – a science of 'facts' and their interrelations; second, in making a still more radical move in intellectual mid-course, by moving from an empirical to an existential position.

sort of Parkinsonism appeared, which had a clear and specific cause: this encephalitic or post-encephalitic Parkinsonism,[6] unlike the idiopathic illness, could affect people of any age, and could assume a form and a severity much graver and more dramatic than ever occurred in the idiopathic illness. A third great cause of Parkinsonism has been seen only in the last twenty years, and is an unintended (and usually transient) consequence or 'side-effect' of the use of phenothiazide and butyrophenone drugs – the so-called 'major tranquillizers.' It is said that in the United States alone there are two million people with Parkinsonism: a million with idiopathic Parkinsonism or Parkinson's disease; a million with drug-induced Parkinsonism; and a few hundred or thousand patients with post-encephalitic Parkinsonism – the last survivors of the great epidemic. Other causes of Parkinsonism – coal-gas poisoning, manganese poisoning, syphilis, tumours, etc. – are excessively rare, and are scarcely likely to be seen in a lifetime of practice by the ordinary physician.

Parkinson's disease has been called the 'shaking palsy' (or its Latin equivalent – *paralysis agitans*) for some centuries. It is necessary to say at the outset that the shaking or tremor is by no means a constant symptom in Parkinsonism, is never an isolated symptom, and is often the least problem which faces the Parkinsonian patient. If tremor is present, it tends to occur at rest and to disappear with movement or the intention to move;[7] sometimes it is confined to the hand, and has a characteristic 'pill-rolling' quality or (in Gowers's words) a quality 'similar to that by which Orientals beat their small drums'; in other, and especially in post-encephalitic patients, tremor may be extremely violent, may affect any or every part of the body, and tends to be increased by effort, nervousness, or fatigue. The second commonly mentioned symptom of Parkinsonism, besides tremor, is stiffness or

---

[6] The term 'post-encephalitic' is used to denote symptoms which have come on *following* an attack of *encephalitis lethargica,* and as a direct or indirect consequence of this. The onset of such symptoms may be delayed until many years after the original attack.

[7] There are many actors, surgeons, mechanics, and skilled manual workers who show severe Parkinsonian tremor at rest, but not a trace of this when they concentrate on their work or move into action.

rigidity; this has a curious plastic quality – often compared to the bending of a lead pipe – and may be of intense severity.[8] It must be stressed, however, that neither tremor nor rigidity is an essential feature of Parkinsonism; they may both be completely absent, especially in the post-encephalitic forms of disease with which we shall especially be concerned in this book. The essential features of Parkinsonism, which occur in every patient, and which reach their extremest intensity in post-encephalitic forms of disease, relate to disorders of movement and 'push.'

The first qualities of Parkinsonism which were ever described were those of *festination* (hurry) and *pulsion* (push). Festination consists of an acceleration (and with this, an abbreviation) of steps, movements, words, or even thoughts – it conveys a sense of impatience, impetuosity, and alacrity, as if the patient were very pressed for time; and in some patients it goes along with a *feeling* of urgency and impatience, although others, as it were, find themselves hurried against their will.[9] The character of movements associated with festination or pulsion are those of quickness, abruptness, and brevity. These symptoms, and the peculiar 'motor impatience' (akathisia) which often goes along with them, were given full weight by the older authors: thus Charcot speaks of the 'cruel restlessness' suffered by many of his patients, and Gowers of the 'extreme restlessness . . . which necessitates . . . every few minutes some slight change of posture.' I stress these aspects – the alacrity and pressure and precipitation of movement – because they represent, so to speak, the less familiar 'other side' of Parkinsonism, Parkinsonism-on-the-boil, Parkinsonism in its expansile and explosive aspect, and as such have peculiar relevance to many of the 'side-effects' of L-DOPA which patients exhibit.

---

[8] It was observed by Charcot, and is observed by many Parkinsonian patients themselves, that rigidity can be loosened to a remarkable degree if the patient is suspended in water or swimming (see below the cases of Hester Y., Rolando P., Cecil M., etc.). The same is also true, to some extent, of other forms of stiffness and 'clench' – spasticity, athetosis, torticollis, etc.

[9] Thus festination *('scelotyrbe festinans')* is portrayed by Gaubius in the eighteenth century: 'Cases occur in which the muscles, duly excited by the impulses of the will, do then, with an unbidden agility, and with an impetus not to be repressed, run before the unwilling mind.'

The opposite of these effects – a peculiar slowing and difficulty of movement – are more commonly stressed, and go by the general and rather uninformative name of 'akinesia.' There are many different forms of akinesia, but the form which is exactly antithetical to hurry or pulsion is one of active *retardation* or *resistance* which impedes movement, speech, and even thought, and may arrest it completely. Patients so affected find that as soon as they 'will' or intend or attempt a movement, a 'counter-will' or 'resistance' rises up to meet them. They find themselves embattled, and even immobilized, in a form of physiological conflict – force against counter-force, will against counter-will, command against countermand. For such embattled patients, Charcot writes: 'There is no truce' – and Charcot sees the tremor, rigidity, and akinesia of such patients as the final, futile outcome of such states of inner struggle, and the tension and tiredness of which Parkinsonian patients so often complain as due to the pre-emption of their energies in such senseless inner battles. It is these states of push and constraint which one patient of mine (Leonard L.) would always call 'the goad and halter.'[10] The appearance of passivity or inertia is deceiving: an obstructive akinesia of this sort is in no sense an idle or restful state, but (to paraphrase de Quincey) '. . . no product of inertia, but . . . resulting from mighty and equal antagonisms, infinite activities, infinite repose.'[11]

[10] Analogous concepts are used by William James, in his discussion of 'perversions' of will (*Principles,* 2, xxvi). The two basic perversions delineated by James are the 'obstructive' will and the 'explosive' will; when the former holds sway, the performance of normal actions is rendered difficult or impossible; if the latter is dominant, abnormal actions are irrepressible. Although James uses these terms with reference to neurotic perversions of the will, they are equally applicable to what we must term Parkinsonian perversions of the will: Parkinsonism, like neurosis, is a *conative* disorder, and exhibits a formal analogy of conative structure.

[11] At this point we must introduce a fundamental theme which will re-appear and re-echo, in various guises, throughout this book. We have seen Parkinsonism as sudden starts and stops, as odd speedings and slowings. Our approach, our concepts, our terms have so far been of a purely mechanical or empirical type: we have seen Parkinsonians as bodies, but not yet as *beings* . . . if we are to achieve any understanding of *what it is like to be Parkinsonian,* of the actual nature of Parkinsonian existence (as opposed to the parameters of Parkinsonian motion), we must adopt a different and complementary approach and language.

We must come down from our position as 'objective observers,' and meet our patients face-to-face; we must meet them in a sympathetic and imaginative en-

In some patients, there is a different form of akinesia, which is not associated with a feeling of effort and struggle, but with one of continual repetition or perseveration: thus Gowers records the case of one patient whose limbs '. . . when raised remained so for several minutes, and then slowly fell' – a form of akinesia which he correctly compares to catalepsy; this is generally far more common and far more severe in patients with post-encephalitic forms of Parkinsonism.[12]

---

counter: for it is only in the context of such a collaboration, a participation, a relation, that we can hope to learn anything about *how they are.* They can tell us, and show us, what it is like being Parkinsonian – they can tell us, but nobody else can.

Indeed we must go further, for if – as we have reason to suspect – our patients may be subject to experiences as strange as the motions they show, they may need much help, a delicate and patient and imaginative collaboration, in order to formulate the almost-unformulable, in order to communicate the almost-incommunicable. We must be co-explorers in the uncanny realm of being-Parkinsonian, this land beyond the boundaries of common experience; but our quarry in this strange country will not be 'specimens,' data, or 'facts,' but images, similitudes, analogies, metaphors – whatever may assist to make the strange familiar, and to bring into the thinkable the previously unthinkable. What we are told, what we discover, will be couched in the mode of 'likeness' or 'as if,' for we are asking the patient to make *comparisons* – to compare being-Parkinsonian with that mode-of-being which we agree to call 'normal.'

All experience is hypothetical or conjectural, but its intensity and form vary a great deal: thus patients able to achieve some detachment, or patients only partially or intermittently affected, will describe their experiences in metaphorical terms; whereas patients who are continually and completely engulfed by their experience will tend to describe it in hallucinatory terms. . . . Thus, images such as 'Saturnian gravity' are used with great frequency by patients. One patient (Helen K.) was asked how it felt to be Parkinsonian: 'Like being stuck on an enormous planet,' she replied. 'I seemed to weigh tons, I was crushed, I couldn't move.' A little later she was asked how she had felt on L-DOPA (she had become very flighty, volatile, mercurial): 'Like being on a dotty little planet,' she said. 'Like Mercury – no, that's too big, like an asteroid! I couldn't stay put, I weighed nothing, I was all over the place. It's all a matter of gravity, in a way – first there's too much, then there's too little. Parkinsonism is gravity, L-DOPA is levity, and it's difficult to find any mean in between.' Such comparisons are also used, in reverse, by patients with Tourette's (Sacks, 1981).

[12] Arrest (akinesia) or profound slowing (bradykinesia) are equally evident in other spheres – they affect *every* aspect of life's stream, including the stream of consciousness. Thus, Parkinsonism itself is not 'purely' motor – there is, for example, in many akinetic patients, a corresponding 'stickiness' of mind or bradyphrenia, the thought stream as slow and sluggish as the motor stream. The thought stream, the stream of consciousness, speeds up in these patients with

These characteristics – of impulsion, of resistance, and of perseveration – represent the active or positive characteristics of Parkinsonism. We will later have occasion to see that they are to some extent interchangeable, and thus that they represent different phases or forms or transformations of Parkinsonism. Parkinsonian patients also have 'negative' characteristics – if this is not a contradiction in terms. Thus some of them, Charcot particularly noted, would sit for hours not only motionless, but apparently without any impulse to move: they were, seemingly, content to do nothing, and they lacked the 'will' to enter upon or continue any course of activity, although they might move quite well if the stimulus or command or request to move came from another person – *from the outside.* Such patients were said to have an absence of the will – or 'aboulia.'

Other aspects of such 'negative' disorder or deficiency in Parkinsonian patients relate to feelings of tiredness and lack of energy, and of certain 'dullness' – an impoverishment of feeling, libido, motive, and attention. To a greater or less degree, all Parkinsonian patients show alteration of 'go,' impetus, initiative, vitality, etc., closely akin to what may be experienced by patients in the throes of depression.[13]

Thus Parkinsonian patients suffer simultaneously (though in varying proportions) from a pathological absence and a pathological presence. The former cuts them off from the fluent and appropriate flow of normal movement (and – in severe cases – the flow of normal perception and thought), and is experienced as a 'weakness,' a tiredness, a deprivation, a destitution; the latter constitutes a preoccupation, an abnormal activity, a pathological

---

L-DOPA, often speeding too far, into a veritable tachyphrenia, with thoughts and associations almost too fast to follow. Again, there is not merely motor, but a perceptual inertia in Parkinsonism: a perspective drawing of a cube or a staircase, for example, which the normal mind perceives first this way and then that, in alternating perceptual configurations or hypotheses, may be absolutely frozen in one configuration for the Parkinsonian; it will unfreeze as he 'awakens' and may then be thrust, with the continuing stimulation of L-DOPA, in the opposite direction, with a near-delirium of perceptual hypotheses alternating many times a second.

[13] A special form of negative disorder, not described in the classical literature, is depicted with Hester Y. (see pp. 111–112).

organization, which, so to speak, distends or inflates their behaviour in a senseless, distressing, and disabling fashion. Patients can be thought of as *engorged* with Parkinsonism – with pathological excitement ('erethism') – as one may be engorged with pain or pleasure or rage or neurosis. The notion of Parkinsonism as exerting a pressure on the patient seems to be supported, above all, by the phenomenon of *kinesia paradoxa* which consists of a sudden and total (though transient) disappearance or deflation of Parkinsonism – a phenomenon seen most frequently and most dramatically in the most intensely Parkinsonian patients.[14]

---

[14] Thus one may see such patients, rigid, motionless, seemingly lifeless as statutes, abruptly called into normal life and action by some sudden exigency which catches their attention (in one famous case, a drowning man was saved by a Parkinsonian patient who leapt from his wheelchair into the breakers). The return of Parkinsonism, in circumstances like these, is often as sudden and dramatic as its vanishing: the suddenly 'normal' and awakened patient, once the call-to-action is past, may fall back like a dummy into the arms of his attendants.

Dr Gerald Stern tells me of one such patient at the Highlands Hospital in London who was nicknamed 'Puskas' after the famous footballer of the 1950s. Puskas would often sit frozen and motionless *unless* he were thrown a ball; this would instantly call him to life, and he would leap to his feet, swerving, running, dribbling the ball, with a truly Puskas-like acrobatic genius. If thrown a matchbox he would catch it on the tip of one foot, kick it up, catch it, kick it up again, and in this fashion, juggling the matchbox on one foot, hop the entire length of the ward. He scarcely showed any 'normal' activity; only this bizarre and spasmodic super-activity, which ended, as it started, suddenly and completely.

There is another story of the post-encephalitic patients at Highlands. Two of the men had shared a room for twenty years, but without any contact or, apparently, any feeling for each other; both were totally motionless and mute. One evening, while doing rounds, Dr Stern heard a terrific noise coming from this room of perpetual silence. Rushing to it with a couple of nurses, he found its inmates in the midst of a violent fight, throwing each other around and shouting obscenities. The scene, in Dr Stern's words, was 'not far short of incredible – none of us ever *imagined* these men could move.' With some difficulty the men were separated and the fight was stopped. The moment they were separated, they became motionless and mute again – and have remained so for the last fifteen years. In the thirty-five years they have shared a room, this is the *only* time they 'came alive.'

This mixture of akinesia and a sort of motor genius is very characteristic of post-encephalitic patients; I think of one such, not at Mount Carmel, who sits motionless until she is thrown three oranges (or more). Instantly she starts juggling them – she can juggle up to seven, in a manner incredible to see – and can continue doing so for half an hour on end. But if she drops one, or is interrupted for a moment, she suddenly becomes motionless again. With another such patient (Maurice P.), who came to Mount Carmel in 1971, I had no idea

It is scarcely imaginable that a profound deficiency can suddenly be made good, but it is easy to conceive that an intense pressure might suddenly be relieved, or an intense charge discharged. Such conceptions are always implicit, and sometimes explicit, in the thinking of Charcot, who goes on, indeed, to stress the close analogies which could exist between the different forms or 'phases' of Parkinsonism and those of neurosis: in particular Charcot clearly saw the formal similarity or analogy between the three clearly distinct yet interchangeable phases of Parkinsonism – the compliant-perseverative, the obstructive-resistive, and the explosive-precipitate phases – with the plastic, rigid, and frenzied forms of catatonia and hysteria. These insights were reinforced during the 1920s, by observation of the extraordinary amalgamations of Parkinsonism with other disorders seen in the encephalitis epidemic. They were then completely 'forgotten,' or thrust out of the neurological consciousness. The effects of L-DOPA – as we shall see – compel us to reinstate and elaborate the forgotten analyses and analogies of Charcot and his contemporaries.

---

that he was *able* to move, and had long regarded him as 'hopelessly akinetic,' until, one day, as I was writing up my notes, he suddenly took my ophthalmoscope, a most intricate one, unscrewed it, examined it, put it together again, and gave a stunning imitation of me examining an eye. The entire 'performance,' which was flawless and brilliant, occupied no more than a few seconds.

Less abrupt and complete, but of more therapeutic relevance, is the *partial* lifting of Parkinsonism, for long periods of time, in response to interesting and activating situations, which *invite* participation in a non-Parkinsonian mode. Different forms of such therapeutic activation are exemplified throughout the biographies in this book, and explicitly discussed on p. 59, and in an Appendix: Parkinsonian Space and Time, p. 339.

THE SLEEPING-SICKNESS
(*ENCEPHALITIS LETHARGICA*)

In the winter of 1916–17, in Vienna and other cities, a 'new' illness suddenly appeared, and rapidly spread, over the next three years, to become world-wide in its distribution. Manifestations of the sleeping-sickness[15] were so varied that no two patients ever presented exactly the same picture, and so strange as to call forth from physicians such diagnoses as epidemic delirium, epidemic schizophrenia, epidemic Parkinsonism, epidemic disseminated sclerosis, atypical rabies, atypical poliomyelitis, etc., etc. It seemed, at first, that a thousand new diseases had suddenly broken loose, and it was only through the profound clinical acumen of Constantin von Economo, allied with his pathological studies on the brains of patients who had died, and his demonstration that these, besides showing a unique pattern of damage, contained a sub-microscopic, filter-passing agent (virus) which could transmit the disease to monkeys, that the identity of this protean disease was established. *Encephalitis lethargica* – as von Economo was to name it – was a Hydra with a thousand heads.[16]

---

[15] The term 'sleeping-sickness' is used in America to designate both the African, parasite-borne, endemic disease *(trypanosomiasis)* and the epidemic, virus-borne, *encephalitis lethargica;* in England, however, the latter is often called 'sleepy-sickness.'

[16] Thus there arose the most baffling clinical and epidemiological perplexities. The first recognition in England that new and strange disease-syndromes were everywhere afoot, dates from the first weeks of 1918, and one may recapture the excitement of these early reports by looking at *The Lancet* for April 20th of that year and the extraordinary report put out by the Stationery Office in October 1918 (see His Majesty's Stationery Office, 1918). There had been earlier reports – from France, Austria, Poland, and Romania – as far back as the winter of 1915–16, but these were apparently unknown in England, due to the difficulties of disseminating information in wartime. One may see from the HMSO Report

Although there had been innumerable smaller epidemics in the past, including the London sleeping-sickness of 1672–3, there had never been a world-wide pandemic on the scale of that which started in 1916–17. In the ten years that it raged, this pandemic took or ravaged the lives of nearly five million people before it disappeared, as mysteriously and suddenly as it had arrived, in 1927.[17] A third of those affected died in the acute stages of the sleeping-sickness, in states of coma so deep as to preclude arousal, or in states of sleeplessness so intense as to preclude sedation.[18]

---

that confusion reigned, and how reports of the new and unidentified disease came in under the most various of names: botulism, toxic ophthalmoplegia, epidemic stupor, epidemic lethargic encephalitis, acute polioencephalitis, Heine-Medin disease, bulbar paralysis, hystero-epilepsy, acute dementia, and sometimes just 'an obscure disease with cerebral symptoms.' This chaos continued until the great clarifying and unifying work of von Economo, after whom we properly name this disease.

Cruchet, in France, described forty cases of 'subacute encephalomyelitis' ten days before von Economo; neither knew of the other's work, for Paris and Vienna were on opposite sides in the War and, as was often remarked in later years, communication about the disease was slower than communication of the disease itself. Questions of priority were fanned, not only by the discoverers themselves but by forces of national animus and pride; for some years the French literature spoke of 'Cruchet's disease' while the German literature spoke of 'von Economo's disease.' The rest of the world, neutrally, spoke of *encephalitis lethargica*, epidemic encephalitis, chronic encephalitis, etc. Indeed, almost every individual neurologist had their own name for it: for Kinnier Wilson it was 'mesencephalitis,' for Bernard Sachs it was 'basilar encephalitis.' For the public, it was simply 'sleepy sickness.'

[17] There was some coincidence and overlap of the great encephalitis pandemic with the world-wide 'flu' pandemic – as thirty years earlier the Italian *'nona'* was preceded by a virulent if local influenza epidemic. It is probable, but not certain, that the influenza and the encephalitis reflected the effects of two different viruses, but it seems possible, and even probable, that the influenza epidemic in some way paved the way for the encephalitis epidemic, and that the influenza virus potentiated the effects of the encephalitis virus, or lowered resistance to it in a catastrophic way. Thus, between October 1918 and January 1919, when half the world's population was affected by the influenza or its consequences, and more than twenty-one million people died, the encephalitis assumed its most virulent form. If the sleeping-sickness was mysteriously 'forgotten,' the same is true of the great influenza (which had been the most murderous epidemic since the Black Death of the Middle Ages). In the words of H. L. Mencken, written in 1956: 'The epidemic is seldom mentioned, and most Americans have apparently forgotten it. This is not surprising. The human mind always tries to expunge the intolerable from memory, just as it tries to conceal it while current.'

[18]Absolute inability to sleep (agrypnia), in such patients, even without other symptoms, proved fatal in ten to fourteen days. The plight of such patients (in

Patients who suffered but survived an extremely severe somno-lent/insomniac attack of this kind often failed to recover their original aliveness. They would be conscious and aware – yet not fully awake; they would sit motionless and speechless all day in their chairs, totally lacking energy, impetus, initiative, motive, appetite, affect, or desire; they registered what went on about them without active attention, and with profound indifference. They neither conveyed nor felt the feeling of life; they were as insubstantial as ghosts, and as passive as zombies: von Economo compared them to extinct volcanoes. Such patients, in neurologi-cal parlance, showed 'negative' disorders of behaviour, i.e. no behaviour at all. They were ontologically dead, or suspended, or 'asleep' – awaiting an awakening which came (for the tiny frac-tion who survived) fifty years later.

If these 'negative' states or *absences* were more varied and severe than those seen in common Parkinson's disease, this was even truer of the innumerable 'positive' disorders or pathological *presences* introduced by the sleeping-sickness: indeed, von Economo, in his great monograph, enumerated more than five hundred distinct forms or varieties of these.[19]

---

whom the cerebral mechanisms for sleep had been destroyed) showed, for the first time, that sleep was a physiological necessity. Sometimes these insomniac states were accompanied by intense drive, driving those affected into a veritable frenzy of body and mind, a state of ceaseless excitement and movement, until their death (from exhaustion) a week or ten days later. Although terms like 'mania' and 'catatonic excitement' were sometimes used, these wild states more closely resembled rabies (for which they were sometimes mistaken).

Above all they resembled the states of intense cerebral excitement, with tremendous pressure of thought and movement, which may be seen in acute ergot poisoning: an amazing picture of this, as it affected an entire French village convulsed by accidental ergot poisoning (due to contamination of their bread), is given by John G. Fuller in *The Day of St. Anthony's Fire.* His picture of those affected, unable to sleep, talking excitedly all day and all night, making faces, making noises, constantly, compulsively moving and ticcing, driven by a rush and energy which gave no respite, until death from exhaustion came a week later, immediately made me think of those who were stricken by a hyperkinetic-insomniac form of *encephalitis lethargica.*

[19] The enormous range of post-encephalitic symptoms – particularly its unique disturbances of sleep, of sexuality, of affect, of appetite – fascinated physiologists as well as physicians, and led, in the 1920s and 1930s, to the founding of behavioural neurology as a science. Yet in this booming, buzzing confusion (which McKenzie called a 'chaos'), there seemed to von Economo to be three

Parkinsonian disorders, of one sort or another, were perhaps the commonest of these disorders, although their appearance was often delayed until many years after the acute epidemic. Post-encephalitic Parkinsonism, as opposed to ordinary or idiopathic Parkinsonism, tended to show less in the way of tremor and rigidity – indeed, these were sometimes completely absent – but much severer states of 'explosive' and 'obstructive' disorders, of akinesia and akathisia, push and resistance, hurry and impediment, etc., and also much severer states of the compliant-perseverative type of akinesia which Gowers had compared to catalepsy. Many patients, indeed, were swallowed up in states of Parkinsonian akinesia so profound as to turn them into living statues – totally motionless for hours, days, weeks, or years on end. The very much greater severity of these encephalitic and post-encephalitic states revealed that *all* aspects of being and behaviour – perceptions, thoughts, appetites, and feelings, no less than movements – could also be brought to a virtual standstill by an active, constraining Parkinsonian process.

Almost as common as these Parkinsonian disorders, and frequently co-existing with them, were *catatonic* disorders of every sort. It was the occurrence of these which originally gave rise to the notion of an 'epidemic schizophrenia,' for catatonia – until its appearance in the encephalitis epidemic – was thought to be part-and-parcel of the schizophrenic syndrome. The majority of patients who were rendered catatonic by the sleeping-sickness were *not* schizophrenic, and showed that catatonia might, so to speak, be approached by a direct physiological path, and was not

---

main patterns of involvement, or 'types' of disease: somnolent-ophthalmoplegic, hyperkinetic, and myostatic-akinetic (in his terms), corresponding to three main patterns of neuronal involvement (the first of these arising from involvement of the brainstem, of what were later to be delineated as 'arousal-systems' in this area; the last of these – which corresponds to Parkinsonism – to the involvement of the substantia nigra; and the most complex disorders of all – the impulsive and emotional hyperkinetic-tourettic ones – to involvement in the diencephalon and hypothalamus).

Hess's great studies of subcortical function (for which he was later awarded the Nobel Prize) were stimulated in the first place by his wonder at the novel symptoms of the *encephalitis lethargica* (this is described in the preface to his monograph, *Diencephalon,* 1954).

always a defensive manoeuvre undertaken by schizophrenic patients at periods of unendurable stress and desperation.[20]

The general forms or 'phases' of encephalitic catatonia were closely analogous to those of Parkinsonism, but were at a higher and more complex level, and were usually experienced as subjective states which had exactly the same form as the observable behavioural states. Thus some of these patients showed automatic compliance or 'obedience,' maintaining (indefinitely, and apparently without effort) any posture in which they were put or found themselves, or 'echoing' words, phrases, thoughts, perceptions, or actions in an unvarying circular way, once these had been suggested to them (palilalia, echolalia, echopraxia, etc.). Other patients showed disorders of a precisely antithetical kind ('command negativism,' 'block,' etc.) immediately preventing or countermanding any suggested or intended action, speech, or thought: in the severest cases, 'block' of this type could cause a virtual obliteration of all behaviour and also of all mental processes (see the case of Rose R., for example). Such constrained catatonic patients – like constrained Parkinsonians – could suddenly burst out of their immobilized states into violent movements or frenzies: a great many of the tics seen at the time of the epidemic, and subsequently, showed themselves to be interchangeable with 'tics of immobility,' or catatonia (Ferenczi, indeed, called tics 'cataclonia').

An immense variety of involuntary and compulsive movements were seen during the acute phase of the encephalitis, and for a few years thereafter: myoclonic jerks and spasms; states of mobile spasm (athetosis), dystonias and dystonic contortions (e.g. torticollis), with somewhat similar functional organizations to that of Parkinsonian rigidity; desultory, forceless movements dancing from one part of the body to another (chorea); and a

---

[20] Post-encephalitic patients, when they can speak – which in the severest cases was not rendered possible until half a century later, when they were given L-DOPA – are thus able to provide us with uniquely detailed and accurate descriptions of states of catatonic 'entrancement,' 'fascination,' 'forced thinking,' 'thought-block,' 'negativism,' etc., which schizophrenic patients, usually, are unable or unwilling to do, or which they will only describe in distorted, magical, 'schizophrenic' terms.

wide spectrum of tics and compulsive movements at every functional level – yawning, coughing, sniffing, gasping, panting,
breath-holding, staring, glancing, bellowing, yelling, cursing,
etc. – which were enactions of sudden *urges*. [21]

At the 'highest' level the *encephalitis lethargica* presented itself
as neurotic and psychotic disorders of every kind, and a great
many patients affected in this way were originally considered to
have 'functional' obsessional and hysterical neuroses, until the
development of other symptoms indicated the encephalitic aetiology of their complaints. It is of interest, in this connection, that
'oculogyric crises' were considered to be purely 'functional' and
hysterical for several years after their first appearance.

Clearly differentiated forms of affective compulsion were common in the immediate aftermath of the sleeping-sickness, especially erotomanias, erethisms, and libidinal excitement, on the
one hand, and tantrums, rages, and destructive outbursts on the
other. These forms of behaviour were most clearly and undis-
guisedly manifest in children, who sometimes showed abrupt
changes of character, and suddenly became impulsive, provocative, destructive, audacious, salacious, and lewd, sometimes to a
quite uncontrollable degree: such children were often labelled
'juvenile psychopaths' or 'moral aments.'[22] Sexual and destruc-

---

[21] In Thom Gunn's poem 'The Sense of Movement,' there occurs the following
pivotal line:

'One is always nearer by not being still.'

This poem deals with the basic *urge* to *move,* a movement which is always,
mysteriously, *towards.* This is not so for the Parkinsonian: he is *no* nearer for not
being still. He is no nearer to anything by virtue of his motion; and in this sense,
his motion is not genuine movement, as his lack of motion is not genuine rest.
The road of Parkinsonism is a road which leads nowhere; the land of Parkinsonism is paradox and dead end.

[22] Among the many eminent physicians who were deeply concerned with the
changes in character which might be wrought by the sleepy-sickness was Dr
G. A. Auden (father of the poet W. H. Auden). Such changes, Dr Auden
stressed, could not always be regarded as purely deleterious or destructive in
nature. Less zealous to 'pathologize' than many of his colleagues, Dr Auden
noted that some of those affected, especially children, might be 'awakened' into
a genuine (if morbid) brilliance, into unexpected and unprecedented heights
and depths. This notion of a disease with a 'Dionysiac' potential was often

tive outbursts were rarely outspoken in adults, being 'converted' (presumably) to other, more 'allowable,' reactions and expressions. Jelliffe,[23] in particular, who undertook lengthy analysis of some highly intelligent post-encephalitic patients, showed unequivocally how accesses of erotic and hostile feeling could be and were 'converted,' not only into neurotic and psychotic behaviour, but into tics, 'crises,' catatonia, and even Parkinsonism. Adult post-encephalitic patients thus showed an extraordinary ability to 'absorb' intense feeling, and to express it in indirect physiological terms. They were gifted – or cursed – with a pathologically extravagant expressive facility or (in Freud's term) 'somatic compliance.'

Nearly half the survivors became liable to extraordinary crises, in which they might experience, for example, the simultaneous and virtually instantaneous onset of Parkinsonism, catatonia, tics, obsessions, hallucinations, 'block,' increased suggestibility or negativism, and thirty or forty other problems; such crises would last a few minutes or hours, and then disappear as suddenly as they had come.[24] They were highly individual, no two patients

---

discussed in the Auden household, and formed an enduring theme in W. H. Auden's thought. Many other artists at this time, perhaps most notably Thomas Mann, were struck by the world-wide spectacle of a disease which could – however ambiguously – raise cerebral activity to a more awakened and creative pitch: in *Doctor Faustus* the Dionysiac fever is attributable to neurosyphilitic infection; but a similar allegory of extraordinary excitement, followed (and *paid for*) by attrition and exhaustion, could as well apply to post-encephalitic infection.

[23] Smith Ely Jelliffe, a man equally eminent as neurologist and psychoanalyst, was perhaps the closest observer of the sleeping-sickness and its sequelae. This was his summing-up, looking back on the epidemic: 'In the monumental strides made by neuropsychiatry during the past ten years no single advance has approached in importance that made through the study of epidemic encephalitis. No individual group of disease-reactions has been . . . so far-reaching in modifying the entire foundations of neuropsychiatry in general . . . *An entirely new orientation has been made imperative.'* (Jelliffe, 1927)

[24] The astonishing variability of such crises, and their openness to suggestion, were well shown in another patient, Lillian W., whose history is not in this book. Lillian W. had at least a hundred clearly different forms of crisis: hiccoughs; panting attacks; oculogyrias; sniffing attacks; sweating attacks; attacks in which her left shoulder would grow flushed and warm; chattering of the teeth; paroxysmal ticcing attacks; ritualized iterative attacks, in which she would tap one foot

ever having exactly the same sort of crises, and they expressed, in various ways, fundamental aspects of the character, personality, history, perception, and fantasies of each patient.[25] These

___

in three different positions, or dab her forehead in four set places; counting attacks; verbigerative attacks, in which certain set phrases were said a certain number of times; fear attacks; giggling attacks, etc., etc. Any allusion (verbal or otherwise) to any given type of crisis would infallibly call it forth in this patient.

Lillian W. would also have bizarre 'miscellaneous' crises, in which a great variety of phenomena (sniffing, oculogyria, panting, counting, etc., etc.) would be thrown together in unexpected (and seemingly senseless) combinations; indeed new and strange combinations were continually appearing. Although I observed dozens of these complex crises I was almost never able to perceive any physiological or symbolic unity in them, and after a while I ceased to look for any such unity, and accepted them as absurd juxtapositions of physiological oddments, or, on occasion, improvised collages of physiological bric-à-brac. This was also how Mrs W., a talented woman with a sense of humour, regarded her own miscellaneous crises: 'They are just a mess,' she would say, 'like a junk shop, or a jumble-sale, or the sort of stuff you just throw in the attic.' *Sometimes,* however, one could see patterns which were clear-cut but unintelligible, or patterns which seemed to hint, tantalizingly, at some scarcely imaginable unity or significance; and of these crises Mrs W. would say: 'This one's a humdinger, a surrealistic attack – I *think* it's saying something, but I don't know what it is, nor do I know what language it's in.' Some of my students who happened to witness such attacks also received a surrealistic impression: 'That's absolutely wild,' one of them once said. 'It's just like a Salvador Dali!' Another student, fantastically inclined, compared her crises to uncanny, unearthly buildings or music ('Martian churches or Arcturan polyphonies'). Although none of us could agree on the 'interpretation' of Lillian W.'s crises, we all felt them as having a strange fascination – the fascination of dreams, or peculiar art-forms; and, in this sense, if I sometimes thought of Parkinsonism as a relatively simple and coherent dream of the midbrain, I thought of Lillian W.'s crises as surrealistic deliria concocted by the forebrain.

[25] Not infrequently a single, sensational *moment-of-being* is 'caught' by a crisis, and preserved thereafter. Thus Jelliffe (1932) alludes to a man whose first oculogyric crisis came on during a game of cricket, when he had suddenly to fling one hand up to catch a high ball (he had to be carried off the field still entranced, with his right arm still outstretched and clutching the ball). Subsequently, whenever he had an oculogyric crisis, these would be ushered in by a *total replay* of this original, grotesque, and comic moment: he would suddenly feel it was 1919 once again, an unusually hot July afternoon, that the Saturday match was in progress again, that Trevelyan had just hit a probable 'six,' that the ball was approaching him, and that he had to catch it – RIGHT NOW! Similar, dramatic moments-of-being may also be incorporated into epileptic seizures, especially those of psychomotor type; Penfield and Perot, who have provided the most detailed accounts of this, suggest that 'fossilized memories' may be preserved in the cortex – memories which are normally dormant and forgotten, but which can suddenly come to life and be re-activated under special conditions. Such phe-

crises could be greatly influenced, for better or worse, by sugges-tion, emotional problems, or current circumstances. Crises of all sorts became rare after 1930, but I stress them and their charac-teristics because they show remarkable affinities to certain states induced by L-DOPA, not merely in post-encephalitic patients, but in the normally much stabler patients with common Parkinson's disease.

One thing, and one alone, was (usually) spared amid the rav-ages of this otherwise engulfing disease: the 'higher faculties' – intelligence, imagination, judgement, and humour. These were exempted – for better or worse. Thus these patients, some of whom had been thrust into the remotest or strangest extremities of human possibility, experienced their states with unsparing perspicacity, and retained the power to remember, to compare, to dissect, and to testify. Their fate, so to speak, was to become unique witnesses to a unique catastrophe.

THE AFTERMATH OF THE SLEEPING-SICKNESS (1927–67)

⮑ Although many patients seemed to make a complete recov-ery from the sleeping-sickness, and were able to return to their former lives, the majority of them subsequently developed neurological or psychiatric disorders, and, most commonly, Par-kinsonism. Why they should have developed such 'post-encepha-litic syndromes' – after years or decades of seemingly perfect health – is a mystery, and has never been satisfactorily explained.

---

nomena endorse the notion that our memories, or beings, are 'a collection of moments' (see n. 133, p. 256).

These post-encephalitic syndromes were very variable in course: sometimes they proceeded rapidly, leading to profound disability or death; sometimes very slowly; sometimes they progressed to a certain point and then stayed at this point for years or decades; and sometimes, following their initial onslaught, they remitted and disappeared. This great variation of pattern is also a mystery, and seems to admit of no single or simple explanation.

Certainly it could not be explained in terms of microscopically visible disease-processes, as was considered at one time. Nor was it true to say that post-encephalitic patients were suffering from a 'chronic encephalitis,' for they showed no signs of active infection or inflammatory reaction. There was, moreover, a rather poor correlation between the severity of the clinical picture and that of the pathological picture, insofar as the latter could be judged by microscopic or chemical means: one saw profoundly disabled patients with remarkably few signs of disease in the brain, and one saw evidences of widespread tissue-destruction in patients who were scarcely disabled at all. What *was* clear, from these discrepancies, was that there were many other determinants of clinical state and behaviour besides localized changes in the brain; it was clear that the susceptibility or propensity to Parkinsonism, for example, was not a fixed expression of lesions in the 'Parkinsonism-centre' of the brain, but dependent on innumerable other 'factors' in addition.

It seemed, as Jelliffe and a few others repeatedly stressed, as if the *'quality'* of the individual – his 'strengths' and 'weaknesses,' resistances and pliancies, motives and experiences, etc. – played a large part in determining the severity, course, and form of his illness. Thus, in the 1930s, at a time of almost exclusive emphasis on specific mechanisms in physiology and pathology, the strange evolutions of illness in these post-encephalitic patients recalled Claude Bernard's concepts of the *terrain* and the *milieu interne,* and the immemorial ideas of 'constitution,' 'diathesis,' 'idiosyncrasy,' 'predisposition,' etc., which had become so unfashionable in the twentieth century. Equally clear, and beautifully analysed by Jelliffe, were the effects of the external environment, the circumstances and vicissitudes of each patient's life. Thus, post-encephalitic illness could by no means be considered a simple disease, but needed to be seen as an individual creation of the greatest complexity, determined not simply by a primary disease-process, but by a vast host of personal traits and social circumstances: an illness, in short, like neurosis or psychosis, a coming-to-terms of the sensitized individual with his total environment. Such considerations, of course, are of crucial importance in understanding the total reactions of such patients to L-DOPA.

There remain today a few survivors of the encephalitis who, despite Parkinsonism, tics, or other problems, still lead active and independent lives (see for instance the case of Cecil M.). These are the fortunate minority, who for one reason or another have managed to keep afloat, and have not been engulfed by illness, disability, dependence, demoralization, etc. – Parkinson's 'train of harassing evils.'

But for the majority of post-encephalitic patients – in consequence of the basic severity of their illness, their 'weaknesses,' their propensities, or their misfortunes – a much darker future was in store. We have already stressed the inseparability of a patient's illness, his self, and his world, and how any or all of these, in their manifold interactions, through an infinity of vicious circles, can bring him to his nadir of being. How much is contributed by this, and that, and that, and that, can perhaps be unravelled by the most prolonged, intimate contact with individual patients, but cannot be put in any general, universally applicable form. One can only say that most of the survivors went down and down, through circle after circle of deepening illness, hopelessness, and unimaginable solitude, their solitude, perhaps, the least bearable of all.

> As *Sicknes* is the greatest misery, so the greatest misery of sicknes, is *solitude . . . Solitude* is a torment which is not threatened in *hell* itselfe.
>
> DONNE

The character of their illness changed. The early days of the epidemic had been a time of ebullition or ebullience, pathologically speaking, full of movements and tics, impulsions and impetuosities, manias and crises, ardencies and appetencies. By the late twenties, the acute phase was over, and the encephalitic syndrome started to cool or congeal. States of immobility and arrest had been distinctly uncommon in the early 1920s, but from 1930 onwards started to roll in a great sluggish, torpid tide over many of the survivors, enveloping them in metaphorical (if not physiological) equivalents of sleep or death. Parkinsonism, catatonia, melancholia, trance, passivity, immobility, frigidity, apathy: this was the quality of the decades-long 'sleep' which closed over their heads in the 1930s and thereafter. Some patients, indeed, passed into a timeless state, an eventless stasis, which deprived them of all sense of history and happening. Isolated circumstances – fire alarms, dinner-gongs, the unexpected arrival of friends or news – might set them suddenly and startlingly alive for a minute, wonderfully active and agog with excitement. But these were rare flashes in the depths of their darkness. For the most part, they lay motionless and speechless, and in some cases almost will-less and thoughtless, or with their thoughts and feelings unchangingly fixed at the point where the long 'sleep' had closed in upon them. Their minds remained perfectly clear and unclouded, but their whole beings, so to speak, were encysted or cocooned.

Unable to work or to see to their needs, difficult to look after, helpless, hopeless, so bound up in their illnesses that they could neither react nor relate, frequently abandoned by their friends and their families, without specific treatment of any use to them – these patients were put away in chronic hospitals, nursing homes, lunatic asylums, or special colonies; and there, for the most part, they were totally forgotten – the lepers of the present century; there they died in their hundreds of thousands.

And yet some lived on, in diminishing numbers, getting older and frailer (though usually looking younger than their age), inmates of institutions, profoundly isolated, deprived of experience, half-forgetting, half-dreaming of the world they once lived in.

LIFE AT MOUNT CARMEL

༈ Mount Carmel was opened, shortly after the First World War, for war-veterans with injuries of the nervous system, and for the expected victims of the sleeping-sickness. It was a cottage hospital, in these early days, with no more than forty beds, large grounds, and a pleasant prospect of surrounding countryside. It lay close to the village of Bexley-on-Hudson, and there was a free and friendly exchange between the hospital and the village: patients often went to the village for shopping or meals, or silent movies, and the villagers, in turn, frequently visited the hospital; there were dates, and dances, and occasional marriages; and there were friendly rivalries in bowls and football, in which the measured deliberation of the villagers would be met by the abnormal suddenness and speed of movement characteristic of so many encephalitic patients, fifty years ago.[26]

All this has changed, with the passage of years. Bexley-on-Hudson is no longer a village, but a crowded and squalid suburb of New York; the leisurely life of the village has gone, to be replaced by the hectic and harried anti-life of New York; Bexleyites no longer have any time, and rarely spare a thought for the hospital among them; and Mount Carmel itself has grown sick from hypertrophy, for it is now a 1,000-bed institution which

---

[26] This abnormal suddenness and speed of movement, often allied to an odd and unexpected, and sometimes very playful, quality may be of distinct advantage in certain sports. Thus one of my patients, Wilbur F., had been a very successful amateur boxer in his post-encephalitic youth. He showed me some fascinating old newspaper clippings from this time which attributed his success less to strength and skill than to the extraordinary speed and *strangeness* of his movements – movements which, without being illegal, were so odd as to be completely unanswerable. A similar tendency to sudden, 'prankish' moves, allied with great speed and inventiveness, a bizarre sort of 'motor genius,' is sometimes characteristic of Tourette's syndrome (see Sacks, 1981).

has swallowed its grounds; its windows no longer open on pleasant gardens or country, but on ant-nest suburbia, or nothing at all.

Still sadder, and more serious, has been the change in its character, the insidious deterioration in atmosphere and *care*. In its earlier days – indeed, before 1960 – the hospital was both easygoing and secure; there were devoted nurses and others who had been there for years, and most of the medical positions were honorary and voluntary, calling forth the best side, the kindness, of visiting doctors; and though its patients had grown older and frailer, they could look forward to excursions, day-trips, and summer-camps. In the past ten years, and especially the last three years, almost all this has changed. The hospital has assumed somewhat the aspect of a fortress or prison, in its physical appearance and the way it is run. A strict administration has come into being, rigidly committed to 'efficiency' and rules; 'familiarity' with patients is strongly discouraged. Law and order have been ousting fellow-feeling and kinship; hierarchy separates the inmates from staff; and patients tend to feel they are 'inside,' unreachably distant from the real world outside. There are, of course, gaps in this totalitarian structure, where *real* care and affection still maintain a foothold; many of the 'lower' staff – nurses, aides, orderlies, physiotherapists, occupational therapists, speech therapists, etc. – give themselves unstintingly, and with love, to the patients; volunteers from the neighbourhood provide non-professional care; and, of course, *some* patients are visited by relatives and friends. The hospital, in short, is a singular mixture, where freedom and bondage, warmth and coldness, human and mechanical, life and death, are locked together in perpetual combat.[27]

In 1966, when I first went to Mount Carmel, there were still some eighty post-encephalitic patients there, the largest, and

---

[27] We have seen that Parkinsonism and neurosis are innately coercive, and share a similar *coercive structure*. Rigorous institutions are also coercive, being, in effect, *external neuroses*. The coercions of institutions call forth and aggravate the coercions of their inmates: thus one may observe, with exemplary clarity, how the coerciveness of Mount Carmel aggravated neurotic and Parkinsonian tendencies in post-encephalitic patients; one may also observe, with equal clarity, how the 'good' aspects of Mount Carmel – its sympathy and humanity – reduced neurotic and Parkinsonian symptoms.

perhaps the only, such group remaining in the United States, and one of the very few such groups remaining in the world. Almost half of these patients were immersed in states of pathological 'sleep,' virtually speechless and motionless, and requiring total nursing-care; the remainder were less disabled, less dependent, less isolated, and less depressed, could look after many of their own basic needs, and maintain a modicum of personal and social life. Sexuality, of course, was forbidden in Mount Carmel.

Between 1966 and 1969, we brought the majority of our post-encephalitic patients (many of whom had been immured in remote, unnoticed bays of the hospital) into a single, organic, and self-governing community; we did what we could to give them the sense of being *people,* and not condemned prisoners in a vast institution; we instituted a search for missing relatives and friends, hoping that some relationships – broken by time and indolence, rather than hostility and guilt – might thus be reforged; and I myself formed with them such relationships as I could.

These years, then, saw a certain establishment of sympathies and kinships, and a certain melting-away of the rigid staff/inmate dichotomy; and with these, and all other forms of treatment, a certain – but pitifully limited – improvement in their overall condition, neurological and otherwise. Opposing all forms of therapeutic endeavour, and setting a low ceiling on what could be achieved, was the crushing weight of their illness, the Saturnian gravity of their Parkinsonism, etc; and behind this, and mingling with it, all the dilapidations, impoverishments, and perversions of long isolation and immurement.[28]

---

[28] It is of the greatest interest to compare the state of these patients at Mount Carmel with that of the only remaining post-encephalitic community in England (at the Highlands Hospital). Conditions at Highlands – where there are large grounds, free access to and from a neighbouring community, devoted attention, and a much freer and easier atmosphere – are akin to those which obtained at Mount Carmel in its early days. The patients at Highlands (most of whom have been there since the 1920s), although they have severe post-encephalitic syndromes, convey an altogether different appearance from the patients at Mount Carmel. They tend, by and large, to be mercurial, sprightly, impetuous, and hyper-active – with vivid and ardent emotional reactions. This is in the greatest contrast to the deeply Parkinsonian, entranced, grave, or withdrawn appearance

Some of these patients had achieved a state of icy hopelessness akin to serenity: a realistic hopelessness, in those pre-DOPA days:[29] they *knew* they were doomed, and they accepted this with all the courage and equanimity they could muster. Other patients (and, perhaps, to some extent, all of these patients, whatever their surface serenity) had a fierce and impotent sense of outrage: they had been *swindled* out of the best years of life; they were consumed by the sense of time lost, time *wasted;* and they yearned incessantly for a twofold miracle – not only a cure for their sickness, but an indemnification for the loss of their lives. They wanted to be given back the time they had lost, to be magically replaced in their youth and their prime.

These were their expectations before the coming of L-DOPA.

_____

of so many patients at Mount Carmel. It is clear that both groups of patients have the same disease, and it is equally clear that the *form* and evolution of illness have been quite different in the two groups.

It has never been clear to me whether these different forms of illness are due to different pathophysiological 'fates,' or the effects of differing environment and atmosphere: a rather open and cheery atmosphere at Highlands, a rather gloomy and withdrawn atmosphere at Mount Carmel. I favoured the latter interpretation in previous editions, but without clear supporting evidence. I should say that we also have a number of sprightly, impish, witty-ticcy patients at Mount Carmel, strongly reminiscent of their brothers in pathology at Highlands. So perhaps it is 'fate,' not environment. Most likely it is both in interaction. The peculiar *antic* character of such post-encephalitics is extremely characteristic, and often endearing, and earned them the affectionate nickname of 'enkies' in England. The qualities of 'enkieness' were not too striking at Mount Carmel, at first, because so many of the patients were wrapped in deep Parkinsonism when I saw them. They have become much more striking with the lifting of Parkinsonism – the continued stimulation of L-DOPA and (in some cases) a return to the effervescence of their earlier days.

[29] Anticholinergic drugs (hyoscyamine was the first) for the treatment of Parkinsonism had been introduced by Charcot, who used extracts of black henbane *(hyoscyamus niger),* as long ago as 1869 – but they were useful only for treating rigidity and tremor, not for the profound akinesia which post-encephalitic patients tended to have. The same was true of surgical treatments: chemo-pallidectomies and later thalamotomies, were introduced in the 1930s, and found invaluable in treating rigidity and tremor – but were of no help for akinesia. Apomorphine was found in the 1950s to reduce akinesia, but it required injection, and was too brief and too emetic in action, to be of much use. Amphetamines too could reduce akinesia a little, but had prohibitive 'side effects' at the large doses required. Thus akinesia – the single most overwhelming feature of post-encephalitic Parkinsonism – remained untreatable until the advent of L-DOPA.

THE COMING OF L-DOPA

⟳ L-DOPA is a 'miracle-drug' – the term is used everywhere; and this, perhaps, is scarcely surprising, for the physician who pioneered its use – Dr George Cotzias – himself calls L-DOPA 'a true miracle-drug . . . of our age.'[30] It is curious to hear sober physicians, and others, in the twentieth century, speaking of 'miracles,' and describing a drug in millennial terms. And the fervid enthusiasm aroused by reports of L-DOPA, both in the world at large and among physicians who give it and patients who take it – this too is amazing, and suggests that feelings and phantasies of an extraordinary nature are being excited and indulged. The L-DOPA 'story' has been intimately interwoven, for the last six years, with fervours and feelings of a mystical type; it cannot be understood without reference to these; and it would be quite misleading to present it in purely literal and historical terms.

We rationalize, we dissimilate, we pretend: we pretend that modern medicine is a rational science, all facts, no nonsense, and just what it seems. But we have only to tap its glossy veneer for it to split wide open, and reveal to us its roots and foundations,

---

[30] One of the great surprises (or should one say providences?) of nature is that the plant world contains so many substances which have a profound effect upon animals – and yet, apparently, are of no obvious 'use' to the plant. Thus the foxglove *(Digitalis)* contains digitalis glycosides, which are invaluable in the treatment of heart-failure; the autumn crocus *(Colchicum)* contains colchicine, invaluable in the treatment of gout, etc., etc. It is again characteristic that many such 'natural remedies' are discovered at a very early stage of human history, and may form part-and-parcel of a folk-medicine long before their efficacy is allowed by conventional or established medical science. It has recently been established, by chemical analysis, that several species of bean (especially the fava bean) contain large amounts of L-DOPA (of the order of 25 gm. L-DOPA in a pound of beans). There is also a suggestion (which requires careful examination) that such L-DOPA-rich beans may have constituted a 'folk-remedy' for Parkinsonians for many centuries, if not longer. Thus although we ascribe 'The Coming of L-DOPA' to A.D. 1967, it may well have 'come' by 1967 B.C.

its old dark heart of metaphysics, mysticism, magic, and myth. Medicine is the oldest of the arts, and the oldest of the sciences: would one not expect it to spring from the deepest knowledge and feelings we have?

There is, of course, an ordinary medicine, an everyday medicine, humdrum, prosaic, a medicine for stubbed toes, quinsies, bunions, and boils; but all of us entertain the idea of *another* sort of medicine, of a wholly different kind: something deeper, older, extraordinary, almost sacred, which will restore to us our lost health and wholeness, and give us a sense of perfect well-being.

For all of us have a basic, intuitive feeling that once we *were* whole and well; at ease, at peace, at home in the world; totally united with the grounds of our being; and that then we lost this primal, happy, innocent state, and fell into our present sickness and suffering. We had something of infinite beauty and preciousness – and we lost it; we spend our lives searching for what we have lost; and one day, perhaps, we will suddenly find it. And this will be the miracle, the millennium!

We may expect to find such ideas most intense in those who are enduring extremities of suffering, sickness, and anguish, in those who are consumed by the sense of what they have lost, or wasted, and by the urgency of recouping before it is too late. Such people, or patients, come to priests or physicians in desperations of yearning, prepared to believe anything for a reprieve, a rescue, a regeneration, a redemption. They are credulous in proportion to their desperation – the predestined victims of quacks and enthusiasts.

This sense of what is lost, and what must be found, is essentially a metaphysical one. If we arrest the patient in his metaphysical search, and ask him *what it is* that he wishes or seeks, he will not give us a tabulated list of items, but will say, simply, 'My happiness,' 'My lost health,' 'My former condition,' 'A sense of reality,' 'Feeling fully alive,' etc. He does not long for this thing or that; he longs for a *general* change in the complexion of things, for everything to be *all right* once again, unblemished, the way it once was. And it is at this point, when he is searching, here and there, with so painful an urgency, that he may be led into a sudden, grotesque mistake; that he may (in Donne's words) mistake 'the Apothecaryes shop' for 'the Metaphoricall Deity': a mistake which the apothecary or physician may be tempted to encourage.

It is at this point that he, ingenuously, and his apothecary and doctor, perhaps disingenuously, together depart from reality, and that the basic metaphysical truth is suddenly twisted (and replaced by a fantastic, mechanical corruption or falsehood). The chimerical concept which now takes its place is one of the delusions of vitalism or materialism, the notion that 'health,' 'well-being,' 'happiness,' etc. can be reduced to certain 'factors' or 'elements' – principles, fluids, humours, commodities – *things* which can be measured and weighed, bought and sold. Health, thus conceived, is reduced to a *level,* something to be titrated or topped-up in a mechanical way. Metaphysics in itself makes no such reductions: its terms are those of organization or design. The fraudulent reduction comes from alchemists, witch-doctors, and their modern equivalents, and from patients who long *at all costs* to be well.

It is from this debased metaphysics that there arises the notion of a mystical substance, a miraculous drug, something which will assuage all our hungers and ills, and deliver us instantly from our miserable state: metaphorical equivalents of the Elixir of Life.[31]

---

[31] The notion of 'mystical substances' arises from a *reductio ad absurdum* of two world-views which, legitimately employed, have great elegance and power: one is the mosaic or topist view, associated with the philosophies of empiricism and positivism, and the other is a holist or monist view. These derive, respectively, from Aristotelian and Platonic metaphysics. Used with mastery, and a full understanding of their powers and limits, these two world-views have provided a groundwork for fundamental discoveries in physiology and psychology during the past two hundred years.

Mysticism arises by taking analogy for identity – turning similes and metaphors (or 'as' statements) into absolutes (or 'is' statements), converting a useful epistemology into 'absolute truth.' A mystical topism asserts that the world consists of a multitude of points, places, particles, or pieces, without intrinsic relation to each other, but 'extrinsically' related by a 'causal nexus': it asserts this both exclusively and conclusively – it is 'the truth,' 'the whole truth,' and excludes any other 'truth.' Given such a view, one can conceive the possibility of affecting a single point or particle, without the least effect on those surrounding it: one would, for example, be able to *knock out* one point with absolute accuracy and specificity. The therapeutic correlate of such a mysticism is the notion of a *perfect Specific,* which has exactly the effect one wants, and no possibility of any other

Such notions and hopes fully retain today their ancient, magical, mythical force, and – however we may disavow them – show themselves in the very words we use: 'vitamins' (vital amines), and the vitamin-cult; or 'biogenic amines' (life-giving amines) – of which dopamine (the biologically active substance into which L-DOPA is converted) is itself an example.

The notion of such mystical, life-giving, sacramental remedies gives rise to innumerable cults and fads, and to enthusiasms of a particularly extravagant and intransigent type. One sees this in Freud's espousal of the drug cocaine;[32] in the first wild reactions to the appearance of cortisone, when some medical conferences, in the words of a contemporary observer, 'more closely resembled revivalist meetings'; in the present world-wide 'drug-scene';[33] and, not least, in our present enthusiasm for the drug

---

effects. A famous example of such a supposed Specific is the drug arsephenamine, devised by Ehrlich for the treatment of syphilis. Ehrlich's own modest and realistic claims were immediately distorted by absolutist wishes and tendencies – and arsephenamine was soon dubbed 'The Magic Bullet.' *This* sort of mystical medicine, then, is dedicated to the search for more and more 'magic bullets.'

A mystical holism, conversely, asserts that the world is an entirely uniform and undifferentiated mass of 'world-stuff,' 'primal matter,' or plasm. A famous example of such a mystical-holist physiology is exemplified by a dictum ascribed to Flourens: 'The brain is homogeneous like the liver; the brain secretes thought as the liver secretes bile.' The therapeutic correlate of such a monist mysticism is the notion of an all-purpose drug, a Panacea or Catholicon, a Quintessential extract of World-Stuff or Brain-Stuff, absolutely pure bottled Goodness or Godness – de Quincey's 'portable ecstasy corked up in a pink-bottle.'

[32] See Appendix: 'Miracle' Drugs: Freud, William James, and Havelock Ellis, p. 323.

[33] William James (*Varieties,* pp. 304–8) suggests that one of the primary reasons why people turn to alcohol is to achieve a sense of mystic at-oneness, a return to elemental and primal bliss, and that in this partly metaphysical and partly regressive use it exemplifies the deeply felt need for 'mystagogue' drugs; he quotes with approval the familiar maxim that 'the best cure for dipsomania is religiomania.'

We see from history and anthropology that the craving for mystagogues is universal and ancient, and that a wide knowledge of mystagogues is possessed by all races. The use of mystagogues, in the last century, constituted a literary pastime (and at times a necessity), and was part-and-parcel of the development of the Romantic imagination. In our own century, especially in the last twenty years, the use of mystagogues has again become widespread and explicit, Huxley taking mescal to 'cleanse the doors of perception,' and Leary promoting LSD as a 'sacramental' drug. Here – as with L-DOPA – one sees the amalgamation of

L-DOPA. It is impossible to avoid the feeling that here, over and above all legitimate enthusiasms, there is this special enthusiasm, this mysticism, of a magical sort.

We may now pass on to the 'straight' story of L-DOPA, remembering the mystical thread which always winds through it. Parkinson himself looked in vain for the 'seat' or substrate of Parkinsonism, although he tentatively located it in the 'pith' of the lower or medullary parts of the brain. Nor was there any real success in defining the location and nature of the pathological process until a century after the publication of Parkinson's 'Essay.'[34] In 1919 von Economo, and separately Trétiakoff, described the findings of severe damage to the *substantia nigra* (a nucleus in the midbrain, consisting of large pigmented cells) in a number of patients with *encephalitis lethargica* who had shown severe Parkinsonian symptoms. The following year Greenfield, in England, and pathologists elsewhere, were able to define similar, but milder, changes in these cells in patients who had had ordinary Parkinson's disease. These findings, in company with other pathological and physiological work, suggested the existence of a clearly defined *system,* linking the *substantia nigra* to other parts of the brain: a system whose malfunctioning or destruction might give rise to Parkinsonian symptoms. In Greenfield's words:

. . . A general survey has shown *paralysis agitans* in its classical form to be a systemic degeneration of a special type affecting a neuronal system whose nodal point is the *substantia nigra.*

In 1920 the Vogts, with remarkable insight, suggested that this anatomically and functionally distinct system might correspond with a *chemically distinct* system, and that a specific treatment for

---

genuine needs with mystical means, the mistaking of an infinite, metaphorical symbol for a finite, ingestible drug.

[34] There had, in fact, been tentative earlier localizations of a prescient sort, e.g. a famous case, in the 1890s, in which the development of a one-sided Parkinsonism was correlated with the growth of a tuberculoma of one cerebral peduncle; several cases of syphilitic disease of the midbrain, associated with Parkinsonism, etc. The organization of Parkinsonism, indeed, was appreciated, both theoretically and practically, *before* the finding of specific cell-damage: thus two operations for Parkinsonism – cutting the posterior spinal roots, and excising portions of the cerebral cortex – were performed, and found useful, before 1910.

Parkinsonism, and related disorders, might become possible if this hypothetical chemical substance could be identified and administered.

> Studies should answer the question [they wrote], whether the striatal system or parts of it do or do not possess a special disposition towards certain injuring agents . . . Such a positive or negative tendency to react can be assumed to be ultimately due to the specific chemistry of the corresponding centre. The disclosure of the existence of such specific chemistry represents, in turn, at least the first step towards elucidation of its true nature, thereby initiating the development of a biochemical approach to treatment . . .

Thus in the 1920s, there was not merely a vague notion of 'something missing' in Parkinsonism patients (such as Charcot had entertained), but a clear path of research stretching out, pointing towards a prospect of ultimate success.

The most astute clinical neurologists, however, had reservations about this: was there not *structural* damage in the *substantia nigra,* and perhaps elsewhere, damage to nerve-cells and their connections? Could *this* be reversed? Would the administration of the missing chemical substrate be sufficient, or safe, given a marked degree of structural disorganization? Might there not be some danger of over-stimulating or over-loading such cells as were left? These reservations were expressed, with great pungency, by Kinnier Wilson:

> *Paralysis agitans* seems at present an incurable malady *par excellence;* the antidote to the 'local death' of cell-fibre systems would be the equally elusive 'elixir of life' . . . It is worse than useless to administer to the Parkinsonian any kind of nerve tonic to 'whip up' his decaying cells; rather must some form of readily assimilable pabulum be sought, in the hope of supplying from without what the cell itself cannot obtain from within.

Neurochemistry, as a science, scarcely existed in the 1920s, and the project envisaged by the Vogts had to await its slow development. The intermediate stages of this research form a fascinating story in themselves, but will be omitted from consideration here. Suffice it that in 1960 Hornykiewicz, in Vienna, and Barbeau, in Montreal, using different approaches, but almost simultaneously, provided clear evidence that the affected parts of the brain in Parkinsonian patients were defective in the nerve-transmitter *dopamine,* and that the transfer and metabolism of dopamine in these areas was also disturbed. Immediate efforts were made to replenish the brain-dopamine in Parkinsonian patients by giving them the natural precursor of dopamine – laevodihydroxyphenylalanine, or L-DOPA (dopamine itself could not pass into the brain).[35] The results of these early therapeutic efforts were encouraging but inconclusive, and seven more years of arduous research had to be undertaken. Early in 1967, Dr Cotzias and his colleagues, in their now-classic paper, were able to report a resounding therapeutic success in the treatment of Parkinsonism, giving massive doses of L-DOPA by mouth.[36]

The impact of Cotzias's work was immediate and astounding in the neurological world. The good news spread quickly. By March 1967, the post-encephalitic and Parkinsonian patients at Mount Carmel had already heard of L-DOPA: some of them were eager to try it at once; some had reservations and doubts, and wished to see its effects on others before they tried it themselves; some expressed total indifference: and some of course were unable to signal any reaction.

The cost of L-DOPA in 1967 and 1968 was exceedingly high

[35] In contrast, the drug amantadine (introduced as an antiviral agent against influenza A, but discovered serendipitously in 1968 to have anti-Parkinsonian effects as well) acts either by inhibiting dopamine re-uptake, or by increasing its release, or both, effectively increasing the brain's own dopamine. More recently a variety of dopamine agonists (e.g., bromocriptine and pergolide) have been made, which also potentiate dopamine action in the brain; it is hoped that they may have more specific effects than L-DOPA, because their action may be confined to specific receptor sites.

In the past two or three years there have been intriguing trials of tissue transplants – transplanting foetal brain cells, or adult adrenal cells, directly into the brain, where (hopefully) they may survive as living 'dopamine pumps' (see Appendix: Beyond L-DOPA, p. 333).

[36] Cotzias's first work used DL-DOPA, a mixture of the biologically active L-DOPA with its inactive isomer D-DOPA. The separation of these two isomers, in 1966–7, was not easily accomplished, and was exceedingly costly.

(more than $5,000 a pound), and it was impossible for Mount Carmel – a charity hospital, impoverished, unknown, unattached to any university or foundation, beneath the notice of drug-firms, industrial, or government sponsors – to buy L-DOPA at this time. Towards the end of 1968, the cost of L-DOPA started a sharp decline, and in March 1969 it was first used at Mount Carmel.

I could, perhaps, despite its cost, have started a few of our patients on L-DOPA after reading Cotzias's paper. But I hesitated – and hesitated for two years. For the patients under my care were not 'ordinary' patients with Parkinson's disease: they had far more complex pathophysiological syndromes, and their situations were more complex, indeed without precedent – for they had been institutionalised, and out of the world, for decades – in some cases since the time of the great epidemic. Thus even before I started, I was faced by scientific and human complexities, complexities and perplexities of a sort which had not arisen in previous trials of levodopa, or indeed of any treatment in the past. Thus there was an element of the extraordinary, the unprecedented, the unpredictable. I was setting out, with my patients, on an uncharted sea . . .

I did not know what might happen, what might be released – the more so as some of my patients had been violently impulsive and hyperkinetic *before* being enclosed in a straightjacket of Parkinsonism. But as illness and death claimed some of my patients – especially in the fierce summer of 1968 – the need to do something became ever clearer and stronger, finally moving me to start L-DOPA, though with great caution, in March 1969.

Awakenings

FRANCES D.

꧁ Miss D. was born in New York in 1904, the youngest and brightest of four children. She was a brilliant student at high school until her life was cut across, in her fifteenth year, by a severe attack of *encephalitis lethargica* of the relatively rare hyperkinetic form. During the six months of her acute illness she suffered intense insomnia (she would remain very wakeful until four in the morning, and then secure at most two or three hours' sleep), marked restlessness (fidgeting, distractible and hyperkinetic throughout her waking hours, tossing-and-turning throughout her sleeping hours), and impulsiveness (sudden urges to perform actions which seemed to her senseless, which for the most part she could restrain by conscious effort). This acute syndrome was considered to be 'neurotic,' despite clear evidence of her previously well-integrated personality and harmonious family life.

By the end of 1919, restlessness and sleep-disorder had subsided sufficiently to allow resumption and finishing of high school, although they continued to affect Miss D. more mildly for a further two years. Shortly after the end of her acute illness, Miss D. started to have 'panting attacks,' at first coming on two or three times a week, apparently spontaneously, and lasting many hours; subsequently becoming rarer, briefer, milder, and more clearly periodic (they would usually occur on Fridays) or circumstantial (they were especially prone to occur in circumstances of anger and frustration). These respiratory crises (as they clearly were, although they also were termed 'neurotic' at the time) became rarer and rarer, and ceased to occur entirely after 1924. Miss D., indeed, made no spontaneous mention of these attacks when first seen by me, and it was only later, when being questioned in greater detail before the administration of L-DOPA, that she recollected these attacks of half a century previously.

Following the last of her respiratory crises, Miss D. had the first of her oculogyric crises, and these indeed continued to be her sole post-encephalitic symptom for twenty-five years (1924–49), during which time Miss D. followed a varied and successful career as a legal secretary, as an active committee-woman in social and civic affairs, etc. She led a full life, with many friends, and frequent entertaining; she was fond of theatre, an avid reader, a collector of old china, etc. Talented, popular, energetic, well-integrated emotionally, Miss D. thus showed no sign of the 'deterioration' said to be so common after severe encephalitis of the hyperkinetic type.

In the early 1950s, Miss D. started to develop a more sinister set of symptoms; in particular a tendency to freeze in her movements and speech, and a contrary tendency to hurry in her walking, speech, and handwriting. When in 1969 I first asked Miss D. about her symptoms she gave me the following answer: 'I have various banal symptoms which you can see for yourself. But my *essential* symptom is that I cannot start and I cannot stop. Either I am held still, or I am forced to accelerate. I no longer seem to have any in-between states.' This statement sums up the paradoxical symptoms of Parkinsonism with perfect precision. It is instructive, therefore, that in the absence of 'banal' symptoms (e.g. rigidity, tremor, etc., which only became evident in 1963), the diagnosis of Parkinsonism failed to be made, but that a large variety of other diagnoses (such as 'catatonia,' 'hysteria') were offered. Miss D. was finally labeled Parkinsonian in 1964.

Her oculogyric crises, to return to this cardinal symptom, were originally of great severity, coming many times a month and lasting up to fifteen hours each. Within a few months of their onset they had settled down to a fairly strict periodicity, coming 'like clockwork' every fifth day, so much so that Miss D. could plan a calendar for months in advance, knowing that she would inevitably have a crisis every five days, and only very occasionally at other times. The rare departures from this schedule which occurred were usually associated with circumstances of great annoyance or distress. The crises would occur abruptly, without warning, her gaze being forced first downwards or to either side for several minutes, and then suddenly upwards, where it would stay for the remainder of the attack. Miss D. stated that her face would assume 'a fixed angry or scared expression' during these attacks, although she experienced neither rage nor fear while they lasted. Movement would be difficult during a crisis, her voice would be abnormally soft, and her thoughts seemed to 'stick'; she would always experience a 'feeling of resistance,' a force which opposed movement, speech, and thought, during the attack. She would also feel intensely wakeful in each attack, and find it impossible to sleep; as the crises neared their termination, she would start to yawn and become intensely drowsy; the attack would finally end quite suddenly, with restoration of normal movement, speech, and thought (this sudden restoration of normal consciousness Miss D. – a crossword addict – would call 'resipiscence'). In addition to these classical oculogyric crises, Miss D. started to experience a number of variant crises after 1955: forced deviation of gaze became exceptional, being replaced by a fixed and stony stare; some of these staring attacks were of overwhelming severity, completely depriving her of movement and speech, and lasting up to three days. She was admitted to a municipal hospital on several occasions during the 1960s when neighbours had discovered her in these attacks, and she was displayed at staff meetings as a striking case of 'periodic catatonia.' Since 1962, Miss D. has also had brief staring attacks, lasting only a few minutes, in which she is arrested and feels 'entranced.' Yet another paroxysmal symptom has been attacks of flushing and sweating, coming on at irregular intervals, and lasting fifteen to thirty minutes. (Miss D. had completed her menopause in the mid 1940s.) Since 1965, staring and oculogyric crises had become mild and infrequent, and when admitted to Mount Carmel Hospital at the start of 1969, Miss D. had been free of them for more than a year, and continued to be exempt from them until given L-DOPA in June 1969.

Although, as mentioned, rigidity and tremor had appeared in 1963, the most disabling of Miss D.'s symptoms, and the ones which finally necessitated her admission to a chronic disease hospital, were threefold: a progressive flexion-dystonia of the neck and trunk, uncontrollable festination and forced running, backwards or forwards, and uncontrollable 'freezing' which would sometimes arrest her in awkward positions for hours on end. A further symptom of relatively recent onset, for which no local infective aetiology could be found, was urinary frequency and urge; sometimes this urge would coexist with or call forth a 'block' or 'reluctance' of micturition – an intolerable coupling of opposing symptoms.

On admission to Mount Carmel Hospital, in January 1969, Miss D. was able to walk freely using two sticks, or for short distances alone; by June 1969, she had become virtually unable to walk by herself alone. Her posture, which was bent on admission, had become almost doubled-up over the course of the following six months. Transferring from bed to chair had become impossible, as had turning over in bed, or cutting up food. In view of this rather rapid deterioration, and the uselessness of all conventional anti-Parkinsonian drugs, the advent of L-DOPA came at a critical time for Miss D., who seemed about to slip into an accelerating and irrevocable decline.

Before L-DOPA

Miss D. was a tiny, bent woman, so kyphotic that, on standing, her face was forced to gaze at the ground. She was able to raise her head briefly, but it would return within seconds to its habitual position of extreme emprosthotonos, with the chin wedged down on the sternum. This habitual posture could not be accounted for by rigidity of the cervical muscles: rigidity was not more than slightly increased in the neck, and in oculogyric crises her head would be forced backwards to an equally extreme degree.

There was quite severe masking of the face, alertness and emotional expression being conveyed almost exclusively by Miss D.'s quick-glancing, humorous eyes – anomalously mobile in her mask-like face. Spontaneous blinking was rare. Her voice was clear and intelligible, although it was monotonous in volume and timbre, lacked 'personal' intonations and inflections, and could only momentarily be raised above a whispering and hushed hypophonic intensity; at intervals there would be sudden vocal hurries and festinations, accelerated rushes of words sometimes terminating in a verbal 'crash' at the end of a sentence.

Voluntary movement elsewhere, like speech, was characterized by the contradictory features of akinesia and hyperkinesis, either alternating or in paradoxical simultaneity. Most hand movements were marked by akinesia – with feebleness, parsimony, excessive effort, and decay on repetition of the movement. Her handwriting, once started, was large, effortless, and rapid; but if Miss D. became over-excited, her writing would slip out of control, either becoming larger and faster and more violent until it covered the entire paper with eddies and scrawls, or smaller and slower and stickier until it became a motionless point. She could rise from her chair without impediment, but having risen would tend to 'freeze,' often for many minutes, unable to take the first step. At such times she would display an almost cataleptic fixity of posture, almost doubled-over, and resembling a film which had come to a stop. Once a first step was taken – and walking could be inaugurated by a little push from behind, a verbal command from the examiner, or a visual command in the form of a stick, a piece of paper, or something definite to step over on the floor – Miss D. would teeter forward in tiny rapid steps. Six months previously, on her admission, when walking had been altogether easier, festination had represented a most serious problem, always tending to end (like her verbal stampedes and accelerating scrawls) in catastrophe. In remarkable contrast was her excellent ability to climb stairs stably and steadily, each stair providing a stimulus to a step; having reached the top of the stairs, however, Miss D. would again find herself 'frozen' and unable to proceed. She often remarked that 'if the world consisted entirely of stairs,' she would have no difficulty getting around whatever.[37] Pulsion in all directions (propulsion, lateropulsion, retropulsion) could all be elicited with dangerous ease. Severe and protracted freezing would also tend to occur when any switch of activity was necessitated: this was most obvi-

---

[37] See Appendix: Parkinsonian Space and Time, p. 339.

ous in her walking, when she had to turn, but also showed itself, on occasion, when she had to shift her glance from one place to another, or her attention from one idea to another.

Rigidity and tremor were not particularly prominent in the clinical picture. A coarse (flapping) tremor of the right hand would occur, rather rarely, in response to physical or emotional tension: it tended to come on, most characteristically, with the futile effort and distress of freezing. There was mild hypertonia of the left arm and marked ('hemiplegic') hypertonia of the legs. There was also a suggestion of hyper-reflexia and spasticity on the left side of the body. The clinical picture was completed by a number of spontaneous movements and hyperkineses. The muscles about the mouth exhibited puckering movements and occasional pursings and poutings of the lips. There was occasional grinding of the teeth and masticatory movements. Her head was never held quite still, but bobbed and nodded in an irregular fashion. These mouth and head movements were aggravated, synkinetically, during effort. Every so often, perhaps five or six times an hour, Miss D. would be impelled to take a sudden, deep, tic-like inspiration. A residue of the original restlessness and akathisia could be observed in the incessant fidgeting shown by her right hand, a local restlessness which was stilled only when the hands were otherwise occupied.

Miss D. was exceedingly alert and observant of all that went on about her, but not pathologically vigilant or insomniac. She was clearly of superior intelligence, witty and precise in her speech, and without significant stereotypy or stickiness of thought save, as indicated, in her crises. She was notably exact, orderly, punctual, and methodical in all her activities, but showed no severe obsessional symptoms such as fixed compulsions or phobias.

She had continued to maintain, despite being institutionalized, a healthy self-respect, many interests, and a close attention to her environment, providing a focus of stability and humour and compassion on a large ward of disabled and sometimes very disturbed post-encephalitic patients.

She was started on L-DOPA on 25 June 1969.

Course on L-DOPA

30 June. Although this was only five days after the start of treatment, and Miss D. was receiving no more than 0.5 gm. of L-DOPA daily, she exhibited some general restlessness, increased fidgeting of the right hand, and masticatory movements. The puckering of circumoral muscles had become more pronounced and now showed itself to be a form of compulsive grimace, or tic. There was already an obvious increase of general activity: Miss D. was now always, but always, doing something – crocheting (which had been slow and difficult before administration of the drug), washing clothes, writing letters, etc. She seemed somewhat *driven,* and unable to tolerate inactivity. Miss D. also complained even at this very early stage of 'difficulty in catching the breath,' and showed a tachypnoea of forty breaths to the minute, without variation in the force or rhythm of breathing.

6 July. On the eleventh day of drug-trial, and receiving 2 gm. L-DOPA daily, Miss D. now exhibited a complex mixture of desirable and adverse effects. Among the good effects she showed a sense of well-being and abounding energy, a much stronger voice, less freezing, less postural flexion, and stabler walking with longer strides. Among the adverse effects she showed aggravation of her former mild chewing and biting movements, so that she incessantly chewed on her gums, which had become very sore; increased fidgeting of her right hand, to which was now added a tic-like flexion and extension of the forefinger; finally, and most distressing to her, a disintegration of the normal automatic controls of breathing. Her breathing had now become rapid, shallow, and irregular, and was broken up by sudden violent inspirations two or three times a minute, each of which would follow a sudden, powerful, and fully conscious though uncontrollable *urge* to breathe. Miss D. remarked at this time: 'My breathing is no longer automatic. I have to think about each breath, and every so often I am *forced* to gasp.'

In view of these adverse symptoms, the dosage was reduced on this day. Over the ensuing ten days, on a dose of 1.5 gm. L-DOPA daily, Miss D. maintained the desirable effects of the drug and showed less restlessness, chewing, and pressure of activity. Her respiratory symptoms, however, persisted, growing more pronounced daily, finally differentiating, around 10 July, into clear-cut respiratory crises.[38] These attacks would start, without any warning whatever, with a sudden inspiratory gasp, followed by forced breath-holding for ten to fifteen seconds, then a violent expiration, and finally an apnoeic pause for ten to fifteen seconds. In these early and relatively mild attacks there were no associated symptoms or autonomic disturbances (e.g. tachycardia, hypertension, sweating, trembling, apprehension, etc.). This strange and distorted form of breathing could be interrupted for a minute or two by a strong effort of will, but would then resume its bizarre and imperative character. Her crises would last between one and three hours, finally subsiding over a period of about five minutes, with resumption of normal, automatic, unconscious breathing of even rate, rhythm, and force. The timing of these attacks was of interest, for it bore no constant relationship to the times at which L-DOPA was administered. Thus, for the first five days of respiratory crises, attacks occurred invariably in the evening and at no other times. On 15 July, for the first time, an attack occurred in the afternoon (at 1 p.m., an hour after L-DOPA had been given): on 16 July, for the first time, an attack occurred very early in the morning, before the first daily dose of L-DOPA had been taken. Subsequently, two or three attacks would occur every day, al-

---

[38] Respiratory crises were common in the acute phases of the encephalitis, and the subject of many important studies (Turner and Critchley, 1925, 1928; Jelliffe, 1927), but were scarcely seen after 1929. I myself had never seen one until Frances D. had her first attack, and I was quite bewildered when I saw it: was this a form of asthma, acute heart failure, a sort of seizure? Or was it hysterical hyperventilation, or a respiratory response to acidosis . . . Various possibilities, none too plausible, went through my mind, and it was only when *she* said, 'This is exactly what I used to get, back in '19,' that I realized that I was seeing a resurrection of this remarkable 'fossil' symptom. By the end of 1969, however, the majority of our post-encephalitic patients were having respiratory disturbances of one sort and another (see Sacks et al., 1970a). These strange disorders, convulsive in character, and physiological in origin, often came to associate themselves with emotional needs and contexts, to become, as Jelliffe put it, an idiosyncratic form of 'respiratory behaviour.'

One of Frances D.'s respiratory crises is to be seen in the documentary film of *Awakenings,* and one was given dramatic portrayal by Robert De Niro during the filming of *Awakenings.*

though the evening attacks continued to be the longest and severest.

On 16 July, I observed that the attacks were now assuming a most frightening intensity. A violent and protracted gasp (which looked and sounded as desperate as that of a nearly drowned man finally coming to the surface for a lungful of air) would be followed by forced breath-holding for up to fifty seconds, during which time Miss D. would struggle to expel breath through a closed glottis, in so doing becoming purple and congested from the futile effort; finally the breath would be expelled with tremendous violence, making a noise like the boom of a gun. No voluntary control whatever was possible at this time; in Miss D.'s words: 'I can no more control it than I could control a spring tide. I just ride it out, and wait for the storm to clear.' During this crisis speech was, of course, quite impossible, and there was a clear increase of rigidity throughout the body. The pulse-rate was raised to 120, and the blood-pressure rose from its normal 130/75 to 170/100. Twenty mg. of Benadryl, given intravenously, failed to alter the course of this attack. Despite what I would have imagined was a terrifying experience, and an expression of terror on her face, Miss D. denied that any alteration of thinking or special apprehension had been experienced during the crisis. Greatly concerned about the possible effects of so violent an attack in an elderly patient, I was disposed at this time to discontinue the L-DOPA. But, at Miss D.'s insistence, in view of the real benefits she was obtaining from the drug, and in the hope that her respiratory instability might decrease, I contented myself with reducing its dosage to 1.0 gm. daily.

Despite this small dosage, Miss D. continued to have respiratory crises of varying severity, two or more commonly three times a day. Within two or three days, these had established a routine – a crisis at 9 a.m., a crisis at noon, and a crisis at 7.30 p.m. – which remained fixed despite chance and systematic alterations of the times at which she would receive L-DOPA. We had also come to suspect, by 21 July, that her respiratory crises were readily conditionable: on this day our speech-therapist stopped to talk to Miss D. at five in the afternoon (normally a crisis-free time), and inquired whether she had had any crises recently;

before Miss D. could begin to frame an answer, she was impelled to gasp violently and launch into an unexpected crisis which seemed suspiciously like an answer to the question.

By now a therapeutic dilemma was becoming clear. There was no doubt of the enormous benefit derived from L-DOPA: Miss D. was looking, feeling, and moving far better than she had done in twenty years; but she had also become overexcitable and odd in her behaviour, and in particular seemed to be experiencing a revival or revocation of an idiosyncratic respiratory sensitivity (or behaviour) which had lain dormant in her for forty-five years. There was also, even in her first month of treatment, a number of minor 'side-effects' (a term which I found it increasingly difficult to give any meaning to), with the promise (or threat) of others lurking *in posse* – as I imagined it – in an as-yet unactualized state. Could we find a happy medium, an in-between state and dosage which would greatly assist Miss D. *without* calling forth her respiratory symptoms and other 'side-effects'?

Once more (on 19 July) the dosage was reduced – to a mere 0.9 gm. of L-DOPA daily. This reduction was promptly followed, that very day, by the occurrence of an oculogyric crisis – Miss D.'s first such in almost three years. This was disconcerting, because we had already observed, in several other post-encephalitic patients, a situation in which any given therapeutic dose of L-DOPA evoked respiratory crises, and any lessening of this dose oculogyric crises, and we feared that Miss D., too, might have to walk a tightrope between these two disagreeable alternatives.

Although the reported experience of others encouraged us to suppose that one could 'balance' or 'titrate' patients by finding exactly the right dose of L-DOPA, our experience with Miss D. – at this time – suggested that she could no more be 'balanced' than a pin on its point. Her oculogyric crisis, which was severe, was at once followed by a second and third oculogyric crises; with increase of the L-DOPA to 0.95 gm. a day, *these* crises ceased, but respiratory crises returned; with diminution of L-DOPA to 0.925 gm. a day (we were forced, at this stage, to encapsulate L-DOPA ourselves, in order to allow these infinitesimal increments and decrements of dose), the reverse switch occurred; and at a dose of 0.9375 gm. a day, she experienced *both* forms of crisis, in alternation, or simultaneously.

It became clear, at this time, that Miss D.'s crises, which were now occurring several times a day, showed a close association not only with overall psycho-physiological state, mood, and circumstance, but with certain specific dynamics, and in this way acted like migraines, and even like hysterical symptoms. If Miss D. had had a poor night and was tired, crises were more likely; if she was in pain (an ingrown toenail was troubling her at this time), she tended to have a crisis; if she became excited, she was especially prone to have a crisis, whether the excitement was fearful, angry, or hilarious in character; when she became frustrated, she exhibited crises; and when she desired attention from the nursing staff, she developed a crisis. I was slow to realize, while noting the causes of Miss D.'s crises, that the most potent 'trigger' of all was me, myself: I had indeed observed that as soon as I entered her room, or as soon as she caught sight of me, she usually had a crisis, but assumed that this was due to some other cause I had failed to notice, and it was only when an observant nurse giggled and remarked to me, 'Dr Sacks, *you* are the object of Miss D.'s crises!', that I belatedly tumbled to the truth. When I asked Miss D. if this could be the case, she indignantly denied the very possibility, but blushed an affirmative crimson. There was, finally, one other psychic cause of her crises which I could not have known of had Miss D. not mentioned it to me: 'As soon as *I think of getting a crisis,*' she confessed, 'I am apt to get one. And if I try to think of not getting a crisis, I get one. And if I try to think about not thinking about my crises, I get one. Do you suppose they are becoming an obsession?'

In the final week of July, Miss D.'s well-being was compromised not only by these crises, but by a number of other symptoms and signs, which increased in number and variety from day to day, and almost from hour to hour – a pathological blossoming, or ebullience, which could not be stopped, and which could scarcely be modified, however we subdivided or timed the daily dose. Her respiratory crises, in their most florid form, became quite frightening to watch. Her breath-holding increased in duration to almost a minute; her expirations became complicated by stridor, forced retching, and forced phonations ('Oouuggh!'). At times, the rhythm would be broken by a run of forty or fifty quick dog-like pants. Now, for the first time, Miss D. started to experience some apprehension during these attacks, and maintained that it was 'not a normal fear,' but 'a special, strange sort of fear' which seemed to flood over her, and which was wholly unlike anything she had ever experienced before. I repeatedly suggested to her that the L-DOPA should be stopped, but Miss D. fiercely insisted that it must not be stopped, that everything would 'work itself out,' and – on one occasion – that stopping the drug would be 'like a death-penalty.' In this way, and in others, Miss D. indicated that she was no longer (or, at least, not always) her usual, reasonable self, but that she was moving towards a state of passion, intransigence, obstinacy, and obsession.

On 23 July, she experienced a new symptom. She had just washed her hands (she now felt a 'need' to wash them thirty times daily), and was about to walk to supper, when she suddenly found that she could not lift her feet from the ground, and that the more she fought to do so, the more they 'attached themselves' to the ground. Her feet were 'released,' quite suddenly and spontaneously, after about ten minutes. Miss D. was alarmed, annoyed, and amused at this novel experience: 'It's like my feet rebelled against me,' she said. 'It's like they had a will of their own. I was glued there, you know. I felt like a fly caught on a strip of fly-paper.' And later that evening she added, musingly: 'I have often read about people being *rooted to the spot,* but I never knew what it meant – not until today.'

Other impulsions and transfixions appeared in the ensuing days, usually quite abruptly, and without the slightest warning. Miss D. would lift a tea-cup to her mouth, and find herself unable to put it down; she would reach for the sugar-bowl, and find her hand 'stuck' to the bowl; when doing crosswords, she would find herself staring at a particular word, and be unable to shift either her gaze or her attention from it; and, most disquietingly (not only for herself but for others), she would at times feel 'compelled' to gaze into someone else's eyes: 'Whenever I do this,' she explained, disarmingly, 'it stops me getting an oculogyric crisis.' Her inclination to munch and gnaw grew greater and

greater: she would chew and over-chew her food, with a growling noise, like a dog with a bone, and in the absence of food
would bite her lips, or gnash her teeth. It was extraordinary to
see such activity in this refined and elderly lady, and Miss D.
herself was very conscious of the incongruity: 'I am a quiet person,' she expostulated on one occasion. 'I could be a distinguished maiden-aunt. And now look at me! I bite and chew like
a ravenous animal, and there's nothing I can do about it.' It
seemed, indeed, during these last days of July, that Miss D. was
being 'possessed' or taken over by a mass of strange and almost
sub-human compulsions; and she herself confided this dark
thought to her diary, although she forbore to express it aloud.

And yet – there were good days, or at least one good day. On
28 July, during an eagerly awaited and greatly enjoyed day-trip
to the country, Miss D. spent the entire day without so much as
a hint of respiratory abnormality, oculogyria, or any other of her
myriad abnormalities. She returned from this in a most radiant
mood, and exclaimed: 'What a perfect day – so peaceful – I shall
never forget it! It's a joy to be alive on a day like this. And I do
feel alive, more truly alive than I've felt in twenty years. If this
is what L-DOPA can do, it's an absolute blessing!'

The following day saw the onset of the worst and most protracted crisis of Miss D.'s entire life. Sixty hours were spent in a
state of virtually continuous respiratory crisis. This was accompanied, not only by her 'usual' spasms and compulsions, but by a
host of other symptoms never before experienced. Her limbs and
trunk repeatedly became 'jammed' in peculiar postures, and
fiercely resisted both active and passive attempts to dislodge
them. This absolute constraint was accompanied by a most intense, and almost frenzied, urge to move, so that Miss D., though
motionless, was locked in a violent struggle with herself. She
could not tolerate the idea of bed, and screamed incessantly
unless left in her chair. Every so often she would burst loose from
her 'jammed' state, and catapult forwards for a few steps only to
'jam' once more, as if she had suddenly run into an invisible wall.
She exhibited extreme pressure of speech, and now showed, for
the first time, an uncontrollable tendency to repeat words and
phrases again and again (palilalia). Her voice, normally low-

pitched and soft, rose to a shrill and piercing scream. When she
was jammed in awkward positions she would scream: 'My arms,
my arms, my arms, my arms, please move my arms, my arms,
move my arms . . .' Her excitement seemed to come in waves,
each wave rising higher and higher towards some limitless climax, and with these waves a mixture of anguish and terror and
shame overwhelmed her, to which she gave voice in palilalic
screamings: 'Oh, oh, oh, oh! . . . please don't . . . I'm not myself,
not myself . . . It's not me, not me, not me at all.'

This crescendo of excitement responded only to massive doses
of parenteral barbiturates, and these would allow only a few
minutes of exhausted sleep, with resumption of all symptoms
immediately on waking. Her L-DOPA, of course, had been
stopped with the inauguration of this monstrous crisis.

Finally, on 31 July, Miss D. sank naturally into a deep and
almost comatose sleep, from which she awoke after twenty-four
hours. She had no crises on 2 and 3 August, but was intensely
Parkinsonian (far more than she had ever been before the administration of L-DOPA), and painfully depressed, although she still
showed a ghost of her old pluck and humour: 'That L-DOPA,' she
whispered (for she was now almost voiceless), 'that stuff should
be given its proper name – *Hell*-DOPA!'

1969–72

During August 1969 Miss D. remained in a subterranean state:
'She looks almost dazed at times,' our speech-pathologist, Miss
Kohl, wrote to me, 'like someone who has come back from the
front line, like a soldier with shell-shock.' During this shock-like
period, which lasted about ten days, Miss D. continued to show
an exacerbation of her Parkinsonism so extreme that she could
perform none of the elementary activity of daily life without help
from the nursing staff. For the remainder of the month, she was
less Parkinsonian (though still far more so than she had been
before the administration of L-DOPA), but quite deeply and painfully depressed. She had little appetite ('She seems to have no
appetite for *anything*,' wrote Miss Kohl; 'really no appetite for

living. She was like a blow-torch before, and now she's like a candle guttering out. You would never believe the difference'), and lost twenty pounds, and when I returned to New York in September – having been away for a month – I did in fact momentarily fail to recognize the pale, shrunken, and somehow caved-in figure of Miss D.[39]

Before the summer, Miss D., despite her half-century of illness, had always been active and perky, and had seemed considerably younger than her sixty-five years; now she was not only wasted and far more Parkinsonian than I had ever seen her, but frighteningly *aged,* as if she had fallen through another half-century in the month I was away. She looked like an escapee from Shangri-La.

In the months following my return Miss D. spoke to me at length about this month; her candour, courage, and insight provided a convincing analysis of how and *why* she felt as she did; and since her state (I believe) shares essential qualities and deter-

---

[39] When I returned, indeed, I found the ward in chaos – it was not just Miss D., it was *everybody* in trouble. I had left a fairly calm and healthy ward in August, but when I went back to it in September, a horrifying sight met my eyes. Some of the patients were shaking and grossly Parkinsonian, others had returned to statuesque catatonia, many were ticcing, some were verbigerating, and a dozen or more were plunged back in oculogyric crises. My own first thought, when I saw all this, was that there had been some colossal, terrible mix-up in the pharmacy, that every patient had been given the wrong medication or the wrong dose. My next thought (when a glance at the charts showed their medications to be in order) was that they all had the flu, and possibly a high fever (which I knew could drive such patients into exacerbated pathology). But this was not the case either.

What had happened, then, in the brief month I was away? It took me several days to piece this together. There had been, I found, a drastic, even draconian, change in the hospital administration, with the appointment of a new director; the patient community had been abruptly disbanded, visiting hours had been sharply curtailed, and day passes to leave the hospital had been cancelled without recourse or warning. The protests of patients had been completely ignored – they suddenly found they were denied any say in their own affairs. It was this – their sense of grievance, shock, and impotent rage – which had been given a physiological form, and 'converted' into Parkinsonism, crises, tics (see p. 18).

And indeed, later that autumn, as the patient community was reestablished, and visiting privileges and passes became available again, a dramatic physiological improvement occurred, and many of these 'side-effects of L-DOPA' (so-called) suddenly dwindled or disappeared, though a certain sense of insecurity, all too understandably, persisted.

minants with the 'post-DOPA' states experienced by many other Parkinsonian patients (though, of course, it was notably more severe than the majority of patients experience or can expect to experience) I shall interrupt her 'story' for her analysis of the situation.

Miss D. stressed, first, the extreme feeling of 'let-down' produced by the sudden withdrawal of the drugs: 'I'd done a vertical take-off,' she said. 'I had gone higher and higher on L-DOPA – to an impossible height. I felt I was on a pinnacle a million miles high . . . And then, with the boost taken away, I crashed, and I didn't just crash to the ground, I shot way in the other direction, until I was buried a million miles deep in the ground.'

Secondly, Miss D. spoke (as has every patient of mine who has been through a comparable experience) of the bewilderment, uncertainty, anxiety, anger, and disappointment which assailed her when the L-DOPA 'started to go wrong'; when it produced more and more 'side-effects' which I – *we, her doctors* – seemed powerless to prevent, despite all our reassurances, and all our fiddlings and manipulations with the dosage; and finally, the extremity of her hopelessness when the L-DOPA was stopped, an act which she saw as a final verdict or decree: something which said in effect, 'This patient has had her chance and lost it. We gave her the magic and it failed. We now wash our hands of her, and consign her to her fate.'

A third aspect of the L-DOPA 'situation' was alluded to again and again by Miss D. (especially in a remarkable diary she kept at this time and of which she showed me portions). This was an acute, an almost intolerable exacerbation of certain feelings which had haunted her at intervals throughout her illness, and which rose to a climax during the final days of L-DOPA administration and the period immediately following withdrawal of the drug. These were feelings of astonishment, rage, and terror that *such things could happen to her,* and feelings of impotent outrage that she, Miss D., could do nothing about these things.[40] But

---

[40] I think such feelings haunt *all* patients who find themselves, their very sense of 'self,' grotesquely changed by illness or other circumstances, for they suffer the greatest ontological outrage, the most intense and 'inexplicable' assaults on the citadel of the self.

deeper and still more threatening feelings were involved: some of the 'things' which gripped her under the influence of L-DOPA – in particular, her gnawing and biting compulsions,[41] certain violent appetites and passions, and certain obsessive ideas and images – could not be dismissed by her as 'purely physical' or completely 'alien' to her 'real self,' but, on the contrary, were felt to be in some sense *releases* or *exposures* or *disclosures* or *confessions* of very deep and ancient parts of herself, monstrous creatures from her unconscious and from unimaginable physiological depths below the unconscious, pre-historic and perhaps pre-human landscapes whose features were at once utterly strange to her, yet mysteriously familiar, in the manner of certain dreams.[42]

---

[41] Such gnawing and biting compulsions, along with gnashing and grinding of the teeth, and a great variety of other abnormal or abnormally perseverative mouth-movements, are among the commonest 'side-effects' of L-DOPA. Such movements may be quite irresistible, of great violence, and liable to inflict considerable damage upon the gums, tongue, teeth, etc. (See Sacks et al., 1970d). In addition to local damage, such compulsions – like other forms of compulsive scratching, hurting, tickling, and 'titillation' generally – may evoke an intense and ambivalent mixture of pleasure and pain, and thus form the nucleus of ever more complex hedonic, algolagnic, and sado-masochistic perversions: this vicious cycle is akin to that seen in some patients with Gilles de la Tourette syndrome, and in self-mutilating children with Lesch-Nyhan syndrome.

[42] What we saw in Frances D. we were to see, sometimes far more severely and grotesquely, in many of our post-encephalitic patients at the height of their reactions to L-DOPA. What we saw was like some strange and terrible organic growth, a burgeoning and bursting-forth not merely of simple involuntary movements and excitations, but of tics and mannerisms, bizarre motions and notions, of an increasingly complex, capricious, and compulsive kind; *and more* – entire behaviours, entire repertoires, of a most primitive and even prehuman sort. Many years before, in the acute epidemic, Jelliffe had spoken of 'menagerie noises' as characteristic of many patients; and now, in the summer of 1969, visitors to the hospital would hear such noises – menagerie noises, jungle noises, noises of almost unimaginable bestiality: 'My God!' they would exclaim, incredulous shock on their faces. 'What was *that?* Do you keep wild animals, are you vivisecting, do you have a *zoo* up there?' Dr Purdon Martin, who visited us at that time, said he found this 'an incredible scene. I have seen nothing like it since the days of the acute epidemic.' For myself, I had never seen *anything* like it, and I have since realized that it is only in such patients, and sometimes patients with the severest Tourette's syndrome, that one may see the almost convulsive emergence and eruption of such behaviours.

Such behaviours, which are uncanny to see, are utterly different from mere *imitations,* such as one may see in psychotic and bestial regressions. What we see here are genuine ancestral instincts and behaviours which have been summoned

And she could not look upon these suddenly exposed parts of herself with detachment; they called to her with siren voices, they enticed her, they thrilled her, they terrified her, they filled her with feelings of guilt and punishment, they possessed her with the consuming, ravishing power of nightmare.

Connected with all of these feelings and reactions were her feelings towards me – the equivocal figure who had offered her a drug so wonderful and so terrible in its effects; the devious and Janus-faced physician who had prescribed for her a revivifying, life-enhancing drug, on the one hand, and a horror-producing, life-destroying drug, on the other hand. I had first seemed a Redeemer, promising health and life with my sacramental medicine; and then a Devil, confiscating health and life, or forcing on her something worse than death. In my first role – as the 'good' doctor – she necessarily loved me; in my second role – as the 'wicked' doctor – she necessarily hated and feared me. And yet she dared not express the hate and fear; she locked it within herself, where it coiled and recoiled upon itself, coagulating into the thickness and darkness of guilt and depression. L-DOPA, by virtue of its amazing effects, invested me – its giver, the physician held 'responsible' for these effects – with all too much power over her life and well-being. Invested with these holy and unholy

---

from the depths, the phylogenetic depths which all of us still carry in our persons. The existence of such vestiges should not surprise us. Darwin, in his famous chapter on 'Reversion and Atavism,' writes:

> The fertilized germ of one of the higher animals . . . is perhaps the most wonderful object in nature . . . But on the doctrine of reversion . . . the germ becomes a far more marvellous object, for, besides the visible changes which it undergoes, we must believe that it is crowded with invisible characters, proper to both sexes and to a long line of male and female ancestors separated by hundreds or even thousands of generations from the present time, and these characters, like those written on paper with invisible ink, lie ready to be evolved whenever the organization is disturbed by certain known or unknown conditions.

Among these conditions, and perhaps the clearest examples we may expect to see, are those to be found in certain post-encephalitic patients. In them, we may surmise, amid the multitude of tiny excitatory lesions in the thalamus, hypothalamus, rhinencephalon, and upper brainstem, there must be some that stimulate, or disinhibit, these latent behaviours, and show us that man's descent is indeed a billion years long. This, then, is a second form of 'awakening' – but one of momentous biological significance.

powers, I assumed, in Miss D.'s eyes, an absolute, and absolutely contradictory, sovereignty; the sovereignty of parents, authorities, God. Thus Miss D. found herself entangled in the labyrinth of a torturing transference-neurosis, a labyrinth from which there seemed to be no exit, no imaginable exit, whatsoever.

My own disappearance from the scene (on 3 August) at the height of her anguish was experienced both as an enormous relief and as an irretrievable loss. I had placed her in the labyrinth in the first place; yet was I not the thread to lead her from it?

This, then, was Miss D.'s situation when I returned in September.[43] I *felt* what was happening with her, in a very fragmentary and inchoate way, the moment I laid eyes on her again, but it was, of course, months and even years before my own intuitions, and hers, reached the more conscious and explicit formulations which I have sketched above.

Summer 1972

Three years have passed since these events. Miss D. is still alive and well, and living – living a sort of life. The dramatic quality of summer 1969 is a thing of the past; the violent vicissitudes of that time have never been repeated with her, and in retrospect have some of the unreality and nostalgia of a dream, or of a unique, never-repeated, unrepeatable, and now almost unimaginable historical event. Despite her ambivalences, Miss D. greeted my return with pleasure, and with a gentle, qualified request that the use of L-DOPA should be considered again. The insistence and intransigence had gone out of her manner; I felt that her seemingly subterranean month without L-DOPA had also been a month of deep reflection, and of inner changes and accommodations of great complexity. It had been, I was subsequently to realize, a sort of Purgatory, a period in which Miss D. struggled with her divided and manifold impulses, using all her recently acquired knowledge of herself (and her propensities of

---

[43] And *not only* Miss D.'s situation but more or less the situation of some twenty or thirty other Parkinsonian patients under my care who had been 'running the gauntlet' of L-DOPA that summer.

response to L-DOPA), and all her strength of mind and character, to achieve a new unification and stability, deeper and stronger than anything preceding it. She had, so to speak, been forged and tempered by the extremities she had passed through, not broken by them (as were so many of my patients). Miss D. was a superior individual; she had lived and fought with herself and for herself through half a century of illness, and had (against innumerable odds) been able to maintain a life of her own, outside an institution, until her sixty-sixth year. Her disease and her pathological potentials I had already seen; her mysterious reserves of health and sanity only became apparent to me *after* the summer of 1969, and in the ensuing three years.

The rest of Miss D.'s story is more easily told. I put her back on L-DOPA in September 1969 and she has remained on this, more or less continually, ever since. We observed in Miss D. (as in several other patients) that the concurrent use of amantadine ('Symmetrel') could ameliorate some of the responses to L-DOPA, although these benign effects might become reversed after a few weeks, and we have therefore maintained Miss D. on an intermittent regimen of amantadine added to L-DOPA. We tried, as recommended in the literature, to reduce abnormal excitements and movements by the use of phenothiazides, butyrophenones, and other major tranquillizers, but found in Miss D. (as with all our other patients) that these drugs could only reduce or exacerbate the *total* effects of L-DOPA, i.e. that they did not distinguish between the 'good effects' and the 'side-effects' of L-DOPA – as so many enthusiastic physicians do. We found minor tranquillizers and anti-histamines, etc., virtually without any effect on Miss D., but barbiturates – especially the parenteral use of sodium amytal – a valuable mainstay for severe crises of one sort or another.

The responses to L-DOPA (or rather to L-DOPA – amantadine combinations) have been in every sense *milder* than those of summer 1969: Miss D. has never again been as sensationally well as she was then, nor as sensationally ill. Her Parkinsonism is always present, but considerably less severe than it was in the days before L-DOPA; although every few weeks, however, when the effects of the amantadine – L-DOPA mixture become less benign, she shows disabling exacerbations of Parkinsonism (and other symptoms), followed by disabling 'withdrawal symptoms' (similar to, though milder than, those of August 1969) during the week or so she is taken off amantadine. This cycle of improvements–exacerbation–withdrawal symptoms is repeated about ten times a year. Miss D. dislikes the cycle, but has grown to accept it. She has, indeed, lost all choice in the matter, for if her L-DOPA is stopped altogether she moves into a state which is far more distressing and disabling than her original 'pre-DOPA' state. Her position is therefore this: that *she needs* L-DOPA, *but cannot tolerate it* – fully, or indefinitely.[44]

Miss D.'s crises have become rarer and less severe – occurring now only once or twice a week – but, perhaps more remarkably, they have quite changed their character. In the summer of 1969 (as in the summer of 1919), her crises were at first purely respiratory in character, and only subsequently drew to themselves the innumerable other phenomena described earlier. When, however, Miss D. resumed her crises, in the autumn of 1969, it was only these other phenomena which occurred; their respiratory components (or aspects) had mysteriously vanished, and have never shown themselves again. Her 'new' crises were usually marked by the most extreme palilalia, the same word or phrase sometimes being uttered hundreds of times in succession, variously accompanied by intense excitement, sundry urges, compulsions, exacerbated Parkinsonism, and peculiar states of 'block' or 'prohibition' of movement, etc. One must stress the words 'usually,' 'variously,' and 'etc.,' for though every crisis was unmistakably a crisis, no two crises were exactly the same. Moreover the particular character and course of each crisis, as well as its occurrence-as-a-whole, could be extraordinarily modified by sugges-

---

[44] Miss D. has been a relatively fortunate patient in both these regards. Her need and her intolerance for L-DOPA are both moderate in degree. In other patients – some of whose histories are given later in this book – the need and the intolerance for L-DOPA were both overwhelming, precluding the possibility of any compromise or position of satisfaction whatever. Miss D. was never off L-DOPA long enough to determine the duration of her 'post-DOPA' state; in other patients (to be described later), there is no doubt that L-DOPA led to profound disturbances of reaction and behaviour which lasted for well over a year following its withdrawal.

tion or circumstance: thus the intense affect, which was usually angry or fearful, would become one of merriment and hilarity if Miss D. happened to be watching a funny film or TV show, while her 'block,' so to speak, could be *drawn out* of one limb and *transferred* to another. By far the best treatment of her crises was music, the effects of which were almost uncanny. One minute would see Miss D. compressed, clenched, and blocked, or jerking, ticcing, and jabbering – like a sort of human bomb; the next, with the sound of music from a wireless or a gramophone, the complete disappearance of all these obstructive-explosive phenomena and their replacement by a blissful ease and flow of movement as Miss D., suddenly freed of her automatisms, smilingly 'conducted' the music, or rose and danced to it. It was necessary that the music be *legato; staccato* music (and especially percussion bands) sometimes had a bizarre effect, causing Miss D. to jump and jerk with the beat – like a mechanical doll or marionette.[45]

---

[45] This power of music to integrate and cure, to liberate the Parkinsonian and give him freedom while it lasts ('You are the music/while the music lasts,' T. S. Eliot), is quite fundamental, and seen in every patient. This was shown beautifully, and discussed with great insight, by Edith T., a former music teacher. She said that she had become 'graceless' with the onset of Parkinsonism, that her movements had become 'wooden, mechanical – like a robot or doll,' that she had lost her former 'naturalness' and 'musicalness' of movement, that – in a word – she had been 'unmusicked.' Fortunately, she added, the disease was 'accompanied by its own cure.' I raised an eyebrow: 'Music,' she said, 'as I am unmusicked, I must be remusicked.' Often, she said, she would find herself 'frozen,' utterly motionless, deprived of the power, the impulse, the *thought,* of any motion; she felt at such times 'like a still photo, a frozen frame' – a mere optical flat, without substance or life. In this state, this statelessness, this timeless irreality, she would remain, motionless-helpless, *until music came:* 'Songs, tunes I knew from years ago, catchy tunes, rhythmic tunes, the sort I loved to dance to.'

With this sudden imagining of music, this coming of spontaneous inner music, the power of motion, action, would suddenly return, and the sense of substance and restored personality and reality; now, as Edith T. put it, she could 'dance out of the frame,' the flat frozen visualness in which she was trapped, and move freely and gracefully: 'It was like suddenly remembering myself, my own living tune.' But then, just as suddenly, the inner music would cease, and with this all motion and actuality would vanish, and she would fall instantly, once again, into a Parkinsonian abyss.

Equally striking, and analogous, was the power of *touch.* At times when there was no music to come to her aid, and she would be frozen absolutely motionless in the corridor, the simplest human contact could come to the rescue. One had

By the end of 1970, Miss D. had run the gauntlet of L-DOPA, amantadine, DOPA-decarboxylases, apomorphine (all variously divided and sub-divided), alone or in combination with anti-cholinergics, anti-adrenergics, anti-histamines, and every other adjuvant or blocker which ingenuity could devise. She had been through them all, and she had *had* it. 'That's it!' she said. 'You've thrown the whole pharmacy at me. I've been up, down, sideways, inside-out, and everything else. I've been pushed, pulled, squeezed, and twisted. I've gone faster, and slower, as well as *so* fast I actually stayed in one place. And I keep opening up and closing down, like a human concertina . . .' Miss D. paused for breath. Her words irresistibly depicted a Parkinsonian 'Alice' in a post-encephalitic Wonderland.

---

only to take her hand, or touch her in the lightest possible way, for her to 'awaken'; one had only to walk *with* her and she could walk perfectly, not imitating or echoing one, but in her own way. But the moment one stopped she would stop too.

Such phenomena are very commonly seen in Parkinsonian patients, and usually dismissed as 'contactual reflexes.' Miss T.'s interpretation, and indeed her experience, seemed to be of a more existential, and indeed 'sacramental,' type: 'I can do nothing alone,' she said. 'I can do anything *with* – with music or people to help me. I cannot initiate, but I can fully share. You "normals," you are full of "go," and when you are with me I can partake of all this. The moment you go away I am nothing again.'

Kant speaks of music as 'the quickening art,' and for Edith T. this is literally, vitally, true. Music serves to arouse her own quickness, her living-and-moving identity and will, which is otherwise dormant for so much of the time. This is what I mean when I speak of these patients as 'asleep,' and why I speak of their arousals as physiological and existential 'awakenings,' whether these be through the spirit of music or living people, or through chemical rectification of deficiencies in the 'go' parts of the brain.

I am often asked what music can serve to awaken such patients, and what precisely is going on at such times. Rhythmic impetus has to be present, but has to be 'embedded' in melody. Raw or overpowering rhythm, which cannot be so embedded, causes a pathological jerking; it coerces instead of freeing the patient, and thus has an anti-musical effect. Shapeless crooning ('slush,' Miss D. calls this), without sufficient rhythmic/motor power, fails to move her – either emotionally or motorically – at all. One is reminded here of Nietzsche's definitions regarding the pathology of music: here he sees, first and foremost, 'degeneration of the sense of rhythm.' 'Degenerate' music sickens and forces, 'healthy' music heals and frees. This was precisely Miss D.'s experience; she could never abide 'banging' or 'slush,' and required a firm but 'shapely' music.

Would any music, then, provided it was firm and shapely, serve to get Frances D. going in the right way? By no means. The only music which affected her in

By this time, then, Miss D. clearly saw that L-DOPA had become a necessity to her, and equally clearly that her responses to it had become limited and unspectacular, and would stay this way; she realized that this was now unalterably the case. This decision marked the completion of her 'dis-investment' in L-DOPA, her renunciation of the passionate hopes and yearnings which had dominated her life for more than a year. Thus, denying nothing, pretending nothing, and expecting nothing (though in her diary she continued to express, from time to time, half-serious, half-joking hopes that things might be different), Miss D. turned *away* from her phantasies, and *towards* her reality – a double turning-point which marked her release from the labyrinth which had trapped her for a year. All her relationships, from this point onwards, assumed a much easier and saner and pleasanter quality. Her attitude to L-DOPA became one of detached and humorous resignation, as did her attitude to her own symptoms and disabilities; she ceased to envy the patients who were flying aloft on L-DOPA, or to view with identificatory terror those patients who had done badly on the drug; and, above all, she ceased to see me as a Redeemer/Destroyer holding her fate in my drug-giving hands. The denials, the projections, the identifications, the transferences, the postures, and the impostures of the L-DOPA 'situation' fell away like a carapace, revealing 'the old Miss D.' – the real self – underneath.

In the second half of 1970, then, Miss D. became ready and eager to address herself to what could be done with regard to her Parkinsonism, her relationships, and the business of staying alive and human in a Total Institution.[46] These problems – perhaps – might have been by-passed had L-DOPA been and remained the perfect remedy, had it sustained its first promise; but it had not – for Miss D. She now saw L-DOPA divested of its glamour: as a most useful, and indispensable, adjunct, but no longer as salva-

---

the right way was music she could *enjoy;* only music which moved her 'soul' had this power to move her body. *She was only moved by music which moved her.* The 'movement' was simultaneously emotional and motoric, and essentially autonomous (thus distinguishing it from passive jerkings and other pathology).

[46] This term, and many of the concepts embodied in it, I owe to Goffman's remarkable book *Asylums.*

tion. Now she could be face-to-face with her own resources, and mine, and those of the institution, to make the best of what remained.[47]

---

[47] A brief allusion to some of Miss D.'s 'methods' may be made. In her long years of illness, she had observed her own propensities and symptoms with a minute curiosity, and had devised many ingenious ways of reducing, overcoming, or circumventing these. Thus, she had various ways of 'defreezing' herself if she chanced to freeze in her walking: she would carry in one hand a supply of minute paper balls of which she would now let one drop to the ground: its tiny whiteness immediately 'incited' or 'commanded' her to take a step, and thus allowed her to break loose from the freeze and resume her normal walking pattern. Miss D. had found that regular blinking, or a loud-ticking watch, or horizontal lines or marks on the ground, etc., similarly served to *pace* her, and to prevent the incontinent hastenings and retardations which otherwise marred her ambulation. Similarly in reading, or talking, she learned to emphasize certain words at set intervals, which would serve to prevent verbal hurry, stuttering, impaction, or freezing. In these and a thousand and one other ways, Miss D. – by herself, with me, with other patients, and with an increasingly intrigued staff of nurses, phys-iotherapists, speech-therapists, etc. – filled many productive and enjoyable hours exploring and playing with endless possibilities of self – and mutual help. Such methods are discovered or devised by *all* gifted post-encephalitic and Parkin-sonian patients, and I have learned more from such patients than from a library of volumes.

Ed W. is a highly gifted young patient with 'ordinary' Parkinson's disease, who often finds himself 'frozen,' 'paralysed,' in his chair, and unable to stand. Unable, that is, to stand *directly*. But he has discovered methods of standing – *indirectly*. He might at first make a slight movement of the eyes (nothing else would be possible); then perhaps a certain movement of the neck; then perhaps an in-finitesimal leaning to one side. He has to go through an exceedingly complex motor sequence, which to a large extent he must improvise or re-invent each time, in order to reach a point where – suddenly, and almost explosively – he is able to stand up. He cannot reach this point without the long sequence; but having reached it, he suddenly finds *he knows how to stand up*.

The moment he has stood up, he forgets what he has done – the knowledge of how-to-stand only being present in the moment of standing, the knowledge being contained in the act. But the knowledge of how-to-stand can immediately lead to other knowledge – of how-to-walk, how-to-dance, how-to-jump, what-ever. This motor knowledge, this knowledge of how-to-act, is not known, explic-itly, to any of us; it is *implicit* knowledge, like the knowledge of language or grammar. What seems highly characteristic of Parkinsonism is the loss of access to implicit knowledge, to built-in motor programmes – and the fact that access can sometimes only be regained by a 'trick.'

Many of the symptoms and features of Parkinsonism, especially 'freezing,' are due to getting stuck in a Parkinsonian 'world,' or rather in a Parkinsonian emptiness, or vacuum, or *un*world ('I freeze in empty spaces,' as Lillian T. says in the documentary film of *Awakenings*). This stuckness depends in part on a stuckness, or paralysis, or entrancement of *attention* – on there being, indeed, no

In these ways, then, Miss D. acclimatized herself to the vagaries of L-DOPA, and actively modified the morbid phenomena of her Parkinsonism, catatonia, impulsiveness, etc. But there were other problems, not stemming from herself, which were beyond her power to modify directly: these, essentially, were the problems of living in a Total Institution.

These problems, in their most general terms, were epitomized in the Pascalian antimonies which echoed through her diary: the sense of isolation and the sense of confinement; the sense of emptiness and the sense of pettiness; the sense of being an inmate – put inside by society, cut off from society . . . subjected to innumerable, degrading rules and regulations; the sense of having been reduced to the status of a child or prisoner, of having been lost or ground up in a machine; the sense of enduring frustration, desolation, and impotence.

These inhuman, institutional qualities, though present to some degree from the founding of the hospital, grew suddenly harsher and more absolute in September 1969.[48] One could clearly perceive, in many other patients, how this grim transition greatly

---

proper *object* for attention. The 'cure' for this (if it is possible) is to redirect attention back to the real world (which is full of objects, proper objects for attention). Sometimes it is sufficient for another person to say 'Look!,' 'Look at that!,' or 'Look over there!' to release the transfixed attention, to disimprison the patient from his spellbound, albeit empty, Parkinsonian attention and allow him once again to move freely in the real world. Sometimes the patient can do this for himself – employing his ingenuity, his cerebral cortex, to bypass the subcortical transfixion of attention, to compensate for the subcortical emptiness of attention. This requires the intervention of consciousness and effort (acts which are normally done 'naturally' and unconsciously can no longer be done, in Parkinsonism, without conscious intervention) – in particular, the fixing of attention on a *real* object or percept or image. This is beautifully shown in the film of *Ivan*, and described by Ivan Vaughan in his book. Ivan is able to run several miles – if he can get started. Instead of concentrating on the first step (which increases his freezing) he must divert his attention onto something else – anything, a leaf, a perceptual object; he touches a leaf, and, magically, this serves to 'release' him. Similarly, Ivan may not be able to get up in the morning, by direct willpower; but he has a tree painted on the bedroom wall by his bed. He looks at this, imagines climbing it, using its branches to get himself going; and by doing this he is enabled to climb out of bed.

[48] During this time of acute institutional deterioration, Miss D. would sometimes exclaim: 'My God, they call this place a *sanitorium?* If you ask me, it's becoming a *thanatorium!*'

modified the clinical state, not simply in terms of mood and attitude, but also in terms of crises, tics, impulsions, catalepsies, Parkinsonian phenomena, etc., and, of course, their reactions to L-DOPA.[49]

---

[49] The mode of *Awakenings* is largely biographic – it presents the reactions of individuals receiving L-DOPA. But these individuals, of course, were not isolated; they were all part of a large post-encephalitic community, and very sensitive to, and sometimes very influenced by, others' reactions.

This sensitivity, this influence, went in different directions. It led first, in the spring and summer of 1969, to a state of shared delight and joy. There was not one 'awakening,' there were *fifty* 'awakenings,' at this time, fifty individuals emerging from the decades-long isolation their illness had imposed on them, suddenly and miraculously finding themselves back in the world and alive, surrounded by fifty other Rip van Winkles or Sleeping Beauties.

A camaraderie speedily developed among them – all of them had lived in the same tunnel or dungeon, all of them were now out in the bright light of day. Suddenly released, they fell to dancing and talking together: some of the most charming scenes in the documentary film of *Awakenings* show the newly-awakened patients dancing, enjoying life, convivial, together. They discovered, they delighted in, each other as *people* – where hitherto they had only been contiguous statues on a ward. They shared their memories, their tragedies, their perplexities, their new hopes. They delighted in each other's daily-increasing health and vitality, and strengthened each other in the resolve for a new life. Thus there was not just individual, there was *communal* health, all that summer, and a peculiar excitement, and an elation of shared hope. This reached a height when Aaron E. left the hospital: 'Perhaps all of us can hope to leave it now as well!'

But then in September, there came tribulations of all sorts. Some of this was due to the treacherous 'side-effects' of L-DOPA, the very limited stability of their own nervous systems when excited; some to harsh changes occurring in the hospital at this time (see n. 39, p. 53); and some, no doubt, to their own regressive needs. But what was also all too clear, in the close medium of the ward, was how despondency, and 'side effects,' would spread from one person to another. Everyone, in that summer, was encouraged by everyone else – optimism and hope spread like a contagion. Whereas now every setback in a patient aroused fear in the others, every discouragement discouraged the others – fear and helplessness spread like a contagion through the ward. These patients, above all others, were highly impressionable, not only psychically, but somatically as well – the 'somatic compliance' of which Jelliffe liked to speak. (Such an almost hypnoid impressionability, and tendency to mimesis, here, is biologically as well as psychologically determined; it is characteristic of all the diencephalic syndromes.)

The fear of fluctuations, the fear of tics, seemed to play a part in actually precipitating tics and fluctuations. And as the patients got past the critical point, and advanced further and further along the path of instability, psychic influences became more potent than ever. Happiness, freedom, good relationships stabilised them; stress, isolation, boredom destabilised them: all of these became quite as potent as L-DOPA. Thus the atmosphere of the ward, its mood, became

There is no doubt that Miss D. herself was greatly affected by these changes in her environment; I cannot, however, make any definite judgement as to how much her course on L-DOPA was an inevitable consequence of the drug's action and her individual, built-in reactivity, and how much it may have been modified by the increasingly adverse conditions of her life. I can only represent the total picture, as fairly and fully as I can, and leave such judgements to my readers.

Three things, however, have been unmistakably clear. First, that whenever Miss D. succeeds in expressing her feelings and achieving some change in her environment, *all* her pathological phenomena decrease. Secondly, that whenever Miss D. leaves the hospital for a day's outing (such outings have become increasingly rare since the easy-going days of 1969) *all* her symptoms and signs decrease. Lastly, that since Miss D. has forged a deep and affectionate relationship with two other patients on the ward – i.e. since the early part of 1971 – she has been visibly better in *all* possible ways.

So, finally, we come to the present time, the summer of 1972. Miss D. continues on a modest, intermittent dosage of L-DOPA and amantadine. She is pretty active and can look after her basic needs for nine months in the year, the other three months being occupied with exacerbations of illness and withdrawal symptoms. She has a small crisis perhaps twice a month, which no longer really disturbs her or anyone else. She reads a good deal, crochets like a professional, and does innumerable crosswords far faster than I can. She is most herself when she talks to her friends. She has put most of her petulancies, obstinacies, dependencies, and insistencies quite firmly behind her. She is now very genial (except when she shuts herself up with her diary in her blacker, private moods), and well-liked by everyone round her. One often sees her by the window, a mild old lady approaching seventy, somewhat bowed and fixed in her attitude, crocheting rapidly, and looking at the traffic which roars through Bexley.

She is not one of our star patients, one of those who did

---

all-important – I did not have fifty isolated, insulable patients; I had a *community* which was like a single living organism.

fabulously well on L-DOPA, and stayed well. But she has survived the pressures of an almost life-long, character-deforming disease; of a strong cerebral stimulant; and of confinement in a chronic hospital from which very few patients emerge alive. Deeply rooted in reality, she has triumphantly survived illness, intoxication, isolation, and institutionalization, and has remained what she always was – a totally human, a prime human being.

MAGDA B.

Mrs B. was born in Austria in 1900, and came to the United States as a child. Her childhood was free of any serious illnesses, and her academic and athletic progress at high school was exemplary. In 1918–19, while working as a secretary, she contracted a severe somnolent-ophthalmoplegic form of *encephalitis lethargica,* recovered from this after a few months, but started to show Parkinsonism and other sequelae around 1923.

The course of her illness over the following forty-five years was at first known to me only from exiguous hospital notes, for Mrs B. had been quite unable to speak for many years. In addition to the ophthalmoplegia which failed to resolve after her acute encephalitis, Mrs B.'s chief problems were profound akinesia and apathy, and a variety of autonomic disturbances (profuse salivation, sweating, and repeated peptic ulcerations). She had not been prone to oculogyric or other crises. She showed occasional 'flapping' tremor, but virtually no rigidity, dystonia, or resting ('pill-rolling') tremor.

A note dated 1964 remarks on the 'curious absence of anger or frustration in circumstances which would seem to warrant these reactions.' A note written in 1966, when Mrs B. was seriously ill from concurrent illness, commented upon the absence of any anxiety or fear in response to her situation. During 1968, she was repeatedly subjected to verbal and physical abuses by a mad, hostile dement placed next to her in the ward (the latter would insult and curse her, and occasionally struck her): Mrs B. showed neither motor nor emotional reaction to such intolerable goading. Many other notes, which need not be quoted in detail, similarly attested to her abnormal passivity and calmness. On the other hand, there was no suggestion of depressive or paranoid tendencies, and no evidence of eccentric ideation or behaviour: Mrs B. seemed amiable and appreciative of help, but docile, *bland,* and perhaps incapable of emotional reaction.

Before L-DOPA

Mrs B. was seated, motionless, in her wheel chair, when first seen by me: akinesia was so extreme at this time that she would sit without blinking, or change of facial expression, or any hint of bodily movement, for the greater part of the day. She showed a habitual dropped posture of the head, but was able to combat this for brief periods. There was little or no cervical rigidity. She appeared to have a bilateral nuclear and internuclear ophthalmo-plegia, with alternating exotropia. Mrs B. was sweating very freely, showed a greasy seborrhoeic skin, and moderately in-creased lacrimation and salivation. There were rare attacks of spontaneous lid-clonus or closure, but no spontaneous blinking at all. Mrs B. was virtually aphonic – able to produce a faint 'Ah!' with great effort, but not to articulate a single word audibly: she had been speechless for more than ten years, and severely hypo-phonic for at least fifteen years before this.

She showed profound facial masking – at no time during the initial examinations did any hint of facial expression appear – was scarcely able to open the mouth, to protrude the tongue beyond the lip-margin, or to move it at all within the mouth from side to side. Chewing and swallowing were feeble and slowly per-formed – the consumption of even a small meal would take more than an hour – but there were no signs of bulbar or pseudo-bulbar palsy.

All voluntary movements were distinguished by extreme slowness and feebleness, with almost no involvement of 'background'
musculature, and a tendency to premature arrest of movements
in mid-posture. When raised from her chair – for Mrs B. was
quite unable even to inaugurate the act of rising by herself – she
stood as motionless as a statue, although she was unable to maintain her balance, due to an irresistible tendency to fall backwards.
Stepping was not only impossible, but somehow seemed *unthinkable.* If she closed her eyes, while standing or sitting, she at once
dropped forward like a wilted flower.

Mrs B. was thus profoundly incapacitated, unable to speak and
almost unable to initiate any voluntary motion, and in need of
total nursing care. Added to the motor problems were a striking
apathy and apparent incapacity for emotional response, and considerable drowsiness and torpor for much of the day. Conventional anti-Parkinsonian drugs had been of very little use to her,
and surgery had never been considered. She had been regarded
for many years as a 'hopeless' back-ward post-encephalitic, with
no capacity for rehabilitation. She was started on L-DOPA on 25
June.

Course on L-DOPA

2 July. After one week of treatment (and on a dose of 2 gm.
L-DOPA daily), Mrs B. started *talking* – quite audibly – for the first
time in many years, although her vocal force would decay after
two or three short sentences, and her new-found voice was low-
pitched, monotonous, and uninflected.

8 July. With raising of the dose to 3 gm. L-DOPA daily, Mrs B.
became nauseated, and insomniac, and showed striking dilation
of the pupils, but no tachycardia, lability of blood-pressure, or
akathisia. She now showed considerable spontaneous activity –
ability to shift positions in her chair, to turn in bed, etc. She was
much more alert, and had ceased to show any drowsiness or
'dullness' in the course of the day. Her voice had acquired further
strength, and the beginnings of intonation and inflection: thus
one could now realize that this patient had a strong Viennese
accent, where a few days previously her voice had been monoto-

nous in timbre, and, as it were, *anonymously* Parkinsonian.

Mrs B. was now able to hold a pencil in her right hand, and to make a first entry in her diary: her name, followed by the comment, 'It is twenty years since I have written. I'm afraid I have almost forgotten how to write my name.'

She also showed emotional reaction – anxiety at her sleeplessness and vomiting – and requested me to reduce the new drug, but by no means to stop it. The dose was reduced to 2 gm. daily.

Reduction of the dose alleviated the nausea, insomnia, and mydriasis, but led to a partial loss of vocal and motor power. A week later (15 July), it was possible to restore the larger (3 gm. daily) dose, without causing any adverse effects whatever, and she was subsequently maintained on this dose. On this, Mrs B. had shown a stable and continued improvement. By the end of July, she was able to rise to her feet and stand unaided for thirty seconds, and to walk twenty steps between parallel bars. She could adjust her position in chair or bed to her own comfort. She had become able to feed herself. Diminishing flexion of the trunk and neck could be observed with each passing week, so that by mid-August a striking normalization of posture had occurred.

Previously indifferent, inattentive, and unresponsive to her surroundings, Mrs B. became, with each week, more alert, more attentive, and more interested in what was taking place around her.

At least as dramatic as the motor improvement, and infinitely moving to observe, was the recovery of emotional responsiveness in this patient who had been so withdrawn and apathetic for so many years. With continued improvement of her voice, Mrs B. became quite talkative, and showed an intelligence, a charm, and a humour, which had been almost totally concealed by her disease. She particularly enjoyed talking of her childhood in Vienna, of her parents and family, of schooldays, of rambles and excursions in the country nearby, and as she did so would often laugh with pleasure at the recollection, or shed nostalgic tears – normal emotional responses which she had not shown in more than twenty years. Little by little Mrs B. emerged as a *person,* and as she did so was able to communicate to us, in vivid and frightening terms, what an *unperson* she had felt before receiving L-DOPA.

She described her feelings of impotent anger and mounting depression in the early years of her illness, and the succeeding of these feelings by apathy and indifference: 'I ceased to have any moods,' she said. 'I ceased to care about anything. Nothing *moved* me – not even the death of my parents. I forgot what it felt like to be happy or unhappy. Was it good or bad? It was neither. It was nothing.'[50]

1969–71

Mrs B.'s course on L-DOPA, by and large, was the smoothest and most satisfactory I have seen in *any* patient.[51] Throughout her two years on the drug, she maintained an altogether admirable degree of activity, sanity, and general fullness of living. There was, it is true, some small dropping-off in her level of energy and motility towards the end of the second year, and there were brief outcroppings of morbid activity: these latter will be described in the context they occurred in.

Much of this was associated with her renewal of emotional contact with, and obvious delight in, her daughters and sons-in-law, her grandchildren, and the many other relatives who came to her now she was well, and, so to speak, restored to reality. She remembered every birthday and anniversary, and never forgot to mark them with a letter; she showed herself agreeable and eager to be taken out on car-rides, to restaurants, to theatres, and above all, to the homes of her family, without ever becoming demanding or importunate. She renewed contact with the rabbi and other orthodox patients in the hospital, went to all the religious services, and loved nothing so much as lighting the Shabbas candles. In short, she donned again her former identity, as a 'frum' Viennese lady of good family and strong character. More remarkably, she assumed, with apparent ease, the mantle of old age and

---

[50] 'Thus when God forsakes us, Satan also leaves us' – Sir Thomas Browne.

[51] It is curious that the *only* two patients I have ever seen who showed an almost unqualified excellence of response for the entire two years they were taking L-DOPA (Magda B. and Nathan G.) were not, as might be thought, minimally involved patients with Parkinson's disease, but two of the most profoundly involved post-encephalitics I have ever seen.

'Grannie-hood,' 'bubishkeit,' despite having dropped, as through a vacuum, from her mid-twenties to her late sixties.[52]

She had not, apparently become bitter or virulent in the decades of her illness, and this, perhaps, was connected with her apathy: 'I often felt,' said one of her daughters, 'that Mother *felt* nothing, although she seemed to notice and remember everything. I used to feel terribly sad at her state, without getting too angry – after all, how can you blame or get mad at a *ghost?*'

Mrs B. did develop two brief psychotic reactions while on L-DOPA. The first of these was in relation to her husband, who failed to visit her with the rest of the family. 'Where is he?' she would ask her daughters. 'Why doesn't he come to see me?' Her daughters temporized, explaining he was ill, indisposed, out of town, on a trip, etc. (He had in fact died some five years before.) These many discrepancies alarmed Mrs B., and precipitated a brief delusional episode. During this time, she heard her husband's voice in the corridors, saw his name in the papers, and 'understood' he was having innumerable *affaires.* Seeing what was happening, I asked her daughters to tell her the truth. Mrs B.'s response to this was: 'Ach! you sillies, why didn't you tell me?' followed by a period of mourning, and complete dissipation of her psychotic ideas.

Her other psychosis had reference to a rapidly advancing deterioration of eyesight, which had been 'accepted' with indifference before the L-DOPA. This was especially severe in her

---

[52] It is of much interest and significance that Magda B. seemed to have little or no difficulty in accommodating to the immense time-lapse, the immense 'loss' of time, entailed by her illness. This is in absolute contrast to the following patient (Rose R.), who on 'awakening' after forty-three years, found herself faced with 'a time-gap beyond comprehension or bearing,' 'an intolerable and insoluble anachronism' to which accommodation was completely impossible (see p. 87). Why such a difference? I think this reflects the absolute contrast (discussed in the Prologue) between 'negative' and 'positive' disorders of being. Magda B., engulfed in non-activity, non-being, nothingness, situationlessness, was not, I think, frustrated or tormented like Rose R.; she was becalmed, asleep, on the ocean of life. When Being and activity were given to her, she accepted it as a pure gift, with gratitude and joy; but their absence, prior to her 'awakening,' was *also* accepted, with a placid indifference (and so too, conceivably, might have been a return to inactivity and inexistence, had the L-DOPA lost its effect). However, it is possible that Magda B., once re-awakened to life and hope, could not have borne its loss again.

second year on the drug, when the faces of her children, the face of the *world,* were rapidly becoming dim and ungraspable. Mrs B. rebelled against the diagnosis of 'senile macular degeneration, progressive and incurable,' the more so as this was delivered to her by a specialist she had never seen before, with a curt finality and a marked lack of sympathy, and for some weeks implored us pitifully to restore her sight, and experienced dreams and hallucinations of seeing again perfectly. During this painful period, Mrs B. developed a curious 'touching tic,' continually touching the rails, the furniture, and – above all – various people as they passed in the corridor. I once asked her about this: 'Can you blame me?' she cried. 'I can hardly see anything. If I touch and keep touching, it is to keep me in touch!' As Mrs B. adjusted to her increasing blindness, and as she started to learn Braille (an enterprise *she* had thought of and insisted upon), her anguish grew less, her dreams and demands and hallucinations ceased, and her compulsive touching grew less marked, and *much* less importunate.[53] It should be stressed, perhaps, that the dosage of L-DOPA was not altered in these psychoses, for it was clear that they were reflections of an alterable reality.

In July 1971, Mrs B., who was in good general health and not given to 'hunches,' had a sudden premonition of death, so clear and peremptory she phoned up her daughters. 'Come and see me today,' she said. 'There'll be no tomorrow . . . No, I feel quite well . . . Nothing is bothering me, but I *know* I shall die in my sleep tonight.'

Her tone was quite sober and factual, wholly unexcited, and it carried such conviction that *we* started wondering, and obtained blood-counts, cardiograms, etc., etc. (which were all quite normal). In the evening Mrs B. went round the ward, with a laughter-silencing dignity, shaking hands and saying 'Good-bye' to everyone there.

She went to bed and she died in the night.

---

[53] I am not suggesting that this touching tic was entirely 'psychogenic' or *created* by circumstance. I have seen somewhat similar touching tics in impulse-ridden post-encephalitic patients who were not in Mrs B.'s position. But I do think that a mild, or latent, propensity to tic was 'brought out' by her excitement, and given shape by her circumstances, so that it *became* a reflection or expression of her feelings.

ROSE R.

❧ Miss R. was born in New York City in 1905, the youngest child of a large, wealthy, and talented family. Her childhood and school days were free of serious illness, and were marked, from their earliest days, by love of merriment, games, and jokes. High-spirited, talented, full of interests and hobbies, sustained by deep family affection and love, and a sure sense of who and what and why she was, Miss R. steered clear of significant neurotic problems or 'identity-crises' in her growing-up period.

On leaving school, Miss R. threw herself ardently into a social and peripatetic life. Aeroplanes, above all, appealed to her eager, volant, and irrepressible spirit; she flew to Pittsburgh and Denver, New Orleans and Chicago, and twice to the California of Hearst and Hollywood (no mean feat in the planes of those days). She went to innumerable parties and shows, was toasted and fêted, and rolled home drunk at night. And between parties and flights she dashed off sketches of the bridges and waterfronts with which New York abounded. Between 1922 and 1926, Miss R. lived in the blaze of her own vitality, and lived more than most other people in the whole of their lives. And this was as well, for at the age of twenty-one she was suddenly struck down by a virulent form of *encephalitis lethargica* – one of its last victims before the epidemic vanished. 1926, then, was the last year in which Miss R. really *lived*.

The night of the sleeping-sickness, and the days which followed it, can be reconstructed in great detail from Miss R.'s relatives, and Miss R. herself. The acute phase announced itself (as sometimes happened: compare Maria G.) by nightmares of a grotesque and terrifying and premonitory nature. Miss R. had a series of dreams about one central theme: she dreamed she was imprisoned in an inaccessible castle, but the castle had the form

and shape of herself; she dreamed of enchantments, bewitch-
ments, entrancements; she dreamed that she had become a living,
sentient statue of stone; she dreamed that the world had come to
a stop; she dreamed that she had fallen into a sleep so deep that
nothing could wake her; she dreamed of a death which was
different from death. Her family had difficulty waking her the
next morning, and when she awoke there was intense consterna-
tion: 'Rose,' they cried 'wake up! What's the matter? Your expression, your position . . . You're so still and so strange.' Miss
R. could not answer, but turned her eyes to the wardrobe-mirror,
and there she saw that her dreams had come true. The local
doctor was brisk and unhelpful: 'Catatonia,' he said; *'Flexibilitas
cerea.* What can you expect with the life she's been leading? She's
broken her heart over one of these bums. Keep her quiet and
feed her – she'll be fine in a week.'

But Miss R. was not to recover for a week, or a year, or
forty-three years. She recovered the ability to speak in short
sentences, or to make sudden movements before she froze up
again. She showed, increasingly, a forced retraction of her neck
and her eyes – a state of almost continuous oculogyric crisis,
broken only by sleep, meals, and occasional 'releases.' She was
alert, and seemed to notice what went on around her; she lost
none of her affection for her numerous family – and they lost
none of their affection for her; but she seemed absorbed and
preoccupied in some unimaginable state. For the most part, she
showed no sign of distress, and no sign of anything save intense
concentration: 'She looked,' said one of her sisters, 'as if she were
trying her hardest to remember something – or, maybe, doing
her damnedest to forget something. Whatever it was, it took
all her attention.' In her years at home, and subsequently in
hospital, her family did their utmost to penetrate this absorption,
to learn what was going on with their beloved 'kid' sister. With
them – and, much later, with me – Miss R. was exceedingly
candid, but whatever she said seemed cryptic and gnomic, and
yet at the same time disquietingly clear.[54]

---

[54] I would often ask Miss R. what she was thinking about.
'Nothing, just nothing,' she would say.

When there was only this state, and no other problems, Miss R.'s family could keep her at home: she was no trouble, they loved her, she was simply – elsewhere (or nowhere). But three or four years after her trance-state had started, she started to become rigid on the left side of her body, to lose her balance when walking, and to develop other signs of Parkinsonism. Gradually these symptoms grew worse and worse, until full-time nursing became a necessity. Her siblings left home, and her parents were ageing, and it was increasingly difficult to keep her at home. Finally, in 1935, she was admitted to Mount Carmel.

Her state changed little after the age of thirty, and when I first

---

'But how can you possibly be thinking of nothing?'

'It's dead easy, once you know how.'

How exactly do you think about nothing?'

'One way is to think about the same thing again and again. Like 2 = 2 = 2 = 2; or, I am what I am what I am what I am . . . It's the same thing with my posture. My posture continually leads to itself. Whatever I do or whatever I think leads deeper and deeper into itself . . . And then there are maps.'

'Maps? What do you mean?'

'Everything I do is a map of itself, everything I do is a part of itself. Every part leads into itself . . . I've got a thought in my mind, and then I see something in it, like a dot on the skyline. It comes nearer and nearer, and then I see what it is – it's just the same thought I was thinking before. And then I see another dot, and another, and so on . . . Or I think of a map; then a map of that map; then a map of that map of that map, and each map perfect, though smaller and smaller . . . Worlds within worlds within worlds within worlds . . . Once I get going I can't possibly stop. It's like being caught between mirrors, or echoes, or something. Or being caught on a merry-go-round which won't come to a stop.'

Sometimes, Miss R. told me, she would feel compelled to circumscribe the sides of a mental quadrangle, to seven notes of an endlessly-reiterated Verdi aria: *'Tum – ti-tum – ti-tum – ti-tum,'* a forced mental perambulation which might go on for hours or days. And at other times she would be forced to 'travel,' mentally, through an endless 3-D tunnel of intersecting lines, the end of the tunnel rushing towards her but never reached.

'And do you have any *other* ways of thinking about nothing, Rosie?'

'Oh yes! The dots and maps are *positive* nothings, but I also think of *negative* nothings.'

'And what are those like?'

'That's impossible to say, because they're takings-away. I think of a thought, and it's suddenly gone – like having a picture whipped out of its frame. Or I try to picture something in my mind, but the picture dissolves as fast as I can make it. I have a particular idea, but can't keep it in mind; and then I lose the *general* idea; and then the general idea *of* a general idea; and in two or three jumps my mind is a blank – *all* my thoughts gone, blanked out or erased.'

saw her in 1966, my findings coincided with the original notes from her admission. Indeed, the old staff-nurse on her ward, who had known her throughout, said: 'It's uncanny, that woman hasn't aged a day in the thirty years I've known her. The rest of us get older – but Rosie's the same.' It was true: Miss R. at sixty-one looked thirty years younger; she had raven-black hair, and her face was unlined, as if she had been magically preserved by her trance or her stupor.

She sat upright and motionless in her wheelchair, with little or no spontaneous movement for hours on end. There was no spontaneous blinking, and her eyes stared straight ahead, seemingly indifferent to her environment but completely absorbed. Her gaze, when requested to look in different directions, was full, save for complete inability to converge the eyes. Fixation of gaze lacked smooth and subtle modulation, and was accomplished by sudden, gross movements which seemed to cost her considerable effort. Her face was completely masked and expressionless. The tongue could not be protruded beyond the lip-margins, and its movements, on request, were exceedingly slow and small. Her voice was virtually inaudible, though Miss R. could whisper quite well with considerable effort. Drooling was profuse, saturating a cloth bib within an hour, and the entire skin was oily, seborrhoeic, and sweating intensely. Akinesia was global, although rigidity and dystonia were strikingly unilateral in distribution. There was intense axial rigidity, no movement of the neck or trunk muscles being possible. There was equally intense rigidity in the left arm, and a very severe dystonic contracture of the left hand. No voluntary movement of this limb was possible. The right arm was much less rigid, but showed great akinesia, all movements being minimal, and decaying to zero after two or three repetitions. Both legs were hypertonic, the left much more so. The left foot was bent inwards in dystonic inversion. Miss R. could not rise to her feet unaided, but when assisted to do so could maintain her balance and take a few small, shuffling, precarious steps, although the tendency to backward-falling and pulsion was very great.

She was in a state of near-continuous oculogyric crisis, although this varied a good deal in severity. When it became more severe, her Parkinsonian 'background' was increased in intensity, and an intermittent coarse tremor appeared in her right arm. Prominent tremor of the head, lips, and tongue also became evident at these times, and rhythmic movement of buccinators and corrugators. Her breathing would become somewhat stertorous at such times, and would be accompanied by a guttural phonation reminiscent of a pig grunting. Severe crises would always be accompanied by tachycardia and hypertension. Her neck would be thrown back in an intense and sometimes agonizing opisthotonic posture. Her eyes would generally stare directly ahead, and could not be moved by voluntary effort: in the severest crises they were forced upwards and fixed on the ceiling.

Miss R.'s capacity to speak or move, minimal at the best of times, would disappear almost entirely during her severer crises, although in her greatest extremity she would sometimes call out, in a strange high-pitched voice, perseverative and palilalic, utterly unlike her husky 'normal' whisper: 'Doctor, doctor, doctor, doctor . . . help me, help, help, h'lp, h'lp . . . I am in terrible pain, I'm so frightened, so frightened, so frightened . . . I'm going to die, I know it, I know it, I know it, I know it . . .' And at other times, if nobody was near, she would whimper softly to herself, like some small animal caught in a trap. The nature of Miss R.'s pain during her crises was only elucidated later, when speech had become easy: some of it was a local pain associated with extreme opisthotonos, but a large component seemed to be central – diffuse, unlocalizable, of sudden onset and offset, and inseparably coalesced with feelings of dread and threat, in the severest crises a true *angor animi.* During exceptionally severe attacks, Miss R.'s face would become flushed, her eyes reddened and protruding, and she would repeat, 'It'll kill me, it'll kill me, it'll kill me . . .' hundreds of times in succession.[55]

---

[55] Compare cases cited by Jelliffe: the patient who would cry out in 'anguish' during her attacks, but could give no reason for her fear, or the patient who would feel every attack to be 'a calamity' (see Jelliffe, 1932, pp. 36–42). The same term was often used by Lillian W., especially in relation to those very complex oculogyric crises which she sometimes called 'humdingers' (see p. 19). Even though she had oculogyric crises every week, she would invariably say during each attack, 'This is the worst one I ever had. The others were just bad – *this* is a calamity.' When I would remonstrate, 'But Mrs. W., this is exactly what

Miss R.'s state scarcely changed between 1966 and 1969, and when L-DOPA became available I was in two minds about using it. She was, it was true, intensely disabled, and had been virtually helpless for over forty years. It was her *strangeness* above all which made me hesitate and wonder – fearing what might happen if I gave her L-DOPA. I had never seen a patient whose regard was so turned away from the world, and so immured in a private, inaccessible world of her own.

I kept thinking of something Joyce wrote about his mad daughter: '. . . fervently as I desire her cure, I ask myself what then will happen when and if she finally withdraws her regard from the lightning-lit reverie of her clairvoyance and turns it upon that battered cabman's face, the world . . .'

Course on L-DOPA

But I started her on L-DOPA, despite my misgivings, on 18 June 1969. The following is an extract from my diary.

25 June. The first therapeutic responses have already occurred, even though the dosage has only been raised to 1.5 gm. a day. Miss R. has experienced two entire days unprecedentedly free of oculogyric crises, and her eyes, so still and preoccupied before, are brighter and more mobile and attentive to her surroundings.

1 July. Very real improvements are evident by this date: Miss R. is able to walk unaided down the passage, shows a distinct reduction of rigidity in the left arm and elsewhere, and has become able to speak at a normal conversational volume. Her mood is cheerful, and she has had no oculogyric crises for three days. In view of this propitious response, and the absence of any adverse effects, I am increasing the dosage of L-DOPA to 4 gm. daily.

6 July. Now receiving 4 gm. L-DOPA. Miss R. has continued to improve in almost every way. When I saw her at lunchtime, she was delighted with everything: 'Dr Sacks!' she called out, 'I

---

you said last week!' she would say, 'I know. I was wrong. This one *is* a calamity.' She never got used to her crises in the least – even though she had had them, each Wednesday, for more than forty years.

walked to and from the new building today' (this is a distance of about six hundred yards). 'It's fabulous, it's gorgeous!' Miss R. has now been free from oculogyric crises for eight days, and has shown no akathisia or undue excitement. I too feel delighted at her progress, but for some reason am conscious of obscure forebodings.

7 July. Today Miss R. has shown her first signs of unstable and abrupt responses to L-DOPA. Seeing her 3½ hours after her early-morning dose, I was shocked to find her very 'down' – hypophonic, somewhat depressed, rigid and akinetic, with extremely small pupils and profuse salivation. Fifteen minutes after receiving her medication she was 'up' again – her voice and walking fully restored, cheerful, smiling, talkative, her eyes alert and shining, and her pupils somewhat dilated. I was further disquieted by observing an occasional impulsion to run, although this was easily checked by her.

8 July. Following an insomniac night ('I didn't feel in the least sleepy: thoughts just kept rushing through my head'), Miss R. is extremely active, cheerful and affectionate. She seems to be very busy, constantly flying from one place to another, and all her thoughts too are concerned with movement; 'Dr Sacks,' she exclaimed breathlessly, 'I feel great today. I feel I want to fly. I love you, Dr Sacks, I love you, I love you. You know, you're the kindest doctor in the world . . . You know I always liked to travel around: I used to fly to Pittsburgh, Chicago, Miami, California . . .' etc. Her skin is warm and flushed, her pupils are again very widely dilated, and her eyes constantly glancing to and fro. Her energy seems limitless and untiring, although I get the impression of exhaustion somewhere beneath the pressured surface. An entirely new symptom has also appeared today, a sudden quick movement of the right hand to the chin, which is repeated two or three times an hour. When I questioned Miss R. about this she said: 'It's new, it's odd, it's strange, I never did it before. God knows why I do it. I just suddenly get an *urge,* like you suddenly got to sneeze or scratch yourself.' Fearing the onset of akathisia or excessive emotional excitement, I have reduced the dosage of L-DOPA to 3 gm. daily.

9 July. Today Miss R.'s energy and excitement are unabated, but her mood has veered from elation to anxiety. She is impatient, touchy, and extremely demanding. She became much agitated in the middle of the day, asserting that seven dresses had been stolen from her closet, and that her purse had been stolen. She entertained dark suspicions of various fellow patients: no doubt they had been plotting this for weeks before. Later in the day, she discovered that her dresses were in fact in her closet in their usual position. Her paranoid recriminations instantly vanished: 'Wow!' she said, 'I must have imagined it all. I guess I better take myself in hand.'

14 July. Following the excitements and changing moods of 9 July, Miss R.'s state has become less pressured and hyper-active. She has been able to sleep, and has lost the tic-like 'wiping' movements of her right hand. Unfortunately, after a two-week remission, her old enemy has re-emerged, and she has experienced two severe oculogyric crises. I observed in these not only the usual staring, but a more bizarre symptom – captivation or enthralment of gaze: in one of these crises she had been forced to stare at one of her fellow-patients, and had felt her eyes 'drawn' this way and that, following the movements of this patient around the ward. 'It was uncanny,' Miss R. said later. 'My eyes were spellbound. I felt like I was bewitched or something, like a rabbit with a snake.' During the periods of 'bewitchment' or fascination, Miss R. had the feeling that her 'thoughts had stopped,' and that she could only think of one thing, the object of her gaze. If, on the other hand, her attention was distracted, the quality of thinking would suddenly change, the motionless fascination would be broken up, and she would experience instead 'an absolute torrent of thoughts,' rushing through her mind: these thoughts did not seem to be 'her' thoughts, they were not what she wanted to think, they were 'peculiar thoughts' which appeared 'by themselves.' Miss R. could not or would not specify the nature of these intrusive thoughts, but she was greatly frightened by the whole business: 'These crises are different from the ones I used to get,' she said. 'They are worse. They are completely *mad!*'[56]

---

[56] Jelliffe cites many cases of oculogyric crises with fixation of gaze and attention, and also of crises with reiterative 'autochthonous' thinking. Miss R. never vouchsafed the nature of the 'mad' thoughts which came to her during her crises at this time, and one would suspect from the reticence that these thoughts were of

25 July. Miss R. has had an astonishing ten days, and has shown phenomena I never thought possible. Her mood has been joyous and elated, and very salacious. Her social behaviour has remained impeccable, but she has developed an insatiable urge to sing songs and tell jokes, and has made very full use of our portable tape-recorder. In the past few days, she has recorded innumerable songs of an astonishing lewdness, and reams of 'light' verse all dating from the twenties. She is also full of anecdotes and allusions to 'current' figures – to figures who were current in the mid-1920s. We have been forced to do some archival research, looking at old newspaper-files in the New York Library. We have found that almost all of Miss R.'s allusions date to 1926, her last year of real life before her illness closed round her. Her memory is uncanny, considering she is speaking of so long ago. Miss R. wants the tape-recorder, and nobody around; she stays in her room, alone with the tape-recorder; she is looking at everyone as if they didn't exist. She is completely engrossed in her memories of the twenties, and is doing her best to not-notice anything later. I suppose one calls this 'forced reminiscence,' or incontinent nostalgia.[57] But I also have the feeling that

---

an inadmissible nature, either sexual or hostile. Jelliffe refers to several patients who were compelled to think of 'dirty things' during their crises, and to another patient who experienced during his crises 'ideas of reference to which he pays no attention' (see Jelliffe, 1932, pp. 37–39). Miriam H. would have delusional erotic reminiscences whenever she had an oculogyric crisis (see p. 138).

[57] I saw similar phenomena, and had similar thoughts, regarding another patient (Sam G.), whose story, alas, I didn't tell in the original *Awakenings* (though his face appears on the front cover of the 1976 edition). Sam used to be both a car buff and racing driver, bizarrely helped in the latter by his preternaturally quick reactions and his sudden, 'frivolous' moves. He had to give it up around 1930 due to envelopment in a profound Parkinsonism. 'Awakening,' for him, had some of the 'nostalgic' quality it had for Rose R. In particular, the moment he found himself 'released' by L-DOPA, he started drawing cars. He drew constantly, with great speed, and was *obsessed* by his drawing; if we did not keep him well supplied with paper, he would draw on the walls, on tablecloths, on his bedsheets. His cars were accurate, authentic, and had an odd charm. When he was not drawing, he was talking, or writing – of 'the old days' in the twenties when he was driving and racing – and this too was full of vividness and immediacy, minute, compelling, *living* detail. He would be completely transported as he drew, talked, or wrote, and spoke of 'the old days' *as if they were now;* the days before 1930 were clearly much more present than the real now; he seemed, like Rose R., to be living (or reliving) the past, even though (like her) he was

she feels her 'past' as present, and that, perhaps it has never felt 'past' for her. Is it possible that Miss R. has never, in fact, moved on from the 'past'? *Could she still be 'in' 1926 forty-three years later? Is 1926 'now'?*[58]

---

perfectly 'oriented.' He *knew* that it was 1969, that he was ageing, ill, and in hospital, but felt (and *conveyed*) his racing youth of the twenties. (See also Sacks and Kohl, 1970a.)

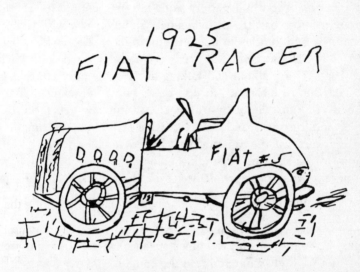

[58] When Rose did 'awaken' with the administration of L-DOPA in 1969, she was extremely excited and animated, but in a way that was strange. She spoke of Gershwin and other contemporaries as if they were still alive; of events in the mid-twenties as if they had just happened. She had obsolete mannerisms and turns of speech; she gave the impression of a 'flapper' come suddenly to life. We wondered if she was disoriented, if she knew where she was. I asked her various questions, and she gave me a succinct and chilling answer: 'I can give you the date of Pearl Harbor,' she said, 'I can give you the date of Kennedy's assassination. I've registered it all – but none of it seems real. I *know* it's '69, I *know* I'm 64 – but I *feel* it's '26, I *feel* I'm 21. I've been a spectator for the last forty-three years.' (There were many other patients who behaved, and even appeared, much younger than their years, as if their personalities, their processes of personal growth and becoming, had been arrested at the same time as their other physical and mental processes.)

Note (1990): Edelman describes how consciousness and memory (which he sees as dependent on continual 'recategorization') are, normally, continually 'updated'; and how this updating depends, in the first place, on *movement,* on free and smooth and orderly movement. The basal ganglia are necessary for this –

28 July. Miss R. sought me out this morning – the first time she had done so in almost two weeks. Her face has lost its jubilant look, and she looks anxious and shadowed and slightly bewildered: 'Things can't last,' she said. 'Something awful is coming. God knows what it is, but it's bad as they come.' I tried to find out more, but Miss R. shook her head: 'It's just a feeling, I can't tell you more . . .'

1 August. A few hours after stating her prediction, Miss R. ran straight into a barrage of difficulties. Suddenly she was ticcing, jammed, and blocked; the beautiful smooth flow which had borne her along seemed to break up, and dam, and crash back on itself. Her walking and talking are gravely affected. She is impelled to rush forward for five or six steps, and then suddenly freezes or jams without warning; she continually gets more excited and frustrated, and with increasing excitement the jamming grows worse. If she can moderate her excitement or her impulsion to run, she can still walk the corridor without freezing or jamming. Analogous problems are affecting her speech: she can only speak softly, if she is to speak at all, for with increased vocal impetus she stutters and stops. I have the feeling that Miss R.'s 'motor space' is becoming confined, so that she rebounds internally if she moves with too much speed or force. Reducing her L-DOPA to 3 gm. a day reduced the dangerous hurry and block, but led to an intensely severe oculogyric crisis – the worst Miss R. has had since starting L-DOPA. Moreover, her 'wiping' tic – which re-appeared on the 28th – has grown more severe and more *complex* with each passing hour. From a harmless feather-light brush of the chin, the movement has become a deep circular gouging, her right index-finger scratching incessantly in tight little circles, abrading the skin and making it bleed. Miss R. has been quite unable to stop this compulsion *directly,* but she can override it by thrusting her tic-hand deep in her pocket and clutching its lining with all of her force. The moment she forgets to do this, the hand flies up and scratches her face.

Edelman calls them 'organs of succession.' The absence of 'updating' in Rose R., and in all our immobilized basal-ganglia–damaged patients, is in striking accordance with this notion.

August 1969

During the first week of August,[59] Miss R. continued to have oculogyric crises every day of extreme severity, during which she would be intensely rigid and opisthotonic, anguished, whimpering, and bathed in sweat. Her tics of the right hand became almost too fast for the eye to follow, their rate having increased to almost 300 per minute (an estimate confirmed by a slow-motion film). On 6 August, Miss R. showed very obvious palilalia, repeating entire sentences and strings of words again and again: 'I'm going round like a record,' she said, 'which gets stuck in the groove . . .' During the second week of August, her tics became more complex, and were conflated with defensive manoeuvres, counter-tics, and elaborate rituals. Thus Miss R. would clutch someone's hand, release her grip, touch something near by, put her hand in her pocket, withdraw it, slap the pocket *three* times, put it back in the pocket, wipe her chin *five* times, clutch someone's hand . . . and move again and again through this stereotyped sequence.

The evening of 15 August provided the only pleasant interlude in a month otherwise full of disability and suffering. On this evening, quite unexpectedly, Miss R. emerged from her crises and blocking and ticcing, and had a brief return of joyous salacity, accompanied with free-flowing singing and movement. For an hour this evening, she improvised a variety of coprolalic limericks to the tune of 'The Sheikh of Araby,' accompanying herself on the piano with her uncontractured right hand.

Later this week, her motor and vocal block became absolute. She would suddenly call out to Miss Kohl: 'Margie, I . . . Margie, I want . . . Margie! . . .', completely unable to proceed beyond the first word or two of what she so desperately wanted to say. When she tried to write, similarly, her hand (and thoughts) suddenly stopped after a couple of words. If one asked her to try and say what she wanted, softly and slowly, her face would go blank, and her eyes would shift in a tantalized manner, indicating, per-

---

[59] The following is based on notes provided by our speech-pathologist, Miss Marjorie Kohl. I myself was away during August.

haps, her frantic inner search for the dislimning thought. Walking became impossible at this time, for Miss R. would find her feet completely stuck to the ground, but the impulse to move would throw her flat on her face. During the last ten days of August, Miss R. seemed to be totally blocked in all spheres of activity; everything about her showed an extremity of tension, which was entirely prevented from finding any outlet. Her face at this time was continually clenched in a horrified, tortured, and anguished expression. Her prediction of a month earlier was completely fulfilled: something awful *had* come, and it was as bad as they came.

1969–72

Miss R.'s reactions to L-DOPA since the summer of 1969 have been almost non-existent compared with her dramatic initial reaction. She has been placed on L-DOPA five further times, each with an increase of dose by degrees to about 3.0 gm. per day. Each time the L-DOPA has procured *some* reduction in her rigidity, oculogyria, and general entrancement, but less and less on each succeeding occasion. It has *never* called forth anything resembling the amazing mobility and mood change of July 1969, and in particular has never recalled the extraordinary sense of 1926-ness which she had at that time. When Miss R. has been on L-DOPA for several weeks its advantages invariably become over-weighed by its disadvantages, and she returns to a state of intense 'block,' crises, and tic-like impulsions. The form of her tics has varied a good deal on different occasions: in one of her periods on L-DOPA her crises were always accompanied by a palilalic verbigeration of the word 'Honeybunch!' which she would repeat twenty or thirty times a minute for the entire day.

However deep and strange her pathological state, Miss R. can invariably be 'awakened' for a few seconds or minutes by external stimuli, although she is obviously quite unable to generate any such stimuli or calls-to-action for herself.[60] If Miss A. – a fellow-patient with dipsomania – drinks more than twenty times an hour at the water fountain, Miss R. cries, 'Get away from that

---

[60] See Appendix: The Electrical Basis of Awakenings, p. 327.

fountain, Margaret, or I'll clobber you!' or 'Stop sucking that spout, Margaret, we all know what you really want to suck!' Whenever she hears my name being paged she yells out, 'Dr Sacks! Dr Sacks!! They're after you again!' and continues to yell this until I have answered the page.

Miss R. is at her best when she is visited – as she frequently is – by any of her devoted family who fly in from all over the country to see her. At such time she is all agog with excitement, her blank masked face cracks into a smile, and she shows a great hunger for family gossip, though no interest at all in political events or other current 'news'; at such times she is able to say a certain amount quite intelligibly, and in particular shows her fondness for jokes and mildly salacious indiscretions. Seeing Miss R. at this time one realizes what a 'normal' and charming and alive personality is imprisoned or suspended by her ridiculous disease.

On a number of occasions I have asked Miss R. about the strange 'nostalgia' which she showed in July 1969, and how she experiences the world generally. She usually becomes distressed and 'blocked' when I ask such questions, but on a few occasions she has given me enough information for me to perceive the almost incredible truth about her. She indicates that in her 'nostalgic' state she *knew* perfectly well that it was 1969 and that she was sixty-four years old, but that she *felt* that it was 1926 and she was twenty-one; she adds that she can't really imagine what it's like being older than twenty-one, because she has never really experienced it. For most of the time, however, there is 'nothing, absolutely nothing, no thoughts at all' in her head, as if she is forced to block off an intolerable and insoluble anachronism – the almost half-century gap between her age as felt and experienced (her *ontological* age) and her actual or *official* age. It seems, in retrospect, as if the L-DOPA must have 'de-blocked' her for a few days, and revealed to her a time-gap beyond comprehension or bearing, and that she has subsequently been forced to 're-block' herself and the possibility of any similar reaction to L-DOPA ever happening again. She continues to look much younger than her years; indeed, in a fundamental sense, she *is* much younger than her age. But she is a Sleeping Beauty whose 'awakening' was unbearable to her, and who will never be awoken again.

ROBERT O.

⨀ Mr O. was born in Russia in 1905, but came to the United States as an infant. He enjoyed excellent health, and showed unusual scholastic ability (graduating from high school at the age of fifteen), until his seventeenth year, when he developed a somnolent form of *encephalitis lethargica* concomitantly with the flu. He was intensely drowsy, although not stuporous, for six months, but shortly after recovering from this acute illness became aware of abnormalities in his sleeping, mind, and mood.

Between 1922 and 1930, reversal of sleep-rhythm was perhaps the major problem, Mr O. tending to be very sleepy and torpid by day, and very restless and insomniac by night. Other sleep disorders, at this time, included sudden fits of yawning, narcolepsy, somnambulism, somnoloquy, sleep-paralyses, and nightmares.

Emotionally equable before his encephalitis, Mr O. subsequently showed a tendency to rather marked mood-swings (with frequent sudden depressions and occasional elations) which seemed to him to 'come out of the blue,' and to show no obvious connection with the actual circumstances of his external or emotional life. There were also short periods of restlessness and impulsiveness, when he would feel 'driven to move around, or do something,' which again he could not connect with the day-to-day circumstances of living. He also observed, in these early days, that 'something had happened' to his mind. He retained his memory, his love of reading, his accurate vocabulary, his keeness, his wit, but found that he could no longer concentrate for long periods, because 'thoughts dart into my mind, not my own, not intended if you know what I mean,' or, alternatively, because 'thoughts suddenly vanish, smack in the middle of a sentence sometimes . . . They drop out, leaving a *space* like a frame minus

a picture.' Usually, Mr O. was content to ascribe his erratic thinking to the sleeping-sickness, but at other times became convinced
that 'influences' of various sorts were 'fiddling' with his thoughts.

In 1926, or thereabouts, he started to develop twitching and
shaking of both arms, and observed that he had ceased to swing
the left arm when walking. He presented himself for examination
at Pennsylvania Hospital in 1928, at which time the following
features were noted: 'Fine tremor of the fingers and tongue
. . . fibrillary twitchings of the forearm muscles . . . mask-like
expression . . . constant blinking of both eyes.' During the four
years of his outpatient attendance at this hospital, he appeared
mentally clear at all times, but was observed to suffer from periods of depression and occasionally of euphoria.

Despite these symptoms, Mr O. was able to work as a salesman
until 1936, and subsequently to maintain himself independently,
on a small disability pension, until his admission to Mount Carmel
Hospital in 1956. In the years immediately preceding his admission here, Mr O. had become somewhat solitary and seclusive in
his habits, rather eccentric in his speech and thinking, obsessive
almost to stereotypy in his daily activities, and religious.

On admission, Mr O. was able to walk independently, but
showed a mildly flexed posture of the trunk. He showed a coarse
intermittent tremor of the left arm and leg, rigidity and cogwheeling in all limbs, masking of the face, and inability to look
upwards. He asserted, firmly, but pleasantly, that his moods were
dictated by the interactions of protons and neutrons in the atmosphere, and that his neurological problems were the result of a
spinal tap performed in 1930.

In the early 1960s, Mr O. developed two new symptoms,
which his fellow-patients termed 'pulling faces' and 'talking to
hisself.' The grimacing scarcely resembled any normal expression, but looked more like a man being sick, with retching,
protrusion of the tongue, and agonized-looking clenching of the
eyes. The 'talking to hisself' was not really talking either, but a
sort of murmuring-purring sound emitted with each expiration,
rather pleasing to the ear, like the sound of a distant sawmill, or
bees swarming, or a contented lion after a satisfactory meal. It is
interesting that Mr O. had experienced the 'impulse' to make

noises and faces for at least thirty years, but had controlled these successfully until 1960. These symptoms were most marked if he was tired, excited, frustrated, or ill; they *also* became more striking if they excited attention, which led, of course, to the usual vicious circle.

These years also saw the gradual worsening of his rigid-dystonic symptoms, and his hurrying and festination. I saw Mr O. several times between 1966 and 1968 (i.e. before his receiving L-DOPA), and got to know him quite well. He was an odd, charming, rather gnome-like man, full of surprising turns and twists of phrase, some of these very droll, and some of them quite irrelevant to the mainstream of his thought; his 'thought-disorder,' his very original and sometimes shocking views, and his mocking sense of humour, were all inseparably combined – as in many gifted schizophrenics – and all of these joined to give a curiously Gogolian flavour to his thought and conversation. He showed very little affect of any kind as he spoke, and I never saw him 'put out' in any way during the course of these three years. He was, it seemed, never angry, never belligerent, never anxious, never demanding, but he was assuredly not apathetic in the sense of Mrs B. I had the impression, rather, that his affects had been splintered and displaced and dispersed, in some unimaginably complex but clearly protective fashion. He was a very narcissistic man, not too concerned with the world.

His voice was rapid, soft, low-pitched, and gibbering, as if he were very pressed for time and had a secret to confide. He showed extreme rigidity of the trunk, with a rather disabling flexion-dystonia which forced the trunk forward at a sharp angle to his legs. Mr O. was quite unable to straighten up voluntarily – the effort, if anything, increased the dystonia – but did straighten up when he was in bed and asleep. He showed a marked plastic rigidity of the limbs, without dystonic components, and occasional 'flapping' tremor. He was able to rise to his feet easily, and to walk rather swiftly; he had difficulty coming to a halt, and he could not walk slowly. Propulsion and retropulsion were readily called forth. In addition to his grimacing and humming, Mr O. showed a variety of smaller movements of the ears, the eyebrows, the platysma, or chin. He showed a rather unblinking, lizard-like stare, except when grimacing, or during his rare paroxysms of blepharoclonus. But, all-in-all, Mr O. was one of our most active and independent patients, able to look after himself in every way, to walk round the neighbourhood, and to carry out his singular social activities, which were confined to feeding pigeons, giving candies to children, and nattering by the hour with the hoboes down the road.

Hyoscine and other anti-cholinergics helped his rigidity a little; surgery had never been considered. In view of the fact that he could already get around sufficiently, and that he showed tendencies which might be worsened by L-DOPA, I was somewhat hesitant at first to try this with him. But his bent back was 'killing him,' he said, so we felt it was worth trying the L-DOPA for *this*.

Course on L-DOPA

The administration of L-DOPA was started on 7 May. During the first ten days of the trial, with the daily dosage of L-DOPA being progressively raised to 4 gm. daily, neither therapeutic nor adverse effects were observed.

On 19 May (while he was receiving 4 gm. L-DOPA daily), I noticed for the first time some adverse effects of the drug. Grimacing, which had been sporadic previously, had become frequent, and severe in intensity. Mr O.'s voice was more hurried and showed some tendency to block: this was vividly described by Mr O. himself: 'The words clash together: they interrupt one another: they jam the exit.' His walking also had become more hurried, and had developed an urgent, impatient quality: this too was memorably described by Mr O. 'I feel forced to hurry,' he said, 'as if Satan was chasing me.'

On the evening of 21 May, while performing late rounds, I observed Mr O., fast asleep, pursing his lips during sleep and every so often waving his arms or talking during his sleep.

In the hope of reducing his axial rigidity and flexure, I increased the dose of L-DOPA to 6 gm. daily. This did lead to reduction of rigidity in the limbs, and to a lesser extent in the trunk and neck-muscles, but any advantage this might have been to the patient was offset by a further and intolerable increase in forced and involuntary movements. In particular, forced protrusion and propulsion of the tongue now became violent and practically continuous, and was associated with forced gagging and retching. Speech was rendered impossible by continued tongue-pulsions. Other forms of grimacing – especially forced closures of the eyes – had also become incessant; so much so that Mr O. was virtually blind. In view of these intolerable effects, I felt that L-DOPA should be discontinued, and it was accordingly reduced over the course of a week. By 10 June, the L-DOPA had been cut out, and Mr O. had returned to his pre-DOPA status.

1969–72

Mr O. never *voiced* any disappointment as such, or anger, or envy of those round him who had done well on L-DOPA, but he *showed* his feelings in a change of behaviour. He went out less, and stopped feeding the pigeons. He started reading much more – especially Cabbala – and spent hours making 'diagrams' which he kept locked in a drawer. He was never disagreeable, but he became less accessible. And his thinking seemed more scattered, and less benign than before; his wit had always been sharp, but now became mordant, and once in a while it became vitriolic. And yet, there were pleasant times, especially on fine Sunday mornings, when the protons and neutrons were behaving themselves. At such times Mr O. would walk round the block and once in a while he would drop in to see me (my apartment was only a few yards from the hospital); I would give him some cocoa, and he would look through my books, which he handled with scholarly ease and absorption; he seemed, at such times, to enjoy my presence, provided I said nothing and asked him no questions; he too would be silent, exempt from the nagging and pressure of thought.

But his physical state was going downhill, and it seemed to do so much faster than before. He 'deteriorated' much more in 1970 than in the preceding decade. His axial dystonia became almost unbearable, forcing his trunk forwards at right angles to his legs.

Most disquietingly, he started to lose weight – muscle-bulk and strength which he desperately needed. We gave him custards and milk-shakes and second helpings and egg-nogs, until he protested he was being stuffed like a goose; we gave him injections of anabolic steroids; we did innumerable tests to see whether he had hidden cancer or infection – all of which were entirely negative. His urine was full of creatinine, but this was no more than a reflection of his clinical state. He was wasting away in front of our eyes and nothing we could do seemed to stay his cachexia.[61]

Having observed repeatedly that the effects of L-DOPA were extremely variable, even in the same patient, and that its actions on a second trial might be quite different from those originally seen, we decided in 1971 to try it again. Its actions *were* different this time, whether 'better' or 'worse' it is impossible to say. On its second trial, L-DOPA caused none of the grimacing and respiratory difficulties which were so intolerable the first time: these, if anything, rather declined in severity. The plastic rigidity of his limbs was reduced, so much indeed that they became almost flaccid; but the axial dystonia was unchanged or increased.

L-DOPA, the first time, had scarcely affected his *thinking,* but it did so the second time in a disastrous sort of way. Mr O.'s thoughts became faster, more pressured, less controlled, and fragmented. He had shown occasional 'slippages' and odd associations for fifty years past, but now these burst forth in incontinent fashion.

His thinking and speaking became more and more splintered, and full of neologisms; words and even fragments of words broke up, re-assorted, and were given new meanings; he now spoke in

---

[61] It is well known (and was remarked by Parkinson himself) that progressive weight-loss is a most ominous and usually terminal symptom in Parkinsonian patients. In some patients, this is clearly attributable to reduced intake, difficulties in eating, etc. In a number of post-encephalitic patients, on the other hand, one may see the most extreme weight-loss despite normal and even voracious eating, which suggests the possibility of a central cachexia, of patients being consumed in their own metabolic furnace. The opposite – a mysterious fattening and increase of bulk – may also be seen in some of these patients. In a number of cases, the sudden onset of cachexia or its opposite comes on with L-DOPA, and seems to reflect a central effect of this drug. Whether Mr O.'s cachexia had been set off by L-DOPA is open to question.

a very accelerated Bleulerian 'word salad,' brilliant in a way, but very difficult to follow – like *Finnegans Wake* run backwards on tape.

The L-DOPA, of course, was once again stopped, but Mr O.'s acute thought-disorder continued unabated. It continued, in fact, for another twelve months. Yet there was, clearly, a part of him which was not fragmented, but 'together' and vigilant, for he recognized everybody, and the routine of the ward. He was never, for a moment, confused or disoriented, like someone who is demented or in a delirium. The former Mr O., one couldn't help feeling, was still present somewhere, watching and controlling, somewhere *behind* the broken-up ravings.

His weight-loss, throughout this, continued unabated. He lost seventy pounds over a period of two years, and finally became almost too weak to move. He shrivelled to death in front of our eyes.

One other circumstance, perhaps, deserves recording. The week before he died, Mr O. suddenly became quite lucid in his speech and thought; and more than this, he 're-found' feelings which had been scattered and suppressed for fifty years; he ceased to be 'schizophrenic,' and became a simple and direct human being. We had several talks in those final days, the tone of which was set by Mr O. 'Don't give me any guff,' he said. 'I *know* the score. Bob's down to skin and bone. He's *ready* to go.' In his last few days he joked with the nurses, and he asked the rabbi to read him a psalm. A few hours before his death he said: 'I was going to kill myself, in '22 . . . I'm glad I didn't . . . It's been a good game, encephalitis and all.'

HESTER Y.

Mrs Y. was born in Brooklyn, the elder child of an immi-grant couple. She had no illnesses of note in her growing-up years, certainly nothing which suggested *encephalitis lethargica.*

She showed from the first an active intelligence, and an unusu-ally independent and equable character. Her warmth, her cour-age, and her acute sense of humour are affectionately remem-bered by her younger brother: 'Hester' (he said to me, forty years later) 'was always a good sport and a wonderful sister. She had strong likes and dislikes, but she was never unfair. She was always in scrapes, like the rest of us kids, but she was as tough as they come – she took everything in her stride. And she could laugh at everything, especially herself.'

After finishing high school, and a lightning courtship, Mrs Y. married at the age of nineteen. She gave birth to a son the following year, and to a daughter three years after her marriage. She enjoyed ten years of family life before being struck by illness in her thirtieth year. It is clear that Mrs Y. was the fulcrum of her family, giving it balance and stability with her own strength of character, and that when *she* became ill, its foundations were rocked. Her symptoms, at first, were paroxysmal and bizarre. She would be walking or talking with a normal pattern and flow, and then *suddenly,* without warning, would come to a stop – in mid-stride, mid-gesture, or the middle of a word; after a few seconds she would resume speech and movement, apparently unaware that any interruption had occurred. She was considered, at this time, to have a form of epilepsy, so-called 'absences' or *'petit mal* variants.' In the months that followed, these standstills grew lon-ger, and would occasionally last for several hours; she would often be discovered quite motionless, in a room, with a com-pletely blank and vacuous face. The merest touch, at such times, served to dissipate these states, and to permit immediate resumption of movement and speech.[62] The diagnosis, at this period, had been changed to 'hysteria.'

After two years of these paroxysmal and mysterious standstills, unmistakable signs of Parkinsonism appeared, accompanied by indications of catatonia or trance, impeding all movement and speech and thought. As her Parkinsonism and entrancement grew rapidly worse, Mrs Y. became 'strange' and difficult of access – and it was this, more than her physical difficulties, which disquieted, alarmed, and angered her family. This change is described by her brother as follows: 'Hester was vivid in all her reactions, until her thirties when her illness took hold of her. She didn't lose any of her feelings, and she didn't become hostile or cold, but she seemed to get more remote all the time. One could see her being carried away by the illness, like a swimmer sucked out by the tide. She was being sucked away right out of our reach . . .' By her thirty-fifth year, Mrs Y. was virtually immobile and speechless, and totally immured in a deep, far-off state. Her husband and children felt tortured and helpless, and had no idea which way they should turn. It was Mrs Y. herself who finally decided that it would be best for everybody if she were admitted to hospital; she said, 'I'm finished. There's nothing else to do.'

She entered Mount Carmel in her thirty-sixth year. Her entry

---

[62] Some of these strange arrests started to recur after the use of L-DOPA. One very dramatic one stays in my mind. A huge flood occurred one day, which was traced up to the fifth floor, where my post-encephalitic patients were, and to one of the bathrooms there. When we entered, we found Hester standing motionless, with water up to her armpits. When I touched her shoulder, she jumped and said, 'My God! What's *happened?*'

'You tell me,' I said.

'I had just started running my bath,' she answered, 'there was about two inches of water in the bath. The next thing – you touch me, and I see there's this flood.'

As we talked more, the truth was borne in; that she had been 'frozen' at a single perceptual and ontological moment: had stayed motionless at this moment, with (for her) just two inches of water in the bath, throughout the hour or more in which a vast flood had developed.

A similar arrest is seen in the documentary film of *Awakenings,* which comes on while she is doing her hair. Suddenly, she ceases, all movement ceases . . . and after a minute or two, the audience get restless, and look round to see if the projector has stuck. But it is *Hester's* 'projector' which has stuck, jamming her in a 'freeze-frame' two minutes long.

to hospital, the finality implied, broke the morale and coherence
of her husband and children. Her husband visited her twice in
hospital, and found it unbearable; he never came again, and
finally divorced her; her daughter became acutely psychotic, and
had to be institutionalized in a local state hospital; her son left
home and fled 'somewhere out West.' The Y.s – as a family – had
ceased to exist.

Mrs Y.'s life in Mount Carmel was eventless and placid. She
was well liked by other patients and nurses and staff, for her
humour and character somehow 'showed through' her dense
immobility. She was virtually motionless and speechless at all
times, and when I first met her, in 1966, I suddenly realized –
with a profound sense of shock – that it was possible for Parkinsonism and catatonia to reach an *infinite* degree of severity.[63] She

---

[63] When I speak of 'a profound sense of shock' in regard to my first glimpse of
Hester, I do not use the phrase lightly or loosely. Although it is now seven years
ago, I sharply recall the stunned feeling, the sense of amazement which came
over me, as I suddenly realized the *infinite* nature, the *qualitative* infinity, of the
phenomenon which faced me . . . One speaks of infinite anguishes, poignancies,
desires, and joys – and one does so naturally, with no sense of paradox: one
thinks of them as infinities, in the infinitude of the soul, i.e. one conceives them
in a metaphysical sense. But *Parkinsonism* – was this not something categorically
different? Was it not a simple, mechanical disorder of function – a mere excess
or deficiency – something essentially finite, something which could be measured
in the divisions or units of a suitable scale? Was it not, as it were, a commodity
or *thing,* to be weighed and assayed as a grocer weighs butter?
  This is what I had been taught, what I had read, what I thought. And then
I saw Hester, and experienced a sudden jarring of my thinking, a sudden
wrenching from a way of seeing, a frame of reference, to one which was deeply
and shockingly different. When I saw Hester, I suddenly realized that all I had
thought about the finite, ponderable, numerable nature of Parkinsonism was
nonsense. I suddenly realized, at this moment, that Parkinsonism could in no
sense be seen as a thing which increased or decreased by finite increments. It
suddenly came to me that Parkinsonism was a propensity, a tendency – which
had no minimum, no maximum, and no finite units; that it was anumerical; that
from its first, infinitesimal, intimation or twinge, it could proceed by an infinite
multitude of infinitesimal increments to an infinite, and then more infinite, and
still more infinite, degree of severity. And that its 'least part,' so to speak,
possessed (in infinitesimal form) the entire, indivisible nature of the whole.
Given such a concept we would also have to envisage it as irrational (surd),
immeasurable, and incommensurable. Such thoughts carried a disquieting impli-
cation, viz. that if Parkinsonism *per se* was immeasurable, it would never be
possible to find an exact counter-measure, to counter it, cancel it out, or 'titrate'
it (in more than a limited and temporary fashion). This dark thought, which I

certainly gave no impression of deadness or apathy (like Magda B.); no impression of veto or 'block' (like Lucy K.); no impression of aloofness or withdrawal (like Leonard L. and Miron V.); but she did give the impression of an infinite remoteness. She seemed to dwell in some unimaginably strange, inaccessible ultimity, in some bottomlessly deep hole or abyss of being; she seemed crushed into an infinitely dense, inescapable state, or held motionless in the motionless 'eye' of a vortex. This impression was accentuated by her slow rhythmic humming, and by her slowly rotating palilalic responses.[64] She showed an infinite coercion or *consent* of behaviour – a circular, effortless, ceaseless movement, which seemed still because its locus was infinitesimal in size. She was utterly still, intensely still, yet perpetually moving, in an ontological orbit contracted to zero.

One thing, and one only, could slightly reduce the depth of her state, and allow some emergence from the abyss of Parkinsonism. Every afternoon, in physiotherapy, Mrs Y. would be suspended in a warm pool of water, and after an hour of attempted active and passive movement, she would be stirred a little from her

---

endeavoured to banish, first came to me when I saw Hester in 1966, and recurred to me early in 1967, when I first read of the amazing effects of L-DOPA in patients, and of the appearance of 'side-effects' despite the exactest 'titrations' of dosage.

Thus the merest twinge of Parkinsonism (or migraine, or agony, or ecstasy) prefigures the whole, already has, in miniature, the quality of the whole – *is* the beginning of a potentially infinite enlargement. (Once when I asked a patient, a gifted novelist with migraine, how he experienced his attacks, and in particular how they started, he replied, 'It doesn't start with one symptom, it starts as a whole. You feel the whole thing, quite tiny at first, right from the start . . . It's like glimpsing a point, a familiar point, on the horizon, and gradually getting nearer, seeing it get larger and larger; or glimpsing your destination from far off, in a plane, having it get clearer and clearer as you descend through the clouds. The migraine *looms,*' he added, 'but it's just a change of scale – everything is already there from the start.')

Addendum (1990): In the original version of this footnote I tried to explain the infinite quality of Parkinsonism by reference to infinite numbers and sets. Now I see it – along with countless other aspects of Parkinsonism, of L-DOPA effects, and of cerebral function generally – as requiring models or concepts which had not been created in the 1960s, in particular those of chaos and nonlinear dynamics (see Appendix: Chaos and Awakenings, p. 351).

[64] '. . . magnetized by some words of his own speech, his mind was slowly circling round and round in the same orbit.' James Joyce, 'An Encounter.'

infinite akinesia and show a brief ability to move her right arm, and to make small pedalling motions with her legs in the water. But within half an hour, even this capacity would have faded, and she would be totally reverted to entranced akinesia.

In addition to her akinesia, Mrs Y. had developed, over the years, a severe dystonic contracture of the left arm, and a flexion-dystonia of the neck, which almost impacted the chin on the sternum. This, added to her profound akinesia of chewing and swallowing, had made feeding almost insuperably difficult. Akinesia of chewing and swallowing had become so severe, by May of 1969, that Mrs Y. was being fed on a liquid diet, and the necessity of tube-feeding had become imminent. She was started on L-DOPA as a life-saving measure, for we feared she would die from aphagia or starvation. L-DOPA was first administered in orange-juice, on 7 May.

Course on L-DOPA

During the first ten days of L-DOPA administration (7–16 May), during which the daily dosage was gradually increased to 4 gm., no change whatever was to be observed in Mrs Y. Fearing that some or all of the drug was being decomposed by the acid orange-juice in which it was being given, I requested, on 16 May, that it be given in apple sauce instead. The next day Mrs Y. 'exploded' – as the nursing-staff put it. There was no subjective or objective 'warning' whatever. On Saturday 17 May, about half an hour after receiving her morning gram of L-DOPA, Mrs Y. suddenly jumped to her feet, and before incredulous eyes walked the length of the ward. 'What do you think of that, eh?' she exclaimed in a loud, excited voice. 'What do you think of that, what do you think of that, what do you think of that?' When I spoke to an awed staff-nurse, a couple of days later, she told me what she thought of it: 'I've never seen anything like it. Hester's wonderful, it's just like a miracle.'

Throughout the course of this amazing weekend, Mrs Y. walked excitedly all round the hospital, starting conversations with fellow-patients who had never heard her talk before, rejoic-

ing ebulliently in her new-found freedom. Her capacity to chew
and swallow were suddenly increased, and so too was her appetite: 'Don't give me any of that slush!' she exclaimed, when
presented at lunch-time with her usual thin soup. 'I want a steak,
well done!' The steak, duly procured and grilled, was devoured
with great relish, and with no sign of difficulty in chewing or
swallowing. With her right hand suddenly released from its
decades-long constraint, Mrs Y. made the first entries in a notebook I had left with her, and which I had not seriously imagined
that she would ever find a use for.

19 May. Having left Mrs Y., on Friday evening, in her usual
state of profound immobility, I was awed at the change which had
occurred over the weekend. I had, at this time, had relatively
little experience of the dramatic responses to L-DOPA which
occur in some post-encephalitic patients, and such responses as I
had seen had always been preceded by *some* 'warming-up' period
of increasing activity; but Mrs Y.'s 'awakening' had commenced
and been completed in a matter of seconds.[65] Entering her room

---

[65] Her sudden mobilization and 'normalization,' after years of virtually total
immobility, seemed incredible, and indeed impossible, to all who saw it – hence
my awe, and the awe of the staff, our feeling that it was '. . . just like a miracle.'
I had a profound sense of shock when I first saw Hester in 1966, and realized
that she had reached a virtual standstill, physically and mentally; but this was as
nothing compared with the shock I received in 1969, when I saw her moving
and talking with ease and fluency, with all her original patterns of action perfectly
preserved and intact. This sense of shock deepened the more I pondered upon
it, until I realised that almost all my ideas on the nature of Parkinsonism, of
activity, of existence, and of time itself, would have to be completely revised . . .

For if a *normal* person is 'de-activated' for even a short time, he meets profound and peculiar difficulties in re-activation, that is, in resuming his previous
patterns of activity. Thus if one breaks a leg or ruptures one's quadriceps (and
has one's leg further de-activated by enclosure and immobilization in plaster)
one finds that one is *functionally disabled* even when one is anatomically healed:
thus, after such an experience (or, more accurately, after such a hiatus in normal
experience and activity) one finds that one has 'forgotten' how to use the de-
activated limb, and that one must *re-learn* (or re-discover) how to use it all over
again, a process which may take many weeks or months. Indeed, if a limb is
severely de-activated for any length of time, one will lose all sense of its existence. Such observations show us the truth of Leibniz's dictum *'Quis non agit non
existit'* – he who does not act does not exist. Normally, then, we see that a hiatus
in activity leads to a hiatus in existence – we are critically dependent on a
continual flow of impulses and information to and from all the sensory and motor

on Monday morning, I was loudly greeted by a transformed Mrs Y. sitting on the edge of her bed, perfectly balanced, with wide-open shining eyes, a somewhat flushed complexion, and a smile going from one ear to the other. Loudly, delightedly, and somewhat palilalically, she poured into my ears the events of the weekend; her speech was very rapid, slightly pressured, and exultant: 'Wonderful, wonderful, wonderful!' she repeated. 'I'm a new person, I feel it, I feel it inside, I'm a brand-new person. I feel so much, I can't tell you what I feel. Everything's changed, it's going to be a new life now . . .' etc. Similar sentiments were expressed in the diary which Mrs Y. had now started to keep. The first entry, made on Saturday 17 May, read: 'I feel very good. My speech is getting louder and clearer. My hands and fingers move more freely. I can even take the paper off a piece of candy, which I haven't done for years.' The following day she wrote: 'Anyone who reads this diary will have to excuse my spelling and my writing – they must remember that I haven't done any writing for years and years.' And to this she added, very poignantly: 'I would like to express my feelings fully. It is so long since I had any

---

organs of the body. *We must be active or we cease to exist: activity and actuality are one and the same . . .*

What, then, of Hester, who after being totally motionless, and (presumably) de-activated, for many years, jumped up and walked in the twinkling of an eye? We might suppose, as I did at first, that she was not really de-activated during her motionless state; but this hypothesis is refutable on several grounds – clinical observations on the absoluteness of her standstill, her own descriptions of the quality of her experience during standstill (see p. 111), and the electrical silence found in attempts to record electrical activity in her muscles during periods of standstill; all of these observations indicate that she was truly and completely de-activated during her standstills. But it was also apparent that her standstills had *no subjective duration whatever.* There was no 'elapsing of time' for Hester during her standstills; at such times she would be (if the logical and semantic paradox may be allowed) at once action-less, being-less, and time-less . . . Only through such considerations, fantastic as they seemed to me at first, could I comprehend how Hester was able to resume normal activity after years of inactivity, in contrast to an 'ontologically normal' person who would lose or 'forget' action-patterns over a length of time, and would then require a further, and perhaps very considerable length of time before being able to 'remember' or re-learn the lost action-patterns. In Hester, by contrast, it was as if the ontological current, the current of being, could be suddenly 'switched off' and as suddenly 'switched on,' with no loss of action-patterns in between, nor any need to re-learn them subsequently – and this because *for her no time had elapsed.*

feelings. I can't find the words for my feelings. I would like to have a dictionary to find words for my feelings . . .' One feeling at least was straightforward: 'I am *enjoying* my food, I feel ravenous for food. Before I simply ate what was put in my mouth.' Concluding her entries for the weekend, Mrs Y. summed up: 'I feel full of pep, vigour and vitality. Is it the medicine I am taking, or just my new state of mind?' Her handwriting, sustained over three pages of her diary, was large, fluent, and highly legible.

Completely motionless and submerged for over twenty years, she had surfaced and shot into the air like a cork released from great depth; she had exploded with a vengeance from the shackles which held her. I thought of prisoners released from gaol; I thought of children released from school; I thought of spring-awakenings after winter-sleeps; I thought of the Sleeping Beauty; and I also thought, with some foreboding, of catatonics, suddenly frenzied.

Examining Mrs Y. on 19 May, I found a remarkable loosening in her previously locked neck and right arm, while in the left arm and legs tone seemed to be, if anything, even less than normal. Salivation was much reduced, and drooling had ceased. The expiratory hum was no longer evident. She seemed extremely alert, and her eye-movements, swift and frequent, were now accompanied by appropriate head-movements. When asked to clap, an action which had been not only impossible but unthinkable before she received L-DOPA, Mrs Y. could now clap with an exuberant force, although the clapping was performed with her right arm predominantly. She became excited with the act of clapping, and after about fifteen claps, suddenly switched to an alternation of clapping and slapping her thighs, and then to an alternation of clapping and touching her hands behind her head. I was disquieted by these unsolicited variations, not knowing whether to ascribe them to high spirits, or to something more driven and compulsive than this.

20 May. Compulsive tic-like movements made their appearance yesterday. Mrs Y.'s right hand now shows exceedingly quick darting motions, suddenly touching her nose, her ear, her cheek, her mouth. When I asked her why she made these movements, she said: 'It's nothing, it's nothing. They don't mean a thing. It's just a habit, a habit – like my humming's a habit.' Her movements were extraordinarily quick and forceful, and her speech seemed two or three times quicker than normal speech; if she had previously resembled a slow-motion film, or a persistent film-frame stuck in the projector, she now gave the impression of a speeded-up film – so much so that my colleagues, looking at a film of Mrs Y. which I took at this time, insisted the projector was running too fast. Her threshold of reaction was now almost zero, and all her actions were instantaneous, precipitate, and excessively forceful.[66] Mrs Y. had slept poorly the night before, and was to have no sleep at all the following night.

21 May. I was informed by the nursing staff, when I came on the ward, that Mrs Y. had 'flipped' and had become 'terribly excitable' and 'hysterical.' When I entered her room, I found her intensely agitated and akathisic, constantly kicking and crossing

---

[66] If Mrs Y., before L-DOPA, was the most *impeded* person I have ever seen, she became, on L-DOPA, the most *accelerated* person I have ever seen. I have known a number of Olympic athletes, but Mrs Y. could have beaten them all in terms of reaction-time; under other circumstances she could have been the fastest gun in the West. Such velocity and alacrity and impetuosity of movement can only be achieved in pathological states. It is seen, above all, in Gilles de la Tourette (multiple tic) syndrome; in certain hyperkinetic children; and in states of 'amok' and hyperkinetic catatonia, where movements (according to Bleuler) '. . . are often executed with great strength, and nearly always involve unnecessary muscle-groups . . . All actions may be executed with far too much power and energy for the purpose.' And, of course, by a number of drugs. (The subject of pharmacological retardation and acceleration was treated by H. G. Wells in an entertaining and prophetic story, 'The New Accelerator,' written at the close of the last century.)

Such a patient may be wholly unaware of how accelerated (or retarded) he or she is. When I asked my students to play ball with Hester, they would not only find it impossible to catch her throws, but be hit smartly by the returning ball on the still-outstretched palms of their hands. 'You see how quick she is,' I would have to tell them. 'Don't underestimate her – you'd better be ready.' But they could not be ready for her, since their best reaction-times approached an eighth of a second, whereas Hester's was no more than a thirtieth of a second. I would then say to Hester, 'You have to slow down! Count up to ten, and *then* throw it back.' The ball would fly back with scarcely any diminution of delay, and I would say to Hester, 'I asked you to count to ten.' She would reply, in speech *crushed* by the rapidity of utterance, 'But I *did* count to ten.' At such intensely accelerated times, Hester would internally count up to ten (or twenty, or thirty) in a split second, *but without realizing she did it so fast.* (The reverse of this is equally astonishing, and was shown extremely clearly by another patient, Miron V. – see n. 83, p. 162.)

her legs, banging her hands, and uttering sudden high-pitched screams. She could be calmed, to a remarkable extent, by speaking to her in a soft soothing voice, or holding her hands, or by a very gentle pressure on her frenzied limbs. A constraint, in contrast, caused intense frustration, and heightened her agitation and frenzy: thus if one tried to prevent her kicking her legs, an unbearable tension developed which sought discharge in pounding of the arms; if these were constrained, she would lunge with her now-mobilized head from side to side; and if this was constrained she would scream.

For much of this day, Mrs Y. wrote in her diary, covering page after page in a rapid scrawl full of paligraphic repetitions, puns, clangs, and violent, perseverative crossings-out – a script (and mode of thought) as different from her calm, freely flowing writing of the weekend as this had been from the agonizingly obstructed, virtually impossible lettering which was all she could do before L-DOPA had been given. I was at first astonished that Mrs Y. *could* write in face of such emotional and motor agitation, but it was soon evident that writing was a necessity to her at this juncture, and that the ability to express and record her thoughts in this way allowed a vital act of catharsis and self-communion. It also allowed an indirect form of communication with me, for she was prepared to express herself in writing, and show her writings to me, but not to vouchsafe her most intimate thoughts directly to me.

Her writings, at this time, were almost entirely expressions of blame, rage, and terror, mingled with feelings of grief and loss. There were long paranoid tirades against various nurses and nursing-aides who had 'persecuted' and 'tormented' her since she entered the hospital, and vengeful phantasies as to how she would now 'get back' at them. She reverted, again and again, to a former neighbour in the hospital, a hostile dement who two years before had thrown a glass of water all over her. And there were innumerable pages blotted with tears, which bore witness to her grief and her merciless conscience: 'Look at me now,' she wrote in her diary. 'I'm fifty-five, bent double . . . a cripple . . . a hag . . . I used to be so pretty, Dr Sacks; you'd never believe it now . . . I've lost my husband and son . . . I drove them away

'. . . My daughter's crazy . . . It's all my fault. It must be a
punishment for something I did . . . I've been asleep for twenty
years and grown old in my sleep.'

What she did not express in her diary, and which was perhaps
still repressed, were sexual feelings and libidinous substitutes –
the *voracities* which so many other patients showed during climactic excitements induced by L-DOPA. That she was consumed by
such feelings, *under the surface,* was shown by her lascivious-
nightmarish dreams at this time, and the quality of her hallucinations later this day. I was called to see Mrs Y. around eight in the
evening, because she was constantly screaming with ear-splitting
intensity. When I entered her room she flew into a panic, mistook
my fountain-pen for a syringe, and started screaming: 'It's a needle, a needle, a needle, a needle . . . take it away, take it away
. . . don't stick me, don't stick me!', her screams becoming louder
and louder all the time, while she thrashed her legs and her trunk
in an absolute frenzy. She had written in her diary: 'I don't *think*
I am in a concentration-camp??????', the queries growing larger
and more numerous till they covered the entire page; and on the
following page, in huge capital letters, 'PLEASE I AM NOT MAD,
NOT MAD.' Her face was flushed, her pupils dilated, and her
pulse was bounding and exceedingly rapid. When she was not
screaming at this time, she showed gasping and panting, and
violent out-thrustings of her tongue and her lips.

I requested the nurses to give her 10 mg. of thorazine, in-
tramuscularly, and within fifteen minutes her frenzy subsided,
and was replaced by exhaustion, contrition, and sobbing. The
terror, suspicion, and rage went out of her eyes, and were replaced by a look of affection and trust: 'Don't let it happen again,
Dr Sacks,' she whispered. 'That was like a nightmare, but worse.
Must never happen again, never, never, never . . . never again.'
Mrs Y. now consented to my lowering the dose of L-DOPA, which
she had strenuously and violently opposed before: 'It'll be a
death sentence, if you lower it,' she had said in the morning.

22–5 May. I lowered the L-DOPA from 3 gm. to 2 gm. to 1 gm.
a day, but Mrs Y. continued to show excessive arousal, although
there was no return of the intense paranoia which occurred on
the 21st. She decided, on the 22nd, to settle her scores with her

former neighbour, and on the morning of this day threw a jug of water at her, and came back from this chuckling, in a much better mood. When I asked her whether she had been brooding over the matter for the entire two years, she said: 'No, of course not. I didn't care at the time. I didn't give it a thought till I started L-DOPA. And then I got mad, and couldn't stop thinking about it.' She continued, at this time, to write in her diary – indeed she scarcely did anything else at this time, and the moment she stopped writing her agitation and akathisia immediately recurred. There were no more tirades or phantasies of vengeance after she had secured her token-revenge on her token-persecutor, and her writings on the 22nd and 23rd were entirely concerned with the questions of illness and family and sadness and guilt, and by the increasing recognition that 'Fate' – not herself – was responsible for everything. On the 24th she said to me: 'Please stop the L-DOPA. It's too much to handle. Everything has happened far too fast these few days . . . I need to cool off and think everything over.' I stopped her L-DOPA on this day, as requested. Seeing her on the 25th rigid, motionless, speechless again, her eyes lustreless and her head on her chest – I could hardly believe that the entire cycle of triumphant emergence, 'complications,' and withdrawal, had all taken place in the span of a week.

1969–72

It is now forty months since the above notes were written, forty months in which Mrs Y. has continued to take L-DOPA (except on rare occasions, described below), to react to it violently and hyperbolically, and yet to maintain for herself a fuller and more active life than the great majority of our patients at Mount Carmel. Of all the patients I have ever known, Mrs Y. is the most extravagant and unstable in her physiological activity and reactions to L-DOPA; yet she is the 'coolest' and sanest in her emotional attitudes and accommodations to these, and the most resourceful and ingenious in diverting, circumventing, or otherwise 'managing' her preposterous reactions to L-DOPA. With consummate skill and ease Mrs Y. pilots herself through physiological storms of an incredible ferocity and unpredictability, continually negotiating problems which would cause most patients to founder on the spot. Although, in other case histories, I have avoided lists and tabulations, I will here make use of them in order to avoid diffuseness and prolixity.

1. *Sensitivity to L-DOPA and oscillations of response.* Like all post-encephalitic (and Parkinsonian) patients who have been maintained on L-DOPA for any length of time, Mrs Y. has become exceedingly sensitive to it, her average maintenance-dose now being no more than 750 mg. a day. Her reactions to it have become (indeed, they were almost so from the start) entirely all-or-none in character – she either reacts totally, or not at all: she is no more capable of graduated reaction than one is capable of a graduated sneeze. Her reactions, which were very rapid to begin with, have now become virtually instantaneous – she leaps from one physiological extreme to another in the twinkling of an eye, in a flash, in a fraction of a second: she jumps from one state to another as quickly as one jumps from one thought to another. Such transitions – or, more accurately, transiliences – are no longer 'correlated' in any predictable way with the timing of her L-DOPA doses – indeed, she is apt to make somewhere between 30 and 200 abrupt physiological reversals a day. Of all our patients who are 'swingers' or 'yo-yos,' Mrs Y. is the most profound, abrupt, and frequent in her oscillations. The abruptness and totality of these reversals scarcely give one an impression of a gradual, graduated process, but of sudden reorganizations or transformations of *phase.* If her L-DOPA is stopped, she immediately goes into a coma.

2. *Proliferation of responses to L-DOPA.* It has been indicated that within three days of her 'awakening' on L-DOPA, Mrs Y. showed the onset of clear-cut *tics.* These have continually proliferated in number, so much so that I can now recognize more than 300 distinct and individual patterns of tic.[67] Every two or three days,

---

[67] Hester's tics remained relatively simple, but other patients showed a vast spectrum of automatisms and impulsions, passing from low-level stereotypies and myoclonic movements to tics and urges of the most elaborate kind. Those that were accompanied by a strong inner compulsion, and followed by brief relief, included lip smacking, kissing, sucking and blowing tics, forced sniffing,

so to speak, a new tic is 'invented' – sometimes, seemingly, *de novo,* sometimes as an elaboration of an already-existing tic, sometimes as an amalgam or 'conflation' of two or more pre-existing tics, sometimes as a defensive manoeuvre or counter-tic. These tics affect every aspect of action and behaviour, and one may often perceive a dozen or two proceeding *simultaneously,* apparently independently controlled and in complete functional isolation from one another. All of these tics have distinctive styles and rhythms or movements – 'kinetic melodies' (in Luria's term) – and when Mrs Y. is merrily ticcing, she gives the impression of a clock-shop gone mad, with innumerable clocks all ticking and chiming in their own time and tune.[68]

3. *Mutual transformations (or phase-relations) of tics.* Mrs Y. shows several basic phases of tic, the relationships of which are most clearly shown when they are demonstrated with one and the same basic tic-form. Thus a given tic may take an abrupt, precipitate, darting form; a rhythmical clonic form (like her original humming-tic); or a tonic (or catatonic) form – a so-called 'tic of immobility.' The changes between these phases may be quite instantaneous: thus Mrs Y. may be suddenly arrested in 'mid-tic,' i.e. transformed to a cataleptic perseveration of the tic; again one of her 'favourite' tonic tics – a bizarre flexion of the right arm, so that its fingers rest between the shoulder-blades – may immediately 'break up' into precipitate tics.

4. *No reversion to psychosis.* She becomes immensely excited, emotionally as well as motorically, many times a day, and her excitement, at such times, will assume any form which suggests

---

gasping and panting, sudden scratching and touching, shoulder shrugging, head tossing, grimacing, frowning, gaze tics, saluting and swatting tics, compulsive kicking, jumping and stamping, finger snapping, complex respiratory tics, and complex compulsive phonations such as grunting, barking, squealing, and yelling. Vocal tics ranging from brief inchoate vocalizations to complex ejaculate utterances also occurred.

[68] Thus, when looking at (or 'listening to') Hester's tics, of which a dozen might be proceeding simultaneously, one receive no impression of synchrony or symphony, but an impression of polyphony, of many unrelated *tempi* and melodies proceeding independently.

itself or is appropriate: her 'favourite' and most typical excitement is a hilarious excitement *('titillatio et hilaritas'),* and she loves to be told jokes, to be tickled, or to be put in front of comedy-shows on the television at these times. Anguish, rage, and terror are alternatives to hilarity, but shown much less often. She does *not* display voracities and greeds like a number of patients (Rolando P., Margaret A., Maria G., etc.), nor has she shown any significant tendency to possessiveness, grievance, paranoia, or mania. Whether such things are to be ascribed to a difference of 'level' in neural organization, to her equable temper, or to strict self-control, is not clear to me, but it is certain that Mrs Y. – almost alone of our extremely severely affected postencephalitic patients – preserves her 'upper storey' (her personality, relationships, view-of-the-world, etc.) serene and free from the turbulent urges and affects which go on 'beneath' it. She experiences violent drives, but she herself is 'above' them. Her affects are never neuroticized, as her tics are never mannerized.

5. *Organization, 'level,' and non-use of tics.* It is clear that Mrs Y.'s tics are far more complex in form than mere Parkinsonian jerks, jactitations, or precipitations, and also more complex than the desultory, 'quasi-purposeless' choreic and hyperkinetic movements seen in most patients with ordinary Parkinson's disease with long administration of L-DOPA. Mrs Y.'s tics *look* like actions or deeds – and not mere jerks or spasms or movements. One sees, for example, gasps, pants, sniffs, finger-snappings, throat-clearing, pinching movements, scratching movements, touching movements, etc., etc., which could all be part of a normal gestural repertoire, and whose abnormality lies in their incessant, compulsive and 'inappropriate' repetition. One *also* sees bizarre grimaces, gesticulations, and peculiar 'pseudo-actions,' which cannot by any stretch of the word be called 'normal.' These pseudo-actions, sometimes comic, sometimes grotesque, convey a deeply paradoxical feeling, in that they *seem* at first to have a definite (if mysterious) organization and purpose and then one realizes that in fact they do not (like chorea). It is this odd simulacrum of action and meaning, this parody of sense which baffles the mind. (See footnote 24 on Lillian W.'s crises, p. 18.)

On the other hand, Mrs Y. has shown little or no tendency to utilize, rationalize, mannerize, or ritualize her tics – and, in this way, stands in the sharpest contrast to Miron V., Miriam H., etc. The non-use of tics means that Mrs Y. herself can sit quietly (so to speak) 'in the middle' of her tics, paying remarkably little attention to them. It protects her from being 'possessed' or 'dispossessed' or 'taken over' by tics which become mannerisms, affectations, or impostures – as happened, for example, with Maria G. A special form of 'conflation' and 'cleavage' can be observed in Mrs Y.'s alternation of *'macro-tics'* (sudden, incredibly violent and massive movements, or fulgurations, which may bodily throw her off a chair or onto the ground) and *'micro-tics'* (multiple, minor tics, a twinkling or scintillation of innumerable tics). In general, Mrs Y.'s 'style' favours micro-tics, as opposed to other patients who make a specialty of violent, startling macro-tics.[69]

6. *Relationships of tics and behavioural disorder.* It is possible that I am using the term 'tics' too widely, to denote the total physical-mental states which Mrs Y. shows. With continuing use of L-DOPA, she has shown a greater and greater tendency to 'split' into behavioural *fragments* – discrete, differentiated, behavioural forms. Thus she may, in the course of a minute, jump from a peculiar speech-pattern to a peculiar breathing-pattern, to a peculiar respiratory pattern, etc. – each such total-stage affecting different aspects of behaviour. One can easily see that these seemingly senseless 'unphysiological' jumps have a clear behavioural or dramatic unity; they are all reminiscent of or allusions to each other: one could say that they bear to one another a metaphorical relation, and to her total self or behaviour a metonymical relation. They thus follow one another like sequences of 'free associa-

---

[69] One can observe similar 'styles' of ticcing, and 'uses' of tics, in patients with Tourette's syndrome. Some have small, incessant, 'scintillating' tics – others violent, convulsive 'macro-tics'; some regard or treat their tics as meaningless, others endow (and perhaps elaborate) them with meaning. Neurologists speak here of 'simple' versus 'complex' tics, but, it is clear, there is not a dichotomy but an entire spectrum, going from the lowest-level automatisms and twitches to impulsions and behaviours of the most elaborate and bizarre sort (see Sacks, 1982a).

tion,' and – like these – demonstrate, beneath their superficial 'randomness' or senselessness, the referential and epiphanic nature of even such 'primitive' behaviour.

7. *Stationary states and kinematic states.* In addition to the abovementioned disturbances, Mrs Y. *also* has periods when her movements, speech, and thoughts seem virtually normal: her 'attacks' of normality, indeed, have something of the same paroxysmal and unpredictable quality as her behavioural disorders. When she is normal and undriven and unfettered, one can see what a charming and intelligent person she is, and how 'unspoilt' her original, pre-morbid personality. But these normal, free-flowing periods may themselves be interrupted – with great suddenness, and no warning – by sudden cessations of movement/speech/ thought, so that Mrs Y. will suddenly be arrested like a film in a 'freeze-frame.' These still-states may last a second or an hour, and *cannot* be broken by any voluntary action from Mrs Y. herself (indeed such action is impossible and unthinkable at such times). They may cease spontaneously, or with the merest touch or noise from outside, and then Mrs Y. moves immediately again into free-flowing motion/speech/thought.[70] These states have no

---

[70] The fact that the *smallest possible* stimulus – a single photon of light or quantum of energy – suffices to dissipate these still-states shows us that they are totally *inertia-less;* this is further borne out by the fact that there is an *instantaneous* leap from absolute stillness to normal fluent motion. This absolute stillness of these extraordinary states, coupled with their proneness to sudden phasic transformations, suggest an analogy with the 'stationary states' and quantal 'jumps' postulated of atoms and electronic orbits; they suggest, indeed, that we may be dealing with a large-scale model of such micro-phenomena – 'macro-quantal states,' if the term be allowed. Such inertia-less states stand in absolute contrast (and complementarity) to the positive disorders of Parkinsonism, with their intense inertia and resistance to change, their violent warpings of space and field; for *these* suggest miniature models of galactic phenomena, and so might be termed 'micro-relativistic states.'

It was such considerations which led me to write two years ago that 'our data not only show us the inadequacy of classical neurology, but give us the shape of a new neurophysiology of quantum-relativistic type . . . in accordance with the concepts of contemporary physics' (Sacks, 1972). I will go further. It may be said that even if such analogies are permissible or fruitful, the phenomena we are considering are extremely remote from 'ordinary' life, as remote, in their way, as atoms and galaxies. But this, to my mind, is neither interesting nor true. I think that a vast range of familiar biological phenomena – from the forces and

subjective duration whatever: they are identical with the *stand-stills* which started her illness. It is evident, from questioning Mrs Y., that her perceptions of herself and the world have a very 'weird' quality in these standstills. Thus everything seems sharp-edged, flat, and geometric, with a quality like a mosaic or a stained-glass window; there is no sense of space or time at such times.[71] Sometimes these 'stills' form a flickering vision, like a movie-film which is running too slow.[72]

Mrs Y. and other patients who have experienced 'kinematic vision' have occasionally told me of an extraordinary (and seem-ingly impossible) phenomenon which may occur during such periods, viz. the displacement of a 'still' either backwards or forwards, so that a given 'moment' may occur too *soon* or too *late*. Thus, on one occasion, when Hester was being visited by her brother, she happened to be having kinematic vision at about three or four frames a second, i.e. a rate so slow that there was a clearly perceptible difference between each frame. While watching her brother lighting his pipe, she was greatly startled

---

forms of our passions, to the alternations of standstills and jumps in insects – lend themselves equally to analyses of a relativistic and quantal sort; so much so, indeed, that I feel a certain astonishment that relativity and quantality were not 'discovered' by biologists long before their discovery in physics.

[71] 'These states . . . may be described in purely visual terms, while understanding that they may affect *all* thought and behaviour. The still picture has no true or continuous perspective, but is seen as a perfectly flat dovetailing of shapes, or as a series of wafer-thin planes. Curves are differentiated into discrete, discon-tinuous steps: a circle is seen as a polygon. There is no sense of space, or solidity or extension, no sense of objects except as facets geometrically apposed. There is no sense of movement, or the possibility of movement, and no sense of process or forces or field. There is no emotion or cathexis in this crystalline world. There is no sense of absorption or attention whatever. The state is *there,* and it cannot be changed. From gross still vision, patients may proceed to an astonishing sort of microscopic vision or Lilliputian hallucination in which they may see a dust-particle on the counterpane filling their entire visual field, and presented as a mosaic of sharp-faceted faces. From here the patient may proceed to seeing lattices and networks which are no longer identifiable as familiar forms, until finally his entire sensorium may experience only a single point in one of these lattices, which is seen as an infinite concentricity of haloes, dense in the centre and fading at the edge . . .' (Sacks, 1972).

[72] As patients emerge from kinematic vision, the flickering becomes more rapid until, very suddenly, around sixteen frames per second – the so-called 'flicker fusion frequency' – the normal sensation of motion and continuity is restored.

by witnessing the following sequence: first, the striking of a match; second, her brother's hand holding the lighted match, having 'jumped' a few inches from the matchbox; third, the match flaring up in the bowl of the pipe; and fourth, fifth, sixth, etc. the 'intermediate' stages by which her brother's hand, holding the match, jerkily approached the pipe to be lit. Thus – incredibly – Hester saw the pipe actually being lit several frames too soon; she saw 'the future,' so to speak, somewhat before she was *due* to see it.[73]

When cinematic representation achieves a certain critical rate, her sense of vision and of the world suddenly becomes 'normal,' with the movement, space, time, perspective, curvatures, and continuities expected of it. At times of great excitement, Mrs Y. may experience a kinematic 'delirium,' in which a variety of perceptions or hallucinations or hallucinatory patterns may succeed one another with vertiginous speed, several a second; she is quite distressed and disabled while such deliria last, but they are, fortunately, quite rare. Such deliria go with a fragmentation of time and space itself.

---

[73] If we accept Hester's word in the matter (and if we do not listen to our patients we will never learn anything), we are compelled to make a novel hypothesis (or several such) about the perception of time and the nature of 'moments.' The simplest of these, I think, is to take 'moments' as ontological events (i.e. as *our* 'world-moments') and assume that we 'take in' several at a time (as a moving whale continually swallows a swarm of shrimps), or that we keep a small hoard of them 'in stock' at any given time, and in either case 'feed them' into some internal projector, where they become activated and 'real,' one at a time in their proper sequence. Normally, this proceeds correctly and easily; but in certain conditions, it would seem, our ontological moments may be fed to us in the wrong order, so that moments which are chronologically 'past' or 'future' get ectopically displaced, and presented to us as utterly convincing (but inappropriate) 'nows.' Somewhat allied hypotheses (of defective or mistaken 'time-labelling' in the nervous system) have been presented by Efron with regard to the commoner but still uncanny experiences of *déjà vu, jamais vu, presque vu,* etc. These are not associated with kinematic vision, but are apt to occur in states of intense and unusual nervous excitement (as in the singular cases of Martha N. and Gertie C.). All these states of *anachronism,* in company with other time-strangenesses described in this book, indicate how vast is the gulf between abstract and actual, chronological and ontological, in our conceptions and perceptions of time.

Summer 1972

Mrs Y. has become entirely accustomed to all of these strange states, and admits and discusses them freely with me, or with others. Although she lacks the investigative passion and capacities of another patient (Leonard L.), she accepts all of these singular, and potentially terrifying states, with a quite extraordinary equanimity, detachment, and humour. She never feels persecuted or victimized by them, but seems to see them simply *as things which are there,* like her nose, or her name, or New York, or the world. Thus, she is never 'phased out' or 'flipped out' any more – as she was, for a day, when such things first began. She is absolutely 'together' and will stay together, unlike less stable patients (Maria G., Margaret A., etc.) who became fragmented and schizophrenic under the strain of L-DOPA.

A second factor which has allowed Mrs Y. much greater freedom of action than would have seemed possible with her responses has been her skill and ingenuity in preventing, circumventing, or utilizing her 'side-effects' – a skill which she shares with Frances D. particularly. Both of these ladies, with their sharp wits and their bizarre illnesses, have achieved a knowledge and a control of their nervous systems and reactions which not a neurologist anywhere in the world could approach. I scarcely know, here, who teaches whom: I have learned an immense amount from Mrs Y., and she, perhaps, learns something from me.[74] Moreover, Mrs Y. is always active in and out of the hospital – playing bingo, seeing movies, visiting other patients, undertaking half a dozen projects at any time in occupational therapy or workshop, going to concerts, poetry-readings, philosophy

---

[74] A number of such strategies for 'pacing' and controlling post-encephalitic patients are illustrated by Purdon Martin in his excellent book *The Basal Ganglia and Posture.* A detailed theoretical and practical treatment is given in the last chapter ('The Control of Behaviour') of A. R. Luria's remarkable first book *The Nature of Human Conflicts;* he writes there that '. . . the healthy cortex enables [the Parkinsonian patient] to use external stimuli and to construct a compensatory activity for the subcortical automatisms . . . That which was impossible to accomplish by direct will-force becomes attainable when the action is included in another complex system.'

classes, and – her favourite – excursions. She has as full a life as one can have at Mount Carmel.

The final source of Mrs Y.'s strength – as with so many patients – seems to have come from personal relations: in her case the 'discovery' of the son and daughter whom she had not seen in fifteen years or more, a discovery which she expressed a great longing for in her diary, in the dramatic days of May 1969, and which was finally brought about by our untiring social worker. Her daughter, who had spent two decades in and out of mental hospitals since Mrs Y. became ill, is now a frequent and much-loved visitor at Mount Carmel – a reunion which has given deep pleasure and stability to both Mrs Y. *and* her daughter (the latter has steered clear of psychoses since the time of reunion). Equally affecting has been Mrs Y.'s reunion with her son, who after many years of a quasi-psychopathic life 'out West,' has established home and roots in New York once again. Seeing Mrs Y. with her son and her daughter, one realizes the strength of her character and love; one sees what a remarkable person she is, and how solid and real she must have been as a mother. One sees why her children went mad with her illness, and why they are visibly healing as they return to her now.

Thus, despite the innumerable odds against her – the severity and length and strangeness of her illness, her preposterous responses to L-DOPA, and the grim institution which has housed her for years – Mrs Y. has emphatically awoken and returned to reality, in a manner which would have been unthinkable four years ago.

ROLANDO P.

֍ Rolando P. was born in New York in 1917, the youngest son of a newly immigrated and very musical Italian family. He showed unusual vivacity and precocity as a child, acquiring speech and motor skills at an exceptionally early age. He was an active, inquisitive, affectionate, and talkative child, until at thirty months of age his life was suddenly cut across by a virulent attack of *encephalitis lethargica,* which presented itself as an intense drowsiness lasting eighteen weeks, initially accompanied by high fever and influenzal symptoms.

As he awoke from the sleeping-sickness, it became evident that a profound change had occurred, for he now showed a completely masked and expressionless face, and had great difficulty in moving or talking. He would sit for hours completely motionless in his chair, seemingly inanimate except for sudden, impulsive movements of his eyes. If he was set on his feet, he would walk 'like a little wooden doll,' with both arms hanging stiffly at his side; more commonly he would break into a run which would get faster and faster till he crashed into an obstacle and fell like a statue to the ground. He was generally taken to be mentally defective, except by his very observant and understanding mother, who would say: 'My Rolando is no fool – he is as sharp and bright as he ever used to be. He has just come to a stop inside.'

Between the ages of six and ten, he attended ungraded classes at a school for the mentally defective. He had become virtually unable to move or speak by this time, but conveyed to at least one teacher the impression of an intact but imprisoned intelligence: 'Rolando is not stupid,' said a report in 1925. 'He absorbs everything, but nothing can come out.' This impression of him as purely absorptive, as a sort of unfathomable, black, and hungry *hole* was to be echoed over the next forty years by all who observed him closely; it was only superficial observers who thought him vacuous, stupid, or inattentive. But schooling, such as it was, became increasingly difficult, with each passing year, due to an increasing loss of balance, and increasing salivation. In his last year at school, he had to be propped upright with cushions to each side; otherwise he would fall over as helplessly as an upset statue.

From his eleventh to his nineteenth year, he remained at home, propped before the speaker of a large Victrola gramophone, for music (as his father observed) seemed to be the only thing he enjoyed, and the only thing which 'brought him to life.' Animated music would give the boy its animation, and allow him to nod, sing, or gesture in time with it; but as soon as the music came to a stop, he too would come to a stop, and return at once to his stony immobility. He was admitted to Mount Carmel in 1935.

The next third of a century, in a back ward of the hospital, was completely eventless in the most literal sense of this word. Mr P. – who despite his disabilities had grown into a well-proportioned young man – sat in his chair all day like a statue. Every evening, however, between seven and nine, his rigidity and frigidity would thaw out a little, allowing some movement of the arms, some speech, and some emotional expression. At such times he might sing a snatch of opera or embrace his favourite nurses, but – more commonly – he would inveigh against his fate: 'It's a hell of a life,' he would shout; 'I wish I was dead.' Curiously enough, his evening activity would continue during the first portion of his sleep, when he would toss and turn, talk and verbigerate, and show impulsions to walk in his sleep. After midnight these activities would die down, and he would lie like a statue for the rest of the night.

He was submitted to an operation (a left-sided chemopallidectomy) in 1958, which produced some loosening of the rigidity on the right side of his body, but no alteration of his akinesia, or his overall motionless, speechless state.

I examined Mr P. and talked to him several times between 1966 and 1969. He was a powerfully built man at this time, who appeared far younger than his fifty-odd years; he could easily

have passed for half his actual age. He would always be tied in
his wheelchair, to prevent an otherwise irresistible tendency to
fall forwards. He showed great oiliness of the skin, and continual
sweating, lacrimation, and salivation.

His voice was so soft as to be inaudible: sudden effort and
excitement, however, rendered exclamatory speech possible for
a few seconds. Thus, when I asked him whether his salivation
disturbed him much, he exclaimed loudly: 'You bet it does! It's
one hell of a problem!' immediately afterwards relapsing into
virtual aphonia. There was almost no spontaneous blinking of
normal type, which contrasted with the frequency of spontaneous
lid-clonus and forced closure of the eyes: a touch on the face, or
indeed any sudden movement in the field of vision, elicited
forced clonus or closure of the eyelids. Mr P.'s mouth tended to
remain open unless deliberately closed.

He would sit in his chair, with his head bowed forwards and
very little spontaneous movement, for hours on end. He showed
intense rigidity of the neck and trunk muscles, and moderate
rigidity of the limbs, the right side (which was more rigid before
operation) now being slightly less rigid than the left. Cogwheeling was readily elicited at all major joints. The right hand was
cool, the left cold, and both showed trophic changes of the skin
and nails. There was no fixed deformity, and no tremor. There
was very severe akinesia: asked to clench and unclench his hands,
Mr P. could make only a slight finger-flexion, the movement
decaying to zero after three or four repetitions. Asked to clap, Mr
P. could make only three to five claps, the movement subsequently accelerating, becoming minimal in force, and finally
tremulous, before its complete arrest. A sudden violent effort
would enable Mr P. to rise to a standing position, but he was
unable to stand unaided because of an irresistible tendency to fall
backwards. Given much support, he could walk a few feet with
very small, shuffling steps. On resuming his seat he would fall
back rigidly, and statuesquely, without any segmental movements or reflexes. Mr P. was illiterate, but was able, using the left
hand, to reproduce simple geometrical diagrams: these were
much smaller than the originals which he had been requested to
copy, and were produced only with great effort; there was too

much akinesia in the right hand to allow even an attempt at such copying.

He was one of the most profoundly disabled post-encephalitic patients I had ever seen. I had no doubt that he would react to L-DOPA, but many doubts as to what would be his reactions, or his reactions *to* his reactions – for he had been out of the world, in effect, since the onset of his illness before he was three. But I started him on L-DOPA on 14 May 1969.

Course on L-DOPA

On 20 May, Mr P. said that he had an unusual feeling of 'energy,' and an urge to move his legs: this urge was assuaged by 'dancing,' which he did when supported by an orderly. The following day, Mr P. presented quite dramatic changes in his motor status, being able to walk the entire length of the ward (about 80 feet) and back, with only a finger on his back to support him.

By 24 May (the dose of L-DOPA had now reached 3 gm. daily), Mr P. was showing a variety of responses to the drug. His voice, previously almost inaudible, was now clearly audible at ten feet away, and could be maintained at this intensity without apparent effort. His drooling had ceased entirely. He was able to make fists, and to clap and tap his hands with a good deal of force. He was now able to *stride* around the ward, but still required assistance in view of his overwhelming tendency to fall backwards. The rigidity in his arms and legs was much reduced; so much so, indeed, that their tone felt somewhat *less* than normal. His neck and trunk muscles, formerly immovable, were now less rigid, although they did not display the amazing looseness of his arms. His face seemed flushed on this day, and his eyes were abnormally bright and somewhat protuberant. Lid-clonus and lid-closure had ceased to occur. He was also playful, giggly, and somewhat euphoric, and asked me whether he might improve so much as to be released for a day from the hospital. In particular, he showed a surge of sexual excitement, and a sudden development (or 'release') of libidinous phantasies, his desire to go out being partly the wish to have a sexual experience – his first. Motor activity, mood, and general arousal continued to increase over the weekend, Mr P. being loud in his demands for 'a woman – for Chrissake I *deserve* one after all these years!' On 27 May I found him very flushed, boisterous, insomniac, somewhat manic, and frenzied; his movements, previously so meagre and with so little dynamic background, were now violently forceful, and involved as background the whole of his body; he was intensely vigilant and over-alert. His eye-movements (which had been infrequent and unaccompanied by any head-movement) now had an incessant *darting* quality, and were accompanied by equally quick head-movements. His attention was constantly attracted hither and thither, and seemed to be intensified but also short-lived and distractible. Unexpected noises would startle him, and make him jump. Finally, I observed the onset of some akathisia – in particular, a restless shuffling of the legs, and a tendency to pound his bedside table if impatient. In view of this excessive arousal, I reduced his daily dose of L-DOPA from 3 gm. to 2 gm.

This permitted sleep, but he continued to show inordinate arousal. On 29 May, I was struck by the watchful, predatory expression on his face. Movements were now not only forceful but uncontrollable, and would tend to continual acceleration and perseveration, Mr P. being quite unable to halt them, once started.

On the positive side, Mr P. – who had been saddened and ashamed of his illiteracy since his earliest years – expressed a desire to learn reading and writing. He showed remarkable persistence in his efforts, and they were, initially, crowned with success. Unfortunately, his physiological disturbances made this increasingly difficult: he would either read too fast to take in what he read, or get stuck or transfixed on a single letter or word; his handwriting, similarly, would tend either to 'stickiness' and micrographia, or, more commonly, to be broken up into a multitude of impulsive jabbing strokes, which once he had started he could not control.

His akathisia, previously generalized and non-specific, now showed a differentiation into specific impulsions – a restless 'pawing' movement of the right leg (suggestive of a high-spirited, impatient horse), and a tendency to forced chewing and masticatory movements. Sexual and libidinous arousal was still more marked, and the transit of any female personnel across Mr P.'s field of vision would immediately evoke an indescribably lascivious expression, forced lip-licking and lip-smacking movements, dilation of the nostrils and pupils, and uncontrollable watching; he seemed – visually – to grab and grasp the object of his gaze, and to be unable to relinquish it till it passed from his field of vision.

On the evening of the 29th, I happened to see Mr P. asleep, and observed during his sleep an astounding exaltation of motor activities. In particular he showed incessant masticatory movements, waving and saluting movements of the arms, rhythmic ('salaam') flexions of the head on the chest, kicking movements of the legs, muttering, talking, and singing in his sleep. He showed striking echolalia during sleep, immediately repeating my question when I spoke to him. After filming these movements, and taping his speech, I woke Mr P., and as he awoke there was an immediate cessation of all these activities. He himself had the impression of having slept soundly, and had no recollection of his speech or his movements. When he fell asleep once more, Mr P.'s motor activity resumed, and continued until about 1 a.m., at which time it stopped, not to reappear during the night. *Thus, his activities were an accentuation of phenomena already present before L-DOPA was given.* This was also apparent in Mr P.'s daytime cycles, with inordinate activation occurring each evening – a cycle which persisted however the doses of L-DOPA were shifted or timed. Thus, chewing and masticatory movements would start at 6 or 7 o'clock each evening, and persist, even during his sleep, till midnight, at which time they stopped.

Around 10 June, a new symptom appeared, which could be described as a voracity, an oral mania, or a devouring-urge. The taking of a first mouthful at any meal seemed to let loose an irresistible desire to grab, bite, and devour food, as fast as possible. Mr P. found himself impelled to stuff food into his mouth, masticate it violently (the mastications persisting after swallowing each mouthful), and when his plate was finished, to stuff his fingers or a napkin into his still violently and perseveratingly chewing mouth.

In the third week of June (his dose of L-DOPA remaining unchanged), symptoms of a more disquieting nature appeared, with agitation, perseveration, and stereotypy as their hallmarks. Mr P. would spend the greater part of each day rocking to and fro in his chair and chanting rhythmically: 'I'm crazy, I'm crazy, I'm crazy . . . if I don't get out of this fucking place, I'll go crazy, crazy, crazy!' At other times he would hum or sing in a monotonous, perseverative, verbigerative fashion, for hours on end. With each passing day, the perseveration and stereotypy became greater, and by 21 June Mr P.'s conversation was made difficult by continual palilalic repetitions of words. His affect, which was intense at this time, alternated between anxiety (with fears of madness and chaos), hostility, and intense irritability. Whenever he saw another patient look out of a window, he would yell: 'He's going to jump, going to jump, to jump, to jump, t'jump, t'jump, tchump, tchump . . .' His attitudes, previously somewhat passive and dependent and abject, had now switched to goading, truculence, and bellicosity, although these were moderated, and made acceptable, by smiling and joking. Powerful sexual urges continued throughout this time, manifest as repeated erotic dreams and nightmares, as frequent and somewhat compulsive masturbation, and (combined with aggressiveness and perseveration) as a tendency to curse, to excited coprolalia, and verbigerative singsong pornoloquies with obscene refrains.[75]

On 21 June, Mr P. complained that his eyes were being 'caught' by all moving objects, and that he could only 'release' his gaze by holding a hand in front of his eyes. This remarkable phenomenon could easily be observed by others: on one occasion, a fly entered the room and impinged upon his visual attention; his gaze was then 'locked' onto the fly, and was drawn after it, irresistibly, wherever it flew. As the symptom grew more pronounced, Mr P. would find that his entire attention had to be concentrated upon whatever object compelled his gaze: and this phenomenon he called 'fascination,' 'being spellbound,' or

---

[75] This complex of motor, appetitive, and instinctual disorder is reminiscent of that seen in severer cases of Gilles de la Tourette's syndrome (which may combine coprolalia, obscene obsessions, increased libido, self-mutilation, orexia, excessive motor impetus, and multiple tics).

'witchcraft.' During this period, Mr P.'s 'grasp-reflexes' (which had been present, but mild and asymptomatic, before receiving L-DOPA) also became exaggerated, and caused forced grasping and groping of the hands, and a strong tendency for them to 'stick' to whatever they happened to touch.

Yet another symptom which became prominent during June was respiratory instability, which took the form of frequent, sudden, tic-like inspirations, occasional snuffling, and perseverative coughing – all of which, like his masticatory movements, pawing movements, etc., would come on in the evenings, clearly related to an innate rhythmicity, and not to the timing of his L-DOPA doses.

In view of Mr P.'s extreme emotional and motor excitement, and his distressing perseverations and 'stimulus-slavery,' I reduced the dosage of L-DOPA to 1.5 gm. daily: his excitomotor syndrome continued, unabated, and it was therefore decided to try the effects of haloperidol (a total of 1.5 mg. daily) added to the L-DOPA. Agitation and akathisia still persisting, the dose of L-DOPA was reduced still further. I was astonished to find that so small a dose as 1 gm. of L-DOPA daily could still procure a useful activation of speech and movement, although at the expense of increased salivation. A return to the larger dosage at once caused excessive activation. By mid-July, we could predict the responses to L-DOPA with considerable precision, as tabulated below:

1.5 gm. daily	*1 gm. daily*
Great vocal and motor force	Moderate vocal and motor force
Excited, akathisic, insomniac	No excitement, akathisia, insomnia
Very little drooling	Profuse drooling
Prominent tics and perseverations	No tics or perseverations

It was evident that haloperidol had an effect antagonistic *in toto* to that of L-DOPA, and not distinguishable from the effects of reducing L-DOPA dosage, and even on so minimal a dose as 1 gm.

daily, paroxysmal and rhythmical activations were still prone to occur. Particularly striking, even on 1 gm. a day, was the sudden 'awakening' which occurred every evening – to flushed, bright-eyed, quick-glancing, loud-voiced, forceful, lascivious, expansive, manic-catatonic akathisia – a transformation which often occurred in a minute or less; equally acute (and equally difficult to ascribe to any simple, dose-related effect of the drug) was the reverse change – to compacted, contracted, aphonic akinesia. Thus, by mid-July, we came face-to-face with the essential problem in treating any case of very severe post-encephalitic Parkinsonism: how best to achieve a therapeutic compromise in a patient with an exceedingly unstable nervous system, a patient in whom *all* behaviour tended to have an oscillatory, bi-polar, all-or-none quality.

1969–72

In the past three years Mr P. has continued to take 1.0 gm. of L-DOPA daily: if he misses a dose he becomes deeply disabled, and if he misses a day he goes into stupor or coma. In autumn 1969, his days were almost equally divided between excited-explosive states and obstructive-imploded states, and he swung like a yo-yo from one to the other, making each passage within thirty seconds. In his excited states, Mr P. showed an intense desire to talk and move, and an equally intense hunger for all stimulation. Amongst these hungers was the hunger to read, and during these three months he made remarkable strides in this direction, considering he had been Parkinsonian since the age of three; he became able to read headlines and captions in the papers.

Since the beginning of 1970 Mr P.'s reactions to L-DOPA have become less auspicious, in that his Parkinsonian or 'down' periods have come to overshadow his excited-expansive states, and these latter are the only times in which he is really accessible. Very occasionally he shows a 'normal' or *middle* state, but these are only seen once or twice a month and then only last a few seconds or minutes.

A further problem has been the increasing incidence of stuporous or sleep-like states, accompanied by gesticulating and ticcing, gibbering and echolalia. Such states become more severe whether we increase or decrease the L-DOPA. On several occasions, we have tried the effects of amantadine – which, in some patients, reduces pathological responses to L-DOPA and retrieves (if temporarily) its therapeutic effects. In Mr P., unfortunately, amantadine *exacerbates* pathological and stuporous responses.

His best moods and functioning are brought out by his family, when they take him home for occasional weekends or holidays. In particular Mr P. likes the hi-fi and swimming pool at his brother's country home. Very remarkably, Mr P. can swim the length of the pool, and shows a great diminution of his Parkinsonism in the water; he apparently swims with an ease and fluency which he can never achieve when he moves on dry land. Effortless movement is also called forth by music on the hi-fi, especially *opera buffa,* to which he is addicted; the music calls for singing, 'conducting,' and occasional dancing, and at this time also, his symptoms are minimal. But Mr P.'s favourite occupation is to sit on the porch, watching the wild life which teems in the garden, or gazing at the wide prospects of up-state New York. Mr P. is always intensely depressed when he returns from the country, and the sentiments he expresses are always the same: 'What a goddamn relief to get out of this place! . . . I've been shut up in places since the day I was born . . . I've been shut up in illness since the day I was born . . . That's a hell of a life for someone to have . . . Why the hell couldn't I have died as a kid? . . . What's the sense, what's the use, of my fucking life here? . . . Hey, Doc! I'm sick of L-DOPA – what about a *real* pill from the cupboard the nurses lock up? . . . The *euthanazy* pill or whatever it's called . . . I've needed that pill since the day I was born.'

Epilogue

In the first American edition of *Awakenings* I added a postscript to Rolando P.'s history, as follows: 'Early in 1973 Rolando P. pined away and died. As with Frank G. and others, no cause of death could be found at *post mortem*. I cannot avoid the suspicion that such patients died of hopelessness and despair, and that the *ostensible* cause of death (cardiac arrest, or whatever) was merely the means by which a sought-for *quietus* was finally achieved.' This cryptic postscript has given rise to many questions, and I feel it necessary and proper, therefore, to trace the course of Rolando's final decline, and its probable or possible determinants, in a fuller and more explicit way.

Rolando P.'s mother was exceptionally understanding and deeply devoted: thus it was she who would always defend him in his earliest years, when he was usually taken to be mentally defective or mad. Despite progressive age and arthritis she would visit Rolando every Sunday without fail (or else join him when he was invited to his brother's country home). By the summer of 1972, however, Mrs P. had become so disabled by arthritis that she was no longer able to come to the hospital. The cessation of her visits was followed by a severe emotional crisis in her son – two months of grief, pining, depression, and rage, and during this period he lost twenty pounds. Mercifully, however, his loss was mitigated by a physiotherapist we had on the staff, a woman who combined the skills of her craft with an exceptionally warm and loving nature. By September of 1972 Rolando P. had developed a very intimate 'anaclitic' relation with her, leaning on her as he had previously leant on his mother; and the warmth and wisdom of this good woman's heart allowed her to play this motherly role with genuine, unsimulated, unconditional love, and without ever striking any false notes; indeed, her devotion was such that she would often come in on weekends or evenings, giving him the time and love he so needed. Under this benign and healing influence, Rolando's wound began to heal over – he became calmer and better-humoured, gained weight, and slept well.

Unfortunately, at the start of February, his beloved physiotherapist was dismissed from her job (along with almost a third of the hospital staff) as a result of economies dictated by the recent federal budget. Rolando's first reaction was one of stunned shock, associated with denial and unbelief: he would have repeated dreams at this time that everyone had been dismissed *except* his new 'mother,' that she had been enabled to stay by some special means – and he would wake from these sweet-cruel dreams with a smile on his face, followed by a cry of realization and anguish. But if these were his dreams, his conscious reactions were different – they were exceedingly 'sensible,' exceedingly 'rational.' 'These things happen,' he would say with a nod. 'They are very unfortunate, but they can't be helped . . . No use crying over spilt milk, you know . . . One has to *carry on* – life goes on regardless . . .' At this level, then, of consciousness and reason, Rolando seemed determined to bear with his loss and live on 'regardless'; but at a deeper level, so it seemed to me, he had sustained a wound from which he would not recover. He had once been saved by a surrogate mother, but now she had gone, and there was no prospect of another; Rolando had been deeply ill and dependent since his third year of life – he had the mind of a man, but the needs of an infant. I kept thinking of Spitz's famous studies, and I felt that the chances were against his survival.[76]

By the middle of February, Rolando was showing severe mental breakdown, compounded of grief, depression, terror, and rage. He continually pined for his lost love-object; he continually searched for her (and kept 'mistaking' others for her); he had repeated pangs of grief (and psychic pain), in which he would turn pale, clutch his chest, cry aloud, or groan. Admixed with his grief and pining and searching, he had a bewildered and furious sense of betrayal, and would rail wildly at Fate, at the hospital, and at her: sometimes he would revile her as 'a faithless fucking bitch,' and at other times the hospital for 'taking her away'; he lived in a torment of bewailing and reviling.

---

[76] Spitz has provided unforgettable descriptions of the effects of human deprivation on orphaned children. These orphans (in an orphanage in Mexico) were given excellent mechanical and 'hygienic' care, but virtually no *human* attention, warmth, or care. Almost all of them had died by the age of three. Such studies and similar observations upon the very young, the very old, the very ill, and the regressed, indicate that human care is literally vital, and that if it is deficient or absent we perish, the more quickly and surely the more vulnerable we are; and that death, in such contexts, is first and foremost an existential death, a dying-away of the will-to-live – and that this paves the way for physical death. This subject – 'dying of grief' – is discussed with great penetration in Chapter 2 ('The Broken Heart') of C. M. Parkes's book *Bereavement*.

Towards the end of February his state changed again, and he moved into a settled and almost inaccessible corpse-like apathy; he became profoundly Parkinsonian once again, but beneath the physiological Parkinsonian mask one could see a worse mask, of hopelessness and despair; he lost his appetite and ceased to eat; he ceased to express any hopes or regrets; he lay awake at nights, with wide-open, dull eyes. It was evident that he was dying, and had lost the will to live . . .

A single episode (in early March) sticks in my mind: the medical staff, extremely alert for 'organic disease' (but seemingly blind to despairs of the soul), arranged for Rolando to have a battery of 'tests,' and I was on the ward, that morning, when the diagnostic trolley came up, laden with syringes and tubes for blood, and accompanied by a brisk, white-coated technician. At first, passively, apathetically, Rolando let his arm be taken for blood, but then he suddenly burst out in an unforgettable, white-hot passion of outrage. He pushed the trolley and the technician violently away, and yelled: 'Can't you fuckers leave me alone? Where's the sense in all your fucking tests? Don't you have eyes and ears in your head? Can't you see I'm dying of grief? For Chrissake let me die in peace!' These were the last words which Rolando ever spoke. He died in his sleep, or his stupor, just four days later.

MIRIAM H.

◈ Miss H. was born in New York in 1914, the second child of a deeply religious Jewish family. Both of her parents died within six months of her birth – the first of many blows which life was to deal her. She was separated, as an infant, from her older sister, and sent to the old orphanage in Queens, where like Oliver Twist she was fed on thin gruel and threats. She showed considerable precocity from her earliest years, and was 'buried' in books from the age of ten. At the age of eleven she was pushed off a bridge, and sustained fractures of both legs, her pelvis, and back. And at the age of twelve she developed a severe attack of *encephalitis lethargica* – the only one thus attacked in an orphan-age-population exceeding two hundred. For six months she was so torpid that she would sleep night and day unless roused for food and other necessities, and for a further two years suffered from striking and frequent narcolepsies, sleep-paralyses, night-mares, 'daymares,' and sleep-talking. Upon the heels of these sleep-disorders Parkinsonism followed, so that by the age of sixteen Miss H. had developed left-sided rigidity and a shrunken left hand, postural abnormalities, and an excessive rapidity and impetuosity of speech and thought. Her excellent intelligence was unimpaired by illness, and she was able to resume and finish high school. By the age of eighteen she was so disabled that she was transferred to Mount Carmel Hospital. Thus she had no chance to experience the 'outside' world, and could only learn of it from hearsay and books.

Her course, over the next thirty-seven years, was slowly but progressively downhill. In addition to a hemi-Parkinsonian rigid-ity and akinesia, she developed some spasticity and weakness of the left leg, and a shortening and deformity of the right leg, consequent upon her childhood accident. Despite these difficul-ties, and superadded difficulties of balance and marked festina-tion, Miss H. was able to walk, with the aid of two sticks, until 1966. In addition to great vocal hurry and speed, she showed chewing and masticatory movements of pronounced degree. Very distressing to her, and destructive to her self-esteem, were a variety of hypothalamic disorders which gradually over-whelmed her – extreme hirsutism and obesity, a buffalohump and plethora, acne, diabetes, and repeated peptic ulcerations. She was painfully aware, in these years, of her unattractiveness and gro-tesqueness, and this reinforced her solitariness and seclusiveness, so that she buried herself, more and more, in what she could read. In the early years of her illness, Miss H. used to suffer from sudden paroxysms of left-sided pain, associated with anguish and terror, of sudden onset and offset, and lasting some hours; when I asked her about these, many years later, she answered (as she was fond of doing) by a Dickensian example: 'You keep asking me,' she said, 'about the *location* of the pain, and the only answer I can give is that which Mrs Gradgrind gave: "I used to feel there was a pain *somewhere in the room,* but I couldn't positively say that I had got it." Following the subsidence of these attacks, around 1940, Miss H. continued to suffer from an extreme sensitivity to pain on this side of the body.

Until 1945, or thereabouts, Miss H. was prone to stormy depressions and violent furies, but these gradually gave way to a settled and somewhat apathetic depression. Miss H. remarked of this transition: 'I developed a violent temper after the sleepy-sickness, quite uncontrollable, but it got *tamed* with my disease.' There had also been a tendency to impatience and impulsiveness following her encephalitis, with sudden violent screaming when frustrated, but this too had subsided over the years. Miss H. referred with some embarrassment to these screaming attacks: 'It was as if something built up and suddenly burst out of me. Sometimes I didn't feel that I myself was screaming; I used to feel that it was something apart from me, something not controlled by me, which was doing the screaming. And I would feel awful afterwards, and hate myself.'

Apart from these occasional furies and screaming attacks, most of Miss H.'s hating and blaming was inflected inwards upon herself – or upon God. 'At first,' she said, 'I hated everybody, I longed for vengeance. I felt that people round me were somehow responsible for my disease. Then I became resigned to it, and realized that it was a punishment from God.' When I inquired whether she felt she had done anything to deserve the encephalitis, and why she felt she had been stricken in this way, she answered: 'No, I did not feel that I had done anything specially wrong. I am not a bad person. But I have been singled out – I don't know why. God is inscrutable.'

These feelings of inward blame and depression became greatly exacerbated and almost unbearable during the oculogyric crises from which Miss H. suffered. These crises, which started in 1928, would come with great regularity, every Wednesday; so much so that I could always arrange for my students to come on Wednesdays if they wished to witness such a crisis. Nevertheless, the times of these crises were modifiable to some extent: on one occasion I informed Miss H. that my students could not come on Wednesday, but would be coming on Thursday. 'OK,' said Miss H., 'I will put off the crisis to Thursday,' and she did. During her crises, which would last 8–10 hours, Miss H. would be 'compelled to look up at the ceiling,' although there was no associated opisthotonos. She would be unable to wheel her chair, and only able to speak in a whisper. Throughout the crises she would be 'morose . . . sad . . . disgusted with life.' She would be forced to ruminate obsessively upon her miserable position, in hospital for thirty-seven years, without friends or family, ugly, disabled, etc. She would say to herself again and again: 'Why me? What did I do? Why am I being punished? Why have I been cheated of life? What is the use of going on? Why don't I kill myself?' These thoughts, which would repeat themselves in a sort of inner litany, could not be banished from her mind during the crises: they were reiterative, peremptory, overwhelming, and would exclude all other thoughts from her mind. When the crises were over, Miss H. would feel 'relatively cheerful,' that she was herself again, and that perhaps, after all, things were not too bad. In addition to these crises, though sometimes combined with them, Miss H. – an extraordinary calculator – suffered from counting crises. These attacks, which occurred especially at night, consisted of compulsions to count to a particular number (like 95,000), or to raise 7 to the fifteenth power, before she would be allowed to stop thinking and sleep. In particular, like one of Jelliffe's patients, she was sometimes compelled to count in her oculogyric crises, and the crisis would/could not finish till she had reached her goal; if interrupted in her counting, at such times, she would have to return to 1 and start again; as soon as she reached her predetermined goal, her crisis would instantly cease at this moment.[77]

---

[77] It has since become clear that Miriam H. not only has an extraordinary *facility* for figures (and 'figuring' of all kinds), but a strange intermittent *compulsion* as

Despite her many neurological and neuro-endocrinological problems, and despite the feelings of hopelessness which so often oppressed her, Miss H. fought bravely against her disabilities until 1967, being active in ward and synagogue affairs, an active debater in philosophy and other classes held at the hospital, an omnivorous reader, and a close observer of current affairs. Following the exceedingly hot summer of 1967 – during which her anti-Parkinsonian medication was stopped for fear of the hyper-pyrexia and heat-stroke which devastated our post-encephalitic patients that year – Miss H. regressed neurologically and emotionally, becoming intensely rigid in the left arm, chair-ridden,

---

well. At such times Miriam may have to count footsteps, or the numbers of words on book pages, or the frequency of 'e' in book blurbs. Sometimes, watching through a window, she has to 'record' (internally) the number plate of each car, and then submit this to various operations – squaring the number, finding its cube root, comparing it with various 'analogous' numbers. (She is aided in this by a perfect memory – she remembers every number plate, the number of words counted on every page, the frequency of every 'e' in every blurb in the library.)

Sometimes she has to say, write, or spell whole sentences backwards; sometimes to estimate the volume of fellow patients in cubic inches; sometimes to 'divide' their faces into aggregates of geometrical figures. Here she is helped by an eidetic imagery and memory akin to that of Luria's 'Mnemonist'; when she is 'mathematizing' people in this way she considers them 'problems' rather than people. She considers these compulsions absurd, but also finds them irresistible, and accords them what she describes as an 'enigmatic significance.' This feeling is a prime reason, or rationalization, for all her 'absurdities.'

It is very 'important' for her to 'symmetrize' (her word) different scenes and situations: either in actuality, rearranging objects on the tablecloth, for example (though sometimes this is not a simple symmetry, apparent to others, but a 'secret' or enigmatic symmetry, known only to herself); or more often 'mentally' – this is much faster, almost instantaneous, and is *given* reality by her eidetic imagery.

'Arithmomania,' the compulsion to count and compute, was reported frequently in the early days of the epidemic, and was also regarded as a prime symptom in Gilles de la Tourette syndrome. Later – at least I have found this with Miriam, with other post-encephalitics, and with a number of Touretters under my care – one finds that this arithmomania is, as it were, the *surface* of a more fundamental compulsion, which has to do with order and disorder: the *need* to order, disorder, reorder; the *contemplation* of order, disorder, new order. Arithmomania has to do with arithmetical order; other operations may have to do with logical order; 'symmetrizing' with spatial order, and so on. In this sense, what may at first appear to be a very bizarre and specific compulsion must be seen as a *universal* mental need, though given a bizarre exaggeration, or twist (such oddnesses, such twists, are also characteristic of Tourette's – and of autism).

withdrawn, and apathetic: she seemed to have lost all her former motivations, and would sit motionless in her chair all day, staring dully at the wall in front of her. Anti-depressants made very little difference to this state, and resumption of her previous solenaceous medicines diminished her salivation, but were of no use to her in other respects. She was considered to be irreparably damaged, a hopeless 'back-ward' patient at the time L-DOPA was first administered.

Before L-DOPA

When examined in May 1969 – just before the administration of L-DOPA – Miss H. was a grossly obese, heavily bearded, acromegalic and Cushingoid woman sitting motionless, slumped, and apathetic in her wheelchair. Her face was greatly masked and devoid of any play of emotional expression, while the dullness and hopelessness of her appearance and attitudes was shown by the almost opaque spectacles – clearly uncleaned for many

---

I have been able to find a fascinating EEG correlation to Miriam's arithmetical and intellectual 'attacks.' One day, while taking an EEG on her, I asked her to start taking serial 7s from one hundred – one often gives patients such tasks to see their effects on the brain waves (see Appendix: The Electrical Basis of Awakenings, p. 327).

As soon as I asked this, a look of intense, almost furious, concentration appeared; and at the same time, I heard a wild clattering of the EEG recording pens. This lasted for about twenty seconds before Miss H. looked up, with a smile, and said, 'I'm through.'

'Through?' I queried. 'Where did you get to?'

'I got *there,*' she answered, 'minus six hundred!'

She said that when she reached 2, she thought this 'absurd' – it was a number of 'no sense,' reached by fourteen operations; it was imperative that she reached a 'symmetrical' goal with a 'symmetrical' number of operations. Therefore she had proceeded taking 7s away, until she reached 'a nice round number,' *viz* –600, in a hundred operations. When I asked her what the subtracting was like, she said the answers were *'seen,'* that they were 'thrown up . . . clear as a day . . . on a sort of mental blackboard.' When I came to look at the EEG, which I had heard clattering when she was calculating, I saw *spikes* in both occipital (visual) areas; and when I counted these, there were exactly a hundred. Thus, each intellectual operation seemed to correspond with a spike on EEG – the sort of spike one sees in fits. Thus (it would seem) her arithmetic compulsions may also be arithmetical *'convulsions,'* 'epilepsies,' or 'fits.' This particular 'fit,' which entailed one hundred operations, lasted only twenty seconds.

months – which she wore over her protuberant and myopic eyes. When these were removed, the eyes seemed to stare dully at nothing, showing nothing of the alert, attentive movements which are sometimes the only sign of animation in severely akinetic patients. The pupils were small and unequal in size (the left being somewhat larger), but gaze was normal in all directions save for a moderate deficit of convergence. There was no spontaneous blinking, but glabellar tap or visual approach would elicit a protracted forced closure of the eyelids. Her skin was greasy, showed extensive acne and seborrhoeic dermatitis, and sweated profusely, especially on the left side of the body.

Miss H.'s voice was clear and intelligible, although it alternated between vocal blockings and extreme vocal hurry, every clause being jetted out suddenly, and rapidly decaying into aphonia. In addition to this irregularity of speech-force and rhythm, there were occasional expiratory and phonatory tics (grunting) which further interrupted coherent speech. Her breathing was scarcely perceptible, but she showed occasional, impulsive deep inspirations. Salivation was increased, although there was no actual drooling. She was unable to protrude her tongue, and could only move it slowly and tremulously from side to side, writhing her mouth when requested to wag it quickly. She showed intermittent chewing movements when her attention was not actively engaged, and these (I later had occasion to observe) persisted during sleep in the early part of the night. Miss H. showed a striking unilaterality of rigidity and akinesia, the left side of her body being much more severely affected. The left arm was intensely rigid, with dystonic deformity and contracture of the hand, and had almost no capacity for independent movement. The right arm had only slightly increased rigidity, and the right hand was able to make six to seven clenching movements before akinesia set in. There was intense axial rigidity with almost no available movement of the trunk or neck muscles. The entire left side of the body showed a combination of hypalgesia with intense hyperpathia and over-reaction to painful stimuli. The legs showed some spasticity and weakness of upper motor neurone type: all tendon-reflexes were pathologically increased, and plantar responses were extensor on both sides. Miss H. was quite unable to rise from her chair, and even when supported was unable to stand or walk.

It was astonishing to observe, in a patient of such unprepossessing and regressed appearance, the sudden outcroppings of high intelligence, wit, and charm, for these lay buried, most of the time, by extreme withdrawal compounded by 'block'; so much so, indeed, that those who did not know Miss H. well generally took her to be mentally defective.

Course on L-DOPA

The administration of L-DOPA was started on 18 June 1969. No changes were observed in the first week of L-DOPA medication, while the dosage was being slowly increased, and Miss H. made no complaints of nausea, dizziness, or other symptoms commonly experienced in the first days of receiving the drug. The following are extracts from my diary.

27 June. Now on a dose of 2 gm. L-DOPA daily, Miss H. appears more alert, more cheerful, and more interested in her surroundings.

1 July. Miss H. continues to be alert and cheerful, and now, for the first time in many years, takes an interest in her appearance, requesting that she be shaved three times a week, that her skin problems be attended to, and that she might wear a dress each day, rather than a shapeless hospital gown. She has arranged to borrow a novel from the library – she had had no wish to read for more than two years – and has started to keep a diary in a minute, but daily enlarging, handwriting. There is now a quite remarkable dissolution of rigidity in the left arm, and Miss H. has planned a series of exercises to 'limber up' this previously petrified limb. She has become able to open and close the left hand freely, although separate finger movements still remain impossible. In view of this auspicious therapeutic response, and the absence of any adverse effects, I am raising the dosage of L-DOPA from 3 gm. to 4 gm. daily.

9 July. Miss H. has shown further improvement on an increased dose of L-DOPA, although there are now a number of adverse effects also, none of them, fortunately, too serious. Her left arm, aided by physiotherapy, has become more skilful, and discrete finger movements are now possible: this allows Miss H., amongst other things, to handle a knife and fork in a normal fashion, and to take the paper off sweets and chocolates (to which, despite her obesity and diabetes, she is somewhat addicted).

Miss H. has also become more demanding and impatient; she is now able to make her needs known in a loud voice, if need be, and if this is not heeded screams shrilly. These occasional screamings are felt as ego-alien, and are followed at once by contrition and apologies. She continues to show vocal hurry, but her speech pattern is altogether more even and coherent, and has entirely ceased to have any delay after each clause or sentence. Indeed, I have never seen a human being who can speak like Miss H.: she could easily beat any news announcer, because she can talk at 500 words a minute without missing a syllable. Her rapidity of speech, combined with her rapidity of thought and calculation, makes her more than a match for any of my medical students: When I ask her, for example, to take 17s away from 1,012, she performs these serial subtractions as fast as she can speak.

Masticatory movements had become more marked, and were especially gross in the evenings, continuing after Miss H. had fallen asleep, but they neither annoyed nor inconvenienced her. An entirely novel symptom which had developed on the increased dose of L-DOPA was a *tic,* a lightning-quick movement of the right hand to the face, occurring about twenty times an hour. When I questioned Miss H. about this symptom, shortly after its inauguration, she replied that it was 'a nonsense-movement,' which had no purpose that she was aware of, and which she did not wish to make: 'I feel a tension building up in my hand,' she said, 'and after a time it gets too much, and then I *have* to move it.' Within three days of its appearance, however, this tic had become associated with an intention and a use: it had become a mannerism, and was now used by Miss H. to adjust the position of her spectacles. Her spectacles were indeed loose, and prone to slip down over the bridge of her nose: 'You better not get them fixed,' Miss H. remarked, with insight and humour, 'otherwise I will have to find a new use for this hand-movement of mine.' There was no doubt of the relief when this tic became mannerized, when a 'nonsensical' dynamism became an action with reference. Miss H. was always prone to give a rationalization and a referential form to her 'involuntary' movements; she could not stand mere impulses, like Mrs Y. for example.

21 July. Miss H. has continued to show an even and satisfactory therapeutic response – alertness without insomnia, good humour without excitement, excellent function in her left arm, and now, with the aid of physiotherapy, a capacity to stand with assistance for a few seconds, although the spastic weakness in her legs is unchanged.

1 August. 'It has been the best month I have had in years,' says Miss H., summarizing the events of July. Amongst the other desirable effects of L-DOPA has been the cessation of oculogyric crises, which had tormented her regularly for more than forty years.[78] Although equable under normal circumstances, Miss H. now shows the quick temper which characterized her reactions in the early post-encephalitic years.

Throughout August Miss H. maintained her stable and satisfactory improvement, and, with the aid of physiotherapy, became able to stand on her feet and walk a few steps once more. As striking as the neurological and functional improvement, and most obvious to a stranger's eye, was the transformation which had occurred in Miss H.'s cosmetic appearance and behaviour. Two months previously, she had been a pitiful, motionless, apathetic, backward patient, misshapen and unwholesome in appearance, bundled into an anonymous white hospital gown. Now she was neatly dressed, with a style of her own, shaven, powdered, made-up, and permed. Her obesity, her acromegaly, and her slightly masked face could easily be overlooked now with her new poise and smartness, and especially when one was listening to her admirably witty and fluent conversation. The Ugly Duckling was nearly a swan.

---

[78] One of the most welcome effects of L-DOPA in post-encephalitic patients generally was to rid them, for a while, of their disabling and hellish oculogyric crises (such as nearly a quarter of our patients had; see Sacks and Kohl, 1970b).

1969–72

In her fourth month on L-DOPA (September–October 1969) Miss H. started to show respiratory 'side-effects' to L-DOPA (her dose having been maintained at 4.0 gm. a day). The first such effect was hiccup, which would come in hour-long attacks, starting at 6:30 every morning, a little after Miss H. had awoken and *before* her first dose of L-DOPA for the day. Three weeks later a 'nervous' cough and throat-clearing started, associated with a recurrent tic-like feeling of something blocking or scratching her throat; the hiccup disappeared with the onset of throat-clearing and coughing, as if it had been 'replaced' by these symptoms. In late November Miss H. started to develop a tendency to gasping and breath-holding, which in turn 'replaced' the throat-clearing and coughing. From here she proceeded to increasingly severe 'respiratory crises' which had some similarity to those of Miss D.[79] Towards the end of the year Miss H.'s crises grew intolerably severe, and were accompanied not only by a marked increase of pulse and blood pressure, but by intense emotional excitement, blocking of speech, and recrudescence of Parkinsonism and oculogyria.

She further experienced forced and quasi-hallucinatory 'reminiscences' and phantasies during her crises which were responsible for her peculiar facial expression during these and her 'block.' Thus Miss H. would suddenly 'remember' (in her crises) that she had been sexually assaulted by 'a beast' of an elevator-attendant in 1952, and that in consequence of this she now had syphilis; she 'realized' (in her crises) that this horrible story was known to everyone round her, and that the entire ward was whispering about her 'looseness' and its pathological outcome. It was two weeks before Miss H. could bring herself to divulge these thoughts to me; when I asked if the assault had actually happened, etc., she replied: 'Of course not. That's a lot of nonsense. But I'm *forced* to think it when I have one of my crises.' By the end of

---

[79] Miss H. and Miss D. were 'pet enemies' at this time, were unhappy if apart, and spent most of each day sitting opposite one another having crises *at* one another.

December her crises had become virtually continuous one with another, and it was therefore necessary to stop her L-DOPA.

A month went past, during which Miss H. recovered from her crises, but showed a degree of Parkinsonism considerably in excess of her pre-DOPA state. In February 1970, Miss H. said to me, 'I think I'm ready for L-DOPA again. I've done a lot of thinking in the last month and I've worked my way through that sexual nonsense. I will lay you 20–1 I have no more crises again.' I started her back on L-DOPA again, and worked up once more to 4.0 gm. a day.

Miss H. again had good therapeutic efforts, though not as marked as the first time she had taken it. She continued in fair shape until the summer of 1970, when she again started to have 'side-effects' of various kinds. These did not take the form of hiccups, coughs, gasps, or other respiratory symptoms – as Miss H. herself had predicted and wagered; but they took the form of multiple tics. These had a most bizarre form, 'punching' each arm alternatively into the air, as if swatting mosquitoes which buzzed over her head. By July her rate of ticcing was 300 per minute, her arms moving up and down like streaks of lightning, almost too quickly for the eye to follow (these are seen in the documentary film of *Awakenings*). Other activities became impossible at this time and Miss H. herself asked us to re-stop her L-DOPA.

In September 1970, Miss H. said to me, 'Third time lucky! If you give me L-DOPA once again, I promise you no complications this time.' I did so, and Miss H. proved correct. In the last two years she has continued to take 4.0 gm. a day with a clear-cut if unspectacular therapeutic response. She does have an occasional tantrum or crisis, but not too often and never severe. She *has* continued to maintain her 'spectacles-adjusting' mannerism, which seems to absorb or discharge or express her ticcish propensities, or an undue building-up of psychomotor excitement: 'It's my conduit,' Miss H. says. 'You leave it alone.'

In general Miss H. lives as much of a life as is possible with the disabilities she has, and in the situation she is: she makes a point of going to excursions and movies, whenever she can; she is a terror at bingo, at which she invariably wins, because there is no one in the hospital who can match her shrewdness or her lightning-quick thought; and she is warmly devoted to her one remaining sister. For most of the day however, Miss H. is absorbed in reading and writing: she reads with great speed and intentness and devours what she reads – it is always something 'old-fashioned' (usually Dickens) and never contemporary; she thinks a great deal and keeps her thoughts to herself, confiding them to volume after volume of her extensive diaries. Thus, all in all, Miss H. has done well – amazingly so, considering the existence she has led. Against all odds, Miss H. has always managed to be a real *person* and to face reality without denial or madness. She draws on a strength unfathomable to me, a health which is deeper than the depth of her illness.

LUCY K.

◠ Born in New York, in 1924, an only child, Miss K. apparently had no childhood illnesses of note, and in particular no febrile illnesses characterized by lethargy or restlessness. At the age of two, however, she developed a paralysis and divergence of the left eye: this was ascribed to a 'congenital strabismus,' despite its suddenness of onset (over the course of six weeks), and the normality of gaze before its occurrence. Miss K. is described by her mother as having been eager and quick to learn as a child, as having been very 'good' and obedient in early childhood, although developing a 'nasty disposition' (stubbornness, naughtiness, stealing, lying, tantrums, etc.) at about the age of six. She was greatly attached to her father, and it was shortly after his death (when she was eleven) that Parkinsonian symptoms became plainly manifest.

The first physical abnormalities were observed in her walking, which became by degrees stiff and wooden, and particularly unstable when she faced a downwards flight of stairs, which she would be impelled to descend with uncontrollable speed, usually falling to the bottom. Her face had become 'expressionless and shiny – like a doll's face' by the age of fifteen. Concurrently with these motor symptoms, Miss K. developed increasing emotional disorder, becoming inattentive and quarrelsome at school – which she had to leave at the age of fourteen – and more and more parasitically attached to her mother at home. By degrees, she became more withdrawn, losing interest in her friends, her books, and her hobbies, increasingly disinclined to leave the house, and gradually drawn into a closer and more hostile intimacy with her mother – an intimacy uninterrupted by the presence of a father, of other children, of school, of friends, or of any other interests or emotional attachments. She never dated, despite her mother's 'encouragement,' variously maintaining that she despised, hated, or feared the other sex, and that she was 'perfectly happy' at home with her mother. It is evident, from close questioning of the mother, that this domestic bliss was broken by frequent violent quarrels, apparently started either by Lucy or her mother.

Rigidity, first of the left side, then of the right, set in during her early twenties, and by the age of twenty-seven Miss K. could no longer walk and was confined to a wheelchair. Despite mounting and seemingly impossible difficulties, she remained at home, totally dependent upon her mother, who devoted every hour of the day to caring for her. On one occasion, Miss K. was taken to a neurology outpatient clinic where she was given some pills, and where continued outpatient care and possible surgery were advised. Miss K.'s mother threw away the pills, was shocked by the suggestion of surgery, and never took her daughter back to the clinic.

Eventually, in 1964, when total nursing care had become necessary, Miss K. was brought to Mount Carmel Hospital by her mother. At the time of her admission, the picture was one of severe rigidity, akinesia, ophthalmoplegia, and autonomic disturbances, but with a relatively well-preserved and audible voice. Her admission precipitated a month of violent rages and belligerence, which was followed by a marked and sudden withdrawal and deterioration of her neurological status: in particular, Miss K. ceased to speak, to feed herself, to move in bed, or to show any signs of independent functioning.

About six months after Miss K.'s admission, she became greatly attached to a male orderly on the ward who showed her some human concern and kindliness. During the two months that this orderly was on the ward, Miss K.'s voice returned, and she recovered the ability to feed herself, to turn in bed, etc. When he left the ward her state suddenly and profoundly declined once again; and she remained in a severely regressed and incapacitated state after this time.

Between 1965 and 1968 Miss K. presented a picture of extreme uniformity, of an almost inhuman monotony, except on certain occasions of violent 'release.' She remained uncannily motionless, with a tense, an *intense* motionlessness somewhat different from Parkinsonism; and totally speechless, again in a forced, constrained manner different from the aphonia of Parkinsonism.

Sometimes, when watching a movie, she would be swept by an access of terror or pleasure, and this would suddenly 'break' her clenched silence and immobility, and lead to a loud high scream ('Eeehhh!') accompanied by a child-like clapping of the hands, or a sudden raising of them to the face – as in an infant's startle reflex. She was also notorious for her rages, which would come on extremely suddenly, with scarcely a moment's warning: during these she would curse with great violence and fluency in a particularly sarcastic and wounding way, which showed how closely and cleverly she had watched all those around her (when she was immobile and seemingly dead to the world), and how gifted she was in mockery and caricature; at such times she would glare balefully, wave her clenched fists, and occasionally hit out with a good deal of force. The unmistakably murderous quality of these rages, combined with their total unexpectedness, had a peculiarly unnerving effect. These paroxysms of terror or pleasure, of laughter or rage, would rarely last more than a minute or so; they would vanish as abruptly as they had come, and Miss

K. would suddenly revert, without any intermediate stages, to the violent fixity of her 'normal' state.

Her general appearance, during these years, was pathetic – and grotesque. She was heavily and powerfully built, giving the impression of great physical strength clenched in restraint. She looked (like most post-encephalitics) much younger than her age – one could easily have supposed she was in her twenties, not her forties. Her bizarre 'baby-doll' appearance was accentuated by the immense pains her mother took to 'prepare' her every day. Miss K., when 'prepared,' would sit in the hall rigid and motionless in her over-size chair, invested in an embroidered and ambiguous child's or bride's nightgown. Her jet-black hair would be heavily braided, and her face chalky-white from its coating of powder (she suffered from constant sweatings and seborrhoea). Her dystonic, crippled hands (with fingers immovably flexed at the knuckles) were heavily ringed, and had long scarlet nails. Her inverted feet were daintily slippered. She looked like – I could never decide: like a clown, or a geisha, or Miss Haversham, or a robot. But most of all like a baby-doll, in the most absolute and literal sense of the words: a living reflection of her mother's mad whim.

And, indeed, as I progressively came to realize, not only Miss K.'s appearance, but a great deal of her pathology, was inseparably associated with her mother's behaviour, and could not be considered as a thing-in-itself.

Thus her mutism was in part a *refusal* to speak (a block or veto or interdict on speech), which mirrored the warnings of her paranoid mother. 'Don't speak, Lucy,' she would say every day. 'Ssshhh! Not a word! They're against you round here. Give nothing away – not a move, not a word . . . There's nobody here you can trust in the least.' These dire warnings would alternate with hours of crooning, maudlin baby-talk: 'Lucy, my baby, my little living *doll* . . . There's nobody who loves you like me . . . Nobody in the world *could* love you like me . . . For you, little Lucy, I have given my life . . .'

Miss K.'s mother would arrive at hospital very early in the morning, seven days a week, undertake her feeding and total care (despite the efforts of the nursing staff and others to dislodge her from this despotic position), and leave late at night, when Miss K. was finally and safely asleep. She avowed, truthfully, that she was completely devoted to her daughter, and that she had 'sacrificed' the last twenty-five years to looking after her, and 'protecting' her. It was evident, however, that her attitude was deeply contradictory, and involved hatred, sadism, and destructiveness no less than an inordinate love and devotion. This was particularly manifest if I chanced to walk through the ward with my students: Miss K.'s mother, on spotting our group, would suddenly seize her daughter and jerk her into a sitting position, straightening her neck with a vicious crack; she would then beckon us to approach, and would start a cruel goading of the patient: 'Lucy,' she would say, 'which is the best-looking one? That one there? Wouldn't you like to kiss him, wouldn't you like to marry him?' At this stage, a tear would roll down Lucy's face, or she would utter a hoarse roar of fury.

Early in 1969, I suggested L-DOPA, thinking at this time that there was nothing to lose. For Miss K. was not only mute and motionless from 'wilfulness,' refusal, 'block' and negativism, etc., but deeply and distressingly Parkinsonian as well. She showed – insofar as could be detected 'beneath' catatonic rigidity – a severe plastic rigidity of Parkinsonian type, more on the left, and easily elicited cogwheeling at all major joints. Her crippling dystonic contractures ('bilateral hemiplegic dystonia') have already been noted, and were associated with coldness, waxiness, and some atrophy of hands and feet.

She showed paroxysms of 'flapping' tremor on both sides, and occasional massive myoclonic jerks. Particularly severe was her endless salivation, a constant stream of viscid saliva; which not only necessitated the use of a bib and constant mopping – in itself a humiliation – but by its quantity (approaching a gallon each day) continually threatened her with dehydration. Continual tremor of the lips was present, and – when excited – a rhythmical grimace (her mother called it 'snarling') which bared all her teeth.

She showed an alternating exotropia, with widely skewed eyes, which seemed to shine, when open, with anguish and spite (they were concealed, for much of the day, by tonus/clonus of the eyelids, or anableptic rotation – which exposed only sclera). Her eyes, and these alone, were freely mobile, and were painfully eloquent in expressing her feelings. These were extreme, contradictory, and wholly irresoluble. When Miss K. was hostile and negativistic (as she seemed to be, most of the time), all requests elicited 'refusal': a request to look at one caused looking away; a request to show her tongue caused clenching of the jaws; a request to let herself 'go loose' made her rigid with spasm. At other times, more rarely, she would have a tender, submissive and melting expression, and 'gave herself' unreservedly, catatonically, to those who examined her; at such times, the merest intimation elicited *compliance,* or as much as was possible in her disabled state. Even her Parkinsonian rigidity seemed to 'melt' at such times, and her usually rigid limbs could be moved with some ease. Thus Miss K.'s Parkinsonism, catatonia, and psychotic ambivalence formed a continuous spectrum, all interlocked in inseparable relation.

Early in 1969, then, I suggested L-DOPA. I suggested it once and many times subsequently. (My enthusiasm at that time was scarcely qualified, and I tended to simplify the most complex situations.) 'Lucy is helpless,' I said. 'She needs to be cured. L-DOPA, nothing else, can come to the rescue.' Her mother, however, was implacably opposed, and expressed her opinion in front of Miss K.: 'Lucy is best as she is,' she asserted. 'She'll get stirred up, she'll *blow up* if you give her L-DOPA.' And she added, piously: 'If it is God's will that Lucy should die, then she must die.' Miss K., of course, heard this without speaking, but expressed in her eyes a tortured ambivalence – wish-fear, 'yes-no' – of unlimited degree.

1969–72

In 1969, I started to revise my own opinion: I *saw* several 'blow-ups' in other patients on L-DOPA. I became far less eager to press it on Miss K. I ceased to mention it when I saw her or her mother. But as my enthusiasm waned, Miss K.'s increased. She became more stubborn and defiant in relation to her mother, and stiffened herself in board-like rigidity. Their contact became a wrestling together, with Miss K. 'winning' by sheer catatonia.

Late in 1970, her mother came to me. 'I'm exhausted,' she said. 'I can't cope any more. Lucy's killing me with her hate and her badness . . . Why did you ever mention that *cursed* L-DOPA? It's come like a curse between Lucy and me . . . Give her the drug, and we'll see what we'll see!''

I started L-DOPA with a very small dose, and gradually built it up to 3 gm. daily. Miss K. was mildly nauseated; her Parkinsonism and catatonia, if anything, became more severe. But there was nothing else – only a sense of *something* impending. In her fourth week on L-DOPA, she did react, and – as her mother predicted – she 'blew up' completely. It happened very suddenly one morning without warning. The staff-nurse, usually staid, came running to my office: 'Quick!' she said. 'You must come along quickly. Miss Lucy's moving and talking a mile to the minute . . . It suddenly happened a few minutes ago!' Miss K. was sitting up alone in bed (something normally impossible for her), was flushed and animated and waving her arms. I smiled, rather dazedly, and quickly examined her: not a trace of rigidity in her arms or her legs; akinesia quite vanished; free movement except where contractured.

Her voice was loud and clear, and immensely excited: 'Look at me, look at me! I can fly like a bird!' All the nurses were standing around, exclaiming, congratulating, and hugging Miss K. And her mother was also there, saying nothing at all, with an unfathomable expression contorting her features. That evening, when I visited her alone (her mother had gone, and the nurses had cooled down), I went over the examination again. In the course of this I said, 'Will you give me your hand?', and Miss K. said, 'Yes, yes, I'll give you my hand.'

She continued excited, elated, and very active the next day. When I did rounds in the evening, she took the initiative: 'Dr Sacks!' she said, her words tumbling over themselves in her excitement. 'You asked for my hand. It's yours! . . . I want you to marry me and take me away. Take me away from this horrible place . . . And, promise – you'll never let *her* come near me again!'

I calmed her down as best I could, explained I was her doctor, not anything else; that I liked her and would do my best for her, but – Miss K. gave me a long, anguished, and furious glare: 'OK,' she said. 'That's *it*. I hate you, you louse, you rat-fink, you . . .' She sank back exhausted, and said nothing more.

The next morning, Miss K. was totally mute and blocked and rigid, salivating grossly, and shaking with tremor. 'What happened?' asked the nurses. 'She was doing so well. The L-DOPA can't fade as quickly as that.' Her mother, when she came in, broke into a smile: 'I knew it would happen,' she said. 'You pushed Lucy too far.'

We continued the L-DOPA, for another three weeks, even raising the dose to 5.0 gm. a day, but it could have been chalk for the effect it had. Miss K. *had* exploded – and imploded again, contracted herself to an intransigent point, infinitely withdrawn, Parkinsonian and rigid. She had been exposed and extended – and totally rebuffed; and that was *it* – she was having no more; we could fill her with L-DOPA, but react *she would not*. This, at least, was my guess about her feelings and reactions; I could learn nothing directly, because her silence (including her 'motor silence') became absolute. When I stopped the L-DOPA, she showed no further reaction of any type.

In the months that followed, Miss K.'s Parkinsonism continued profound, and she perhaps came to terms, a little, with what had happened on L-DOPA. She never spoke again to me, but occasionally she smiled.

She seemed, from this time on, to be less tense, less emphatic, less rigid in her posture. Some of the *violence* of her feelings seemed to abate. But she grew sadder and more withdrawn, as far as I could judge. I had the feeling of something broken, irremediably, inside her. There were no more curses or outbursts at others, and she now sat at films without attending or reacting. Her eyes lay closed for most of the day – not clenched, just closed. Her behaviour was that of a ghost or a corpse – of someone who'd *had* it, and had done with the world.

She died, quietly and suddenly, in July 1972.

MARGARET A.

◷ Margaret A. was born in New York, in 1908, the youngest daughter of a poor Irish immigrant couple who were intermittently employed. There was nothing in her early years to suggest retardation, major emotional disturbances, or any significant physical illnesses. She was a student of at least average competence, who graduated from high school at the age of fifteen, a good athlete, and apparently easy-going and equable in her emotional life.

In 1925, at the age of seventeen, she developed an acute illness with overwhelming sleepiness and depression. She did indeed sleep almost continuously for ten weeks, although she could be roused from her sopor to be fed, and was exceedingly lethargic, fearful, and depressed for a year after this. This illness was at first ascribed to 'shock' (her father, to whom she was closely attached, had died shortly before the onset of her symptoms), but subsequently recognized as *encephalitis lethargica*.

Following a year of lethargy and depression, she apparently made a complete recovery, working as a secretary and book-keeper, playing tennis, and being sociable and popular among a large group of friends. In 1928–9, however, she developed the first symptoms of a very complex post-encephalitic syndrome.

Among her first symptoms were a tendency to gross tremor of both hands, some slowness of gait and impaired balance, a tendency to drowse during the day and be wakeful at night, a 'monstrous' appetite (which caused her to gain 100 pounds in two years), insatiable thirst and need to drink, and a tendency to sudden brief elations and depressions which seemed to bear little relation to the actual circumstances of day-to-day living. Two other paroxysmal symptoms developed in the early thirties: severe oculogyric crises which would last ten to twelve hours, and come on, characteristically, on Wednesdays, and frequent short staring spells ('crises of fixed regard') which would suddenly arrest her, and hold her 'in a sort of trance state' for a few minutes. Her bulimia and inversion of sleep-rhythm became less marked after 1932–3, but her other symptoms have gradually worsened over the past forty years.

Miss A. was able to continue working in a clerical capacity until 1935, and subsequently lived at home with her mother – apart from a number of brief hospital admissions – until she entered Mount Carmel Hospital in 1958. Miss A. was reluctant to speak of these other brief periods of hospital care: it was evident, from summaries we had received, that the presenting symptoms in each case were those of depression, hypochondriasis and suicidal rumination. Treatment was made difficult by the fact that these periods of depression, for all their severity, would last only a few days, being succeeded by elations and denial of all problems. It was never necessary, apparently, to administer shock-treatment or anti-depressant medication. She would be discharged with the somewhat vague diagnosis of 'Parkinsonism with psychosis,' or 'Parkinsonism with atypical schizophrenia.'

During her first ten years at Mount Carmel, Miss A.'s state very slowly worsened, although she continued to be able to walk without assistance (despite a strong tendency to festination, and a number of falls), to feed herself, to dress herself with some assistance, and at her 'good times' to type. Her thirst and urge to drink continued to be very prominent: her daily input of water varied between 10 and 15 pints, and there was a commensurate output of very dilute urine. She showed strongly marked cycles and paroxysmal alterations of alertness, motor activity, and mood. Thus every day, between 5 and 6:30 p.m., she became overwhelmingly sleepy, and might fall asleep, quite suddenly, while eating or washing, etc. The drowsiness was accompanied by greatly increased blepharoclonus, uncontrollable drooping of the eyelids, and repeated forced closures of the eyes. This drowsiness might be resisted for a few minutes, but would invariably lead to short sleep. There tended to be somewhat milder attacks of drowsiness in the early afternoon, shortly after 1 p.m.; these might occasionally be of almost narcoleptic abruptness. Her motor activity was at its height between 2 and 4:30 p.m., at which time her voice, normally low-pitched and monotonous, would become loud and expressive, and her small-stepped shuffling gait was replaced by striding with exaggerated swinging of the arms, and synkinetic involvement of the trunk-muscles. Her motor capacities were at their lowest ebb in the early morning hours (5–8 a.m.), when she was fully alert but barely able to speak audibly or rise to her feet. She displayed both wakefulness and increased motor activity after seven in the evenings, and had great difficulty going to sleep at 9 p.m., the usual time at which our patients retire. Even after she had fallen asleep around 10 p.m., she displayed unusual motor activity during sleep, in particular turning-and-tossing in bed, sleep-talking, and on occasion sleep-walking. This motor activity would cease around 1 a.m., and for the remainder of the night her sleep would be tranquil. She had no feeling of tiredness in the mornings, and no recollection of talking or other activities during her sleep.

Her depressions and elations both had a rather stereotyped quality. During the former, she would feel that she was 'bad, repulsive . . .' etc., she hated herself and felt that she was hated by the other patients, she felt they despised her for her woebegone expression and for drinking at the water-fountain fifty times a day, that her life was worthless, pitiful, and not worth going on with, and above all she was tormented by the conviction that she was going blind. Her hypochondriacal fears of blindness had an obsessive, reiterative quality: she would repeat to herself innumerable times, 'I am going blind, I know it, I'm really going blind,' etc., and at such times she *could not* be reassured.

On the other hand, when she was in one of her elated moods, she would feel 'gay as a skylark' (a favourite and much-repeated phrase), care-free, pain-free ('I haven't an ache or pain in my whole body – I feel so good, there's nothing, nothing at all the matter with me,' etc.), full of energy, very active, very sociable and inclined to gossip. These changes of mood and attitude, which were very abrupt and extreme were rarely connected with any realistic change in her circumstances: she herself would say, 'I'm often depressed when there's nothing to worry about, and gay as a skylark when there are all sorts of problems.' Sometimes, however, one of her hypochondriacal depressions might come on during the course of an oculogyric crisis (when indeed she could not see, because of extreme upward deviation of the eyes), and outlast it; and on several occasions a depression would switch to elation during a crisis.

In terms of her *general physical and neurological condition* (understanding that this tended to fluctuate a good deal during the course of each day, and according to mood, etc.) Miss A. was a rather thin woman, appearing considerably younger than her sixty-one years, with a rather greasy and notably hirsute skin, but without clear signs of acromegaly, thyroid or other endocrine disturbance. She experienced considerable salivation, having to wipe her mouth clear of saliva every few minutes. Her face appeared rigid and masked, with some tendency (especially during inattention and sleep) to an open-mouthed posture. There was a resting tremor of the lips, and a gross rotary and intromittent tremor of the tongue. Spontaneous blinking was rare, but forced blinking, blepharoclonus, and protracted forced closure of the eyes were readily elicited by glabellar tap, or sudden stimuli in the visual field. When sleepy, she showed incessant attacks of blepharoclonus, and a tendency to 'micro-crises' with forced lid-closure and upward deviation of the globes for several seconds. Her voice was monotonous and uninflected, low in pitch and volume (occasionally decaying into inaudibility), with some tendency to hurry (vocal festination), but no palilalia. The pupils were small (2 mm.), equal, and reactive, the eyes moist from excess lacrimation, and the gaze full in all directions save for a mild convergence-deficit.

She showed extreme rigidity of the axial musculature, with almost no available neck-motion, and mild-moderate rigidity of the limbs. She showed a very gross ('flapping') tremor of the arms when anxious, excited, or standing, but not at other times. Asked to clench her hands repeatedly, the movement would decay in volume after 2–3 repetitions, then accelerate, and after 6–8 repetitions automatize, decompose rhythmically, and be replaced by uncontrollable flapping tremor. Miss A. tended, when sitting or standing, to assume a strongly flexed posture of the trunk, and could only straighten herself for a few seconds. She would usually arise slowly and with difficulty, and shuffle slowly forwards with her arms held flexed, rigid, and motionless by her sides. Propulsion, laterpulsion, and retropulsion could be elicited with extreme ease, and she showed a considerable tendency to pitch forwards, especially if caught in uncontrollable festination. Although very rigid and bradykinetic at the start of an examination, Miss A. showed a remarkable ability to 'activate' and loosen herself by exercise (her functional state before and after physiotherapy were strikingly different), and she could also be activated for a few minutes, even in her most akinetic early-morning period, if she chanced to sneeze. Her mood, if depressed, would show dramatic improvement *pari passu* with her motor activation. Before being placed on L-DOPA, she had had no full-blown oculogyric crises for over a year. She had received a great number of solenaceous and similar drugs, which controlled her salivation and tremor to some extent, but had made little difference to her flexed posture, bradykinesia, instability of gait, hypophonia, crises, or mood-changes. She was started on L-DOPA on 7 May.

Course on L-DOPA

No effects of any kind were experienced or observed until the dosage had been raised to 2 gm. daily. At this dosage (12 May), Miss A. experienced mild nausea and dizziness, and started to show frequent opening of the mouth – the mouth-posture of yawning, although there was no actual yawning; this alternated with occasional clenching of the teeth. Miss A. described both movements as 'automatic' and involuntary.

By 15 May (the dose had now been raised to 3 gm. L-DOPA daily), Miss A. showed striking changes in many ways. Her expression had become alert and keen, and her features more mobile; she had ceased to have drowsy periods or sopors in the course of the day. Her posture was maintained upright without effort. Her rigidity was distinctly reduced. The abnormal mouth-movements had declined in frequency. She described a state of unprecedented energy and well-being.

On 17 May (with raising of the dosage to 4 gm. L-DOPA daily), there was further reduction in rigidity and akinesia – a variety of daily skills were now within her reach, e.g. dressing and undressing, which had been impossible previously without considerable assistance. She could rise to her feet without hesitation, and stride the length of the corridor swinging her arms. Her face was mobile, and she smiled readily. Her eyes were now very wide open all day, and appeared very 'bright.' Forced opening and clenching of the jaws again became prominent with the raising of dosage-level.

On 19 May (still on 4 gm. L-DOPA daily), Miss A. started to show some disconcerting effects from the drug. She felt extremely wakeful and had found it impossible to sleep for two nights running. Her pupils were dilated (5 mm.), though normally reactive. Her legs felt restless, and she had an urge to cross and uncross them, to tap either foot, and generally to move about. She felt a need, even in bed, to perform her physiotherapy exercises over and over again. Her mouth-movements had become exceedingly conspicuous, and had formed the focus of some paranoid anxiety – that other patients, and nursing staff, were 'watching' her, laughing at her, etc. In view of this excessive arousal – akathisia, agitation, agrypnia – the dosage was reduced to 3 gm. daily.

For several days (18–25 May), on a dosage of 3 gm. daily, Miss A. maintained a steady improvement of posture, gait, and voice, and virtual disappearance of her rigidity and akinesia, without any manifestation of the inordinate arousal seen on the larger dose. We entertained hopes that a stable plateau of improvement had been reached.

On 26 May, however, renewed and novel manifestations of arousal were exhibited. Miss A. felt constant thirst and ravenous hunger – she felt impelled to drink at the water-fountain almost incessantly, and her appetite and voracity reminded her of what she had experienced in the early thirties. Her mood became exalted: she felt 'a wonderful flying and floating feeling inside,' became intensely sociable, talked continually, found reasons to run up and down the stairways ('doing errands'), and wished to dance with the nurses. She beamed at me and said she was sure she must be my 'star patient.' Between other activities, she filled twelve pages of her diary with happy, excited, and partly erotic reminiscences. Her sleep was again diminished and disturbed, with a tendency to toss and turn all night after the action of her night-sedative had worn off. On this date we observed the appearance of a new symptom – a rather sudden 'let-down,' with feelings of weakness and drowsiness – coming on between 2½ and 3 hours after each dose of L-DOPA.

The following day (27 May), she showed still greater activity, and felt driven to perform her physiotherapy exercises by the hundred: 'I had such a *storm* of activity,' she complained, 'that it frightened me. I *could not* keep still.' An additional feature seen on this day were sudden *tic-like movements* – lightning-quick impulsions to touch either ear, to scratch her nose, etc.

Two days later (despite reduction of her dosage to 2 gm. L-DOPA daily), her akathisia was still more marked: Miss A. felt 'forced' (her word) to move her arms and legs continually, shuffling her feet, drumming her fingers, picking up objects and immediately putting them down, 'scratching' (despite the feeling that there was nothing to scratch), and making sudden darting movements with her hands to her nose and ears. She said of these sudden tic-like actions: 'I don't know why I make them, there's no reason for it, I just suddenly *have* to make them.' Palilalic repetition of phrases and sentences was also observed for the first time on 29 May, although this occurred only occasionally: her speech in general was pressured and hurried (tachyphemic). Her insomnia continued to be severe, and barely responsive to chloral or barbiturates; her dreams were extremely vivid, with a tendency to nightmares;[80] and her mood, though consistently ex-

---

[80] Alterations in dreaming are often the first sign of response to L-DOPA, in patients with ordinary Parkinson's disease as well as those with post-encephalitic syndromes. Dreaming typically becomes more vivid (many patients remark on their dreaming, suddenly, in brilliant colour), more charged emotionally (with a tendency towards erotic dreams and nightmares), and more prone to go on all night. Sometimes their 'realness' is so extraordinary that they cannot be forgotten or thrown off after waking. One patient, a pious Catholic, was horrified by having vivid dreams of incestuous intercourse with her father – 'I *never* had such dreams before!' she said indignantly – and had to be reassured that these *were* only dreams, for which she need not feel responsible or guilty. Had she not been so reassured, I could not help thinking, such dreams might have paved the way

cited, was labile in affect, with sudden veerings from stormy hypomania to fearfulness and agitated depression. Her intermittent mouth-openings had been replaced by a strong drive to clench her teeth. Thirst and hunger continued to be inordinate, and Miss A. – normally delicate and restrained in her table-manners – felt the urge to tear her food and stuff it into her mouth. Her water-intake increased to 5–6 gallons a day; tests for *diabetes insipidus* were invariably negative, and her drinking seemed rather to be a compulsion or mania.

With further reduction of dosage (down to 1.5 gm. daily), Miss A. remained comparatively stable for a further week: euphoric but not exalted, able to sleep (but only with sedation), very active, sociable, and talkative. At this period akathisia was only seen if she was constrained to sit still, as at mealtimes: at such times, in her own words, her 'muscles would feel impatient,' and she would be forced to shuffle and kick her feet under the table.

During the second week of June, her tendency to festinate became more marked. Her walking would be quite stable, al-

---

to a psychosis. Excessive dreaming of this sort – excessive both in visual and sensory vividness, and in activation of unconscious psychic content; dreaming akin to hallucinosis – is common in fever, and after many drugs (opiates, amphetamines, cocaine, psychedelics); during (or at the start of) certain migraines and seizures; in other organic excitements; and sometimes at the beginning of psychoses.

The style of *drawing* – as of dreaming and imagining – can change profoundly as patients become stimulated by L-DOPA. Asked to draw a tree, the Parkinsonian tends to draw a small, meagre thing, stunted, impoverished, a bare winter tree with no foliage at all. As he 'warms up,' 'comes to,' is animated by L-DOPA, so the tree acquires vigor, life, imagination – and foliage. If he becomes too excited, high, on L-DOPA, the tree may acquire a fantastic ornateness and exuberance, exploding with a florescence of new branches and foliage with little arabesques, curlicues, and whatnot, until finally its original form is completely lost beneath this enormous, this baroque, elaboration. With Irmgard H., a professional artist and painter on ceramics, paintings before L-DOPA were simple and pastoral – children dancing around a tree, etc. As she became animated on L-DOPA these innocent scenes were replaced by bullfights, cockfights, gladiators, boxers – *she* remained calm; all the new drug-aggression flowed into her art. Later still, her images became highly stylized, intricate, with obsessed, repetitive motifs, labyrinthine, until they resembled Louis Wain's crystalline cats. Such drawings are also rather characteristic of Tourette's syndrome – the original form, the original thought, lost in a jungle of embellishment – and in the so-called 'speed-art' of amphetaminism. First the imagination is awakened, then overexcited, to endlessness and excess.

though it had a hurried, urgent quality about it, until she encountered an obstacle, or the necessity for negotiating a corner. This would elicit sudden festination and forward-impetus, so that she started to suffer the first of many falls. Her mood continued to be elevated, but her attitudes were now marked by increasing impatience and demand, and sometimes by stamping if her demands were not met instantly. Her 'let-downs' in the third hour after medication became more sudden and severe: she would seem to pass within two or three minutes from forceful, noisy bustling into a near-speechless akinesia with intense drowsiness. In view of this, it was decided to give her a smaller dose of L-DOPA spaced at shorter intervals.

On 13 June (an exceedingly hot and sultry day) Miss A.'s emotional excitement became manic in quality. She had an uncontrollable urge to dance and sing, and did so continuously while I was trying to examine her. Her thoughts and speech were very pressured and exalted: 'Oh Dr Sacks!' she exclaimed breathlessly, 'I am so happy, so very very happy. I feel so good, so full of energy. So tingly, like my blood is champagne. I am bubbling and bubbling and bubbling inside. Dance with me! . . . No? Well I'll sing to you then –'(sings 'O what a beautiful morning, O what a beautiful day,' with occasional palilalic repetitions).

Added to the manic pressure there appeared to be a considerable element of motor, bulimic, and other drives: she could not sit still, but constantly danced and pranced across the room; she would shuffle her feet, cross and uncross her legs, suddenly belch, straighten her dress, pat her hair, belch again, clap her hands, touch her nose, and belch a third time, exuberantly and without apologies. She looked warm and flushed, had very dilated pupils, and a bounding tachycardia of 120. Her feeding showed insatiable voracity and hurry: she would tear at her food in an animal-like way, grunting with excitement, and stuffing it into her mouth, and when finished gnawed her fingers in an uncontrollable perseveration of greed. I observed too that when she ate, her tongue would shoot out of her mouth as she brought the morsel to her lips: I had the feeling that her tongue was *enticed* out by the food, and that eating evoked voluptuous pleasure.

Other oral automatisms and urges were also in evidence during this peak of excitement: a tendency to tonic protrusion of the lips (*'schnauzkrampf'*), to make sucking noises, and – most astonishingly of all – to *lap* milk from a saucer: the tongue-movement during lapping was amazingly quick and expert, clearly not under voluntary control, and was called by Miss A. 'automatic . . . it just seems to come naturally to me' (compare Maria G.).

On the afternoon of the 13th her excitement and tachycardia became more extreme, and she exclaimed: 'I feel jam-packed with energy like a rocket. I'm going to take off, take off, take off . . .' It was therefore decided to tranquillize her, and to our surprise a minute (10 mg.) dose of parenteral thorazine brought her 'down' in an hour, to an exhausted, drowsy, almost akinetic state. Her dose of L-DOPA was then further reduced, to 1 gm. daily.

The day following this reduction of dose found Miss A. torpid, sad, somewhat rigid, and akinetic. Moreover, she had an oculogyric crisis lasting several hours, her first for more than a year. During her oculogyric crisis, Miss A. sat absolutely motionless. Describing it afterwards she said: 'I had no impulse to move, I don't think I could have moved . . . I had to concentrate on the bit of ceiling I was forced to look at – it filled my mind, I could think of nothing else. And I was afraid, deathly afraid, as I always am in these spells, although I knew there was nothing to be afraid of.'

Following the crisis, L-DOPA was discontinued for two days. Through these two days, Miss A. showed an *exacerbation* of her pre-DOPA state, being intensely rigid, scarcely able to speak or move, and deeply depressed: 'trombone-tremor' of the tongue also recurred at this time, with extreme intensity. A short trial of haloperidol ('Haldol': 0.5 mg. b.i.d.) only served to aggravate these symptoms. On 18 June, therefore, Miss A. was put back on a very modest dose of L-DOPA (750 mg. daily).

In the ensuing week, there was a satisfactory return of speech and motor force, but this was now combined with some disquieting new symptoms. Miss A.'s expression became somewhat blank and confused, although she was at no time disoriented or unaware of her surroundings. She would have to make a notable effort to speak, but the effort notwithstanding she would speak in a whisper quite different in quality from the hypophonia she had shown in her pre-DOPA days. She conveyed to us, in a whisper, that she had the feeling of 'some force, some sort of obstruction' which stopped her speaking loudly, although she was able to whisper to us without impediment. During this period, a different set of abnormal mouth-movements made their appearance: forced protrusions of the lips, propulsion of the tongue, and occasional choreic dartings of the tongue. Most alarming of all, the tendency to festination and hurry, which had come on ten days beforehand and become slowly worse (despite the fluctuations of drug-dosage, and of her other symptoms), now took a frightening paroxysmal form. Where previously she would festinate only on encountering an obstacle in her path, she would now have a sudden, spontaneous urge to run, and would be impelled forward in a frenzy of little, stamping steps, which were accompanied by shrill screams, tic-like movements of the arms, and a terrified expression. This stampede was followed, after a few steps, by an inability to lift her feet, and inevitably she would fall forwards on her face. Sometimes these paroxysms would take an even more acute form, in which she would be impelled to lunge forwards while remaining (in her own words) 'rooted to the spot.' It became necessary, therefore, to have someone accompany her in order to moderate her walking and save her from falling. It at once became apparent that provided Miss A. could be walked (or persuaded to walk) slowly and gently, no problems would arise, but that as soon as she hurried (or was pushed or pulled beyond a given pace), a sudden resistance would develop which 'rooted' her to the spot. This phenomenon appeared analogous to her speech-problems at this time, where an attempted exclamation immediately evoked resistance and 'block,' but a gentle whisper could 'get through' without impediment.

It was clear that these paroxysms, whatever their nature, were terrifying and indeed dangerous, and that some functional instability (or series of instabilities) had arisen, and was perpetuating itself, despite the very nominal dose of L-DOPA which she was receiving. With regret, but feeling that it was necessary, we therefore replaced the drug-capsules by placebo. The speech-block and stampeding attacks persisted, with lessening intensity, for a further forty-four days, and then ceased. Her rigidity, bradykinesia, and other symptoms reverted to their pre-DOPA level. Towards the end of July, therefore, a small dose of L-DOPA was again started (750 mg. daily), and Miss A. now appears (three weeks later) to be enjoying a substantial stable, though limited, improvement (in terms of speech, walking, balance, etc.), without any return of the adverse and paroxysmal effect encountered earlier.

1969–72

In May of 1969 Miss A. reached her high point, her zenith, her 'stardom'; the last three years have seen her decline and fall. In June 1969, Miss A., at the acme of her excitement, started to come apart like the sky-rocket she compared herself to; the last three years have seen a continual increase of her schism or fission. If these problems are to be ascribed to L-DOPA (i.e. to the particular reactivity of this so-excitable, so-fissionable person to L-DOPA), why did we not stop the drug? *We could not:* like Maria G., Hester Y., and other such patients, Miss A. became critically dependent on the continuance of L-DOPA, and by 1970 would move not merely into exacerbated Parkinsonism and depression but into immediate stupor or coma, if it was stopped for a day; thus we were forced to continue the drug. Miss A. herself was well aware of the dilemma: 'It's driving me mad,' she would say; 'but I'll die if you stop it.'

She has indeed lost almost all possibility of a modulated 'middle' state, and has almost nothing in between coma and hypervigilance, Parkinsonism and frenzy, depression and mania, etc.; her responses have become extreme, abrupt, and all-or-none, reflected and rebounding from one behavioural pole to another. *Both* poles, indeed, may simultaneously occur, and Miss A. will declare – within two or three minutes – that she feels wonderful, terrible, can see perfectly, is blind, cannot move, cannot stop moving, etc. Her will is continually vacillating or paralysed; she wants what she fears, and fears what she wants; she loves what she hates, and hates what she loves. She is driven this way and that by intense contradictions, impossible decisions between impossible choices.

In the presence of excitement and perpetual contradiction, Miss A. has split into a dozen Miss A.'s – the drinker, the ticcer, the stamper, the yeller, the swinger, the gazer, the sleeper, the wisher, the fearer, the lover, the hater, etc. – all struggling with each other to 'possess' her behaviour. Her real interests and activities have practically vanished, and have been replaced by absurd stereotypies, continually ground smaller in the mill of her being. She is completely reduced, for most of the time, to a 'repertoire' of a few dozen thoughts and impulsions, increasingly fixed in phrase and form, and repeated, compulsively, again and again. The original Miss A. – so engaging and bright – has been *dispossessed* by a host of crude, degenerate sub-selves – a 'schizophrenic' fission of her once-unified self.

But there are still a few things which bring her together, or which recall her former un-broken self. Music calms her, relieves her distraction, and gives her – if briefly – its coherence and concord; and so too does Nature, when she sits in the garden. But, above all, she is recalled by a single relation, the only one which still preserves for her undivided meaning and feeling. She has a favourite younger sister who lives out-of-state, but who comes to New York once a month to visit her. This sister always takes Miss A. out for the day – to an opera, or a play, or a good meal in the city. Miss A. is radiant when she returns from these excursions, and describes them in detail, with feeling and wit; at such times there is nothing 'schizophrenic' in her thought or her manner, but a return of wholeness and the sense of the world. 'I can't understand,' her sister once said to me, 'why Margaret is called crazy or broken or strange. We had a wonderful day "on the town" together. She was eager and interested in everything and everyone – chock-full of life, and full of enjoyment . . . She was easy and relaxed – none of the pushing and the drinking you all make so much of . . . She talked and laughed the way she used to in the old days, back in the twenties before she got ill . . . She goes mad in your madhouse because she is shut off from life.'

MIRON V.

℘ Miron V. was born in New York in 1908 and had the flu severely in 1918, although he showed no symptoms which were recognized as encephalitic at this time. After high school he started work as a cobbler, and by the age of thirty owned his own shoe-shop, had married, and had fathered a son.

In 1947 Mr V. showed the first signs of a Parkinsonian syndrome associated with restlessness and impulsiveness, tics and mannerisms, and a tendency to periods of staring and 'trance' – an unmistakable post-encephalitic syndrome.[81] He was able to continue work as a cobbler until 1952, and to stay at home until 1955, at which time increasing disability necessitated his admission to hospital. Immediately following his admission to Mount Carmel, Mr V. developed an 'admission psychosis' – an intense paranoia, with hallucinatory images of castration, degradation, abandonment, vengeance, spite, and impotent rage.[82] With the fading of his acute psychosis, ten days later, he passed into a state of intensely exacerbated Parkinsonism and catatonia – a state so intense as to render him virtually speechless and motionless. This state continued unchanged till he was given L-DOPA.

This Parkinsonian-catatonic state was accompanied by a mixture of intense aloofness, negativism, and withdrawal. In the words of his wife, 'Something happened to Miron when he

---

[81] Miron V. thus showed a period of almost thirty years between what must be presumed to have been a sub-clinical attack of *encephalitis lethargica* in 1918 and the development of an indubitable post-encephalitic syndrome. Even longer 'incubation periods' may occur: thus another patient (Hyman H.) had severe manifest sleeping-sickness in 1917, recovered from this completely, but developed an unmistakable post-encephalitic syndrome in 1962.

[82] Such 'admission psychoses' are not uncommon when patients are unwillingly consigned to what is, in effect, a terminal institution like Mount Carmel. I have seen such psychoses in dozens of patients.

stopped working, and then when he left home and went into hospital. He used to be such a warm man . . . He loved his work more than anything in the world . . . And then he changed . . . He came to hate us and to hate everyone and everything. And maybe he hated himself.' Mr V.'s iciness and hostility were deeply disturbing to his family, who 'responded' by refusing to visit him soon after he had been institutionalized, thus completing and compounding a vicious circle of neurotic reaction.

Over the ensuing fourteen years Mr V.'s state remained essentially the same, although he developed extremely profuse seborrhoea and sialorrhoea. I frequently saw him between 1966 and 1969, and was always impressed by his almost absolute immobility, which was such that he might sit fifteen hours in a chair without the least hint of spontaneous movement.[83] He did, how-

---

[83] I noted above that he often seemed to sit, absolutely immobile, for fifteen hours at a stretch, but this is not wholly correct. I would sometimes see him in the morning, silhouetted against a frosted-glass door, with his right hand apparently motionless a few inches from his knee. I might catch sight of him later, towards the middle of the day, with his hand 'frozen' halfway to his nose (just as one sees in Frances M., see insert). Then, a couple of hours later, his hand would be 'frozen' on his glasses or his nose. I assumed that these were meaningless akinetic poses, and it was only much later, when he was awakened and accelerated by L-DOPA, that the almost incredible truth came out. I remembered his strange frozen 'poses,' and I mentioned them to him.

'What do you mean, "frozen poses"? ' he exclaimed. 'I was merely wiping my nose!'

'But Miron, this just isn't possible. Are you telling me that what I saw as frozen poses was your hand in transit to your nose?'

'Of course,' he said. 'What else would they be?'

'But Miron,' I expostulated, 'these poses were many hours apart. Do you mean to tell me that you were taking six hours to wipe your nose?'

'It sounds crazy,' he reflected, 'and scary too. To me they were just normal movements, they took a second. You want to tell me I was taking *hours* instead of seconds to wipe my nose?'

I didn't know what to answer; I was as nonplussed as he. It did, indeed, sound perfectly absurd. However, I had countless still photos of Miron as he was, silhouetted against the door. I put together thirty of these, taken in the course of one day, made cinephoto-size reductions, and ran them through the projector at sixteen frames a second. Now, incredibly, I saw that the 'impossible' was true; using what amounted to time-lapse photography, I saw that the succession of 'poses' did, in fact, form a continuous action. He was, indeed, just wiping his nose, *but doing so ten thousand times slower than normal.* Inconceivably retarded, but not to himself. Conversely: with Hester's almost unintelligibly fast motions and words, which were too fast for the eye or ear to follow, one had to use

ever, show occasional tics and impulsions – sudden 'saluting' tics with either hand, or sudden throat-clearing or 'giggling' noises – in startling contrast to his overall background of complete immobility and silence. Although exceedingly disinclined to speak, Mr V. could say a few words in a very staccato, exclamatory fashion – sufficient to indicate his intelligence, his bitterness, his hopelessness, and his indifferent awareness of everything around him. He could neither rise to his feet nor walk without aid. When I asked him whether he wished to try L-DOPA, he said, 'I don't care . . . It's up to you.'

Mr V.'s response to L-DOPA, in July 1969, had the same sudden and almost magical quality seen in so many other severely affected post-encephalitic patients. Within the course of a single day he regained an almost normal power and pattern of movement and speech. He also showed feelings of amazement and joy, although these were still overcast by his habitual suspicion, coldness, and constraint. Within two weeks of this initial reaction, Mr V.'s state had swung to the opposite extreme: he became exceedingly impulsive and hyperactive, hypomanic, provocative, impudent, and amorous – everything was velocity, audacity, salacity. His previously rare tics now became much commoner, so that he would find occasion to 'adjust' his spectacles, or clear his throat, two or three hundred times an hour.

Mr V.'s reactions, over the next nine months, were all extreme, erratic, and contradictory. He showed abrupt alternations between totally immobile states and dangerously hyperactive impulsive states. He sustained innumerable falls and no less than three hip fractures due to his impetuosity and folly in his hyperactive states.[84] But his attitudes were mixed, and he also showed, during these difficult months, an increasing interest in people

high-speed cinematography, or 'tape-stretching,' to show their millisecond-long, accelerated forms.

[84] If the commonest *secondary* problems stemming from the activation procured by L-DOPA were mouth-movements and mouth-damage, the most serious, by far, were falls and fractures. Thus of some eighty patients (about half post-encephalitic, and half with common Parkinson's disease) put on L-DOPA in Mount Carmel in 1969, more than a third sustained serious (and sometimes multiple) fractures (similar figures are reported from elsewhere in similar situations).

about him, a diminution of hostility and withdrawal, and some affection for his wife and son, who – after a twelve-year gap – started to visit him again. He also became very handy about the ward – he was extraordinarily adept in the use of his hands – and expressed a longing for work of some kind.

The real change came when we set up a last and a cobbler's bench for Mr V. in our Sheltered Workshop, in May 1970. When he was taken to see these he showed an amazement and joy without the least admixture of suspicion or constraint. His old skills returned to him with amazing speed, and so did his admiration and his love for his work. He started to do cobbling and repairs-jobs for more and more of the patients in hospital, and to show a craftsman's skill and love in making new shoes. With this return to his work, and his *relation* with his work, Mr V.'s reactions to L-DOPA became better and stabler: he ceased to have dangerously impulsive 'ups' and ceased to have depressive-Parkinsonian-catatonic 'downs' with anything like the severity with which they had initially occurred. He became far more affable and accessible, and recovered a good deal of his lost self-esteem: 'I feel like a man again,' he once said to me. 'I feel I've got some use and a place in the world . . . A man can't live without that.'

Since the summer of 1970, Mr V. has done extraordinarily well – miraculously well considering the severity and hopelessness of his original state, and the extreme and erratic reactions he first showed on L-DOPA. It cannot be said that his speech and motor patterns are in any sense 'normal' – they still show a good deal of abruptness and freezing – but they are adequate and controllable, and they allow him to do a full day's work at his last every day, to walk round the hospital, to converse fairly freely, and to go home for occasional weekends with his wife. Of the forty or so post-encephalitic patients at Mount Carmel who showed extremely severe Parkinsonian-catatonic syndromes before L-DOPA, Mr V. – finally – has done by far the best; he has been the *only* one among them able to tolerate the continuous administration of L-DOPA without interruption, and to develop such stability after so unstable a start.

GERTIE C.

꧁ Mrs C. was born in New Hampshire in 1908, the youngest daughter of a harmonious and close-knit family. She had a happy childhood without neurotic distresses or difficulties of significance, made friends easily, did well at school, and worked as a typist-stenographer until the age of twenty-five when she married. She continued in seemingly perfect health, enjoying a full social life and bringing up a family of three children, between her marriage and her thirty-eighth birthday. Shortly after this, however, she developed a violent shaking of both hands, which was first ascribed to the rigours of a New York winter, but recognized a few weeks later as Parkinsonian in nature. In the next six years her illness proceeded relentlessly and rapidly, combining tremor, rigidity, akinesia, pulsions, and extremely profuse sweating, salivation, and seborrhoea. By the age of forty-four Mrs C. had been rendered totally immobile and virtually speechless. Her tremor and rigidity could be diminished somewhat by atropine-like drugs, but her disabling akinesia and aphonia showed no response to these. Despite great difficulties and the necessity for nursing assistance round the clock, Mrs C.'s devoted family kept her at home for another ten years (until 1962).

When I first saw Mrs C. in 1966, I found that she had developed dystonic contractures of all her extremities and showed the most intense rigidity of all her musculature. It was just possible for her to whisper with very great effort. It was clear, however, that she followed everything that was said to her perfectly. She did not in the least seem inert, indifferent, and unreactive (like Mrs B.) but conveyed the impression of an intense inner activity which was motionless and enclosed in itself. Her eyes seemed to shine with intense peacefulness, as if she were contemplating a beautiful picture or a landscape. She gave the impression of being *rapt,* not inert.

I started Mrs C. on L-DOPA in the middle of June 1969. She showed remarkable sensitivity to this, and on a dose of no more than 1 gm. a day started to show a striking restoration of her voice and of all movement, and an equally striking reduction of rigidity and salivation.[85] With a further increase of dosage to 1.5 gm. daily Mrs C.'s voice became virtually normal in strength and timbre, and revealed a full and subtle range of intonation and modulation. Her strength had now become such that she could feed herself and turn the pages of a book, although these activities were difficult because of irreversible contractures in the hands. Her mood was calm, happy, and equable, with no hint of anxiety or emotional extravagance. During this halcyon period Mrs C. was able to talk freely for the first time in almost twenty years, and spoke to me at length about the state she had been in for much of this time.

It had been, she explained, a state of 'great inner stillness' and of 'acquiescence'; her attention would dwell for hours on whatever object or thought entered its field; she would feel herself completely 'absorbed' and 'engrossed' by all of her postures, perceptions, and thoughts; she said, 'My mind was like a still pool reflecting itself.' She would spend hours and days and even weeks reliving peaceful scenes from her own childhood – lying in the sun, drowsing in a meadow, or floating in a creek near her home as a child; these Arcadian moments could apparently be extended indefinitely by the still and intent quality of her thought. Mrs C. added that she had always had a vivid imagination and had been able to picture things clearly, but that its vividness was increased by the motionless concentration which accompanied her Parkinsonism. She stressed that her sense of time and duration had

---

[85]Lawrence Weschler, visiting Mount Carmel in 1982, recorded the following conversation with Gertie C.:

> Weschler: 'Do you remember what it was like when you came to?'
> Gertie: 'Oh, yes.'
> Weschler: 'What was it like?'
> Gertie: 'Suddenly I was talking.'
> Weschler: 'Do you remember your first words?'
> Gertie: 'Oh, yes.'
> Weschler: 'What were they?'
> Gertie: ' "Oooh! I'm talking!" '

become profoundly altered during the previous two decades; that although she was aware of what was happening and what the date was, she herself had *no feeling of happening,* but rather the feeling that time itself had come to a stop, and that every moment of her existence was a repetition of itself.

Four weeks after starting L-DOPA her responses became less favourable and she experienced impulses to gasp and swallow, and reversions to Parkinsonism and aphonia, after each dose. Feeling that Mrs C. was moving along into a pathological reaction, I decided to stop the L-DOPA for a few days. With its cessation, Mrs C. at once reverted to severe Parkinsonism, and to this was added a rather deep depression and somnolence which had not been part of the original picture.

Re-starting her on L-DOPA towards the end of July we found it impossible to regain the beautiful response seen in the previous month. In an effort to try to retrieve the original response we added a small dose of amantadine (100 mg. b.i.d.) to the gram of L-DOPA per day she was receiving – a measure we had found useful in a number of other patients. The effect of this addition was absolutely catastrophic. Within three hours of receiving her first amantadine capsule, Mrs C. became intensely excited and deliriously hallucinated. She would cry out, 'Cars bearing down on me, they're crowding me! They're crowding me!' Her voice would rise to a scream of terror, and she would suddenly clutch my arm; at this time she also saw faces 'like masks popping in and out' – which would snap and mock and grin and yelp at her. Occasionally she would smile rapturously and exclaim: 'Look what a beautiful tree, so beautiful!' and tears of pleasure would enter her eyes. But in general this state was one of a disorganized and terrifying hallucinatory paranoia with multiple Lilliputian hallucinations of sight and sound. It was accompanied by a violent rhythmic thrashing of her head from side to side, and by rhythmic tongue-protrusion, screaming, and tic-like movements of the eyes. These hallucinations and movements were at their worst if Mrs C. was left alone or if the room was darkened; a familiar and friendly presence, or speaking to her, or holding her hand could deliver her from apparitions and movements, and restore her to herself for a few seconds or minutes. Although the L-DOPA and amantadine were immediately stopped with the onset of this state, it continued of its own momentum for more than three weeks, during which time only the heaviest doses of sedation or tranquillization could reduce her excitement. In September her delirium suddenly ceased, leaving her exhausted and torpid, although perfectly rational. It was clear from talking to her, and from observing her, that she retained no conscious memory whatever of the extraordinary state which had possessed or dispossessed her in the preceding three weeks.[86]

At the beginning of October we very cautiously tried Mrs C. on L-DOPA again, this time giving her a total dose of only one quarter of a gram daily. This immediately induced a considerable restoration of her voice and strength, but also evoked a new disorder – a tendency to sudden, tic-like jabbings and swattings in the air, as if she were fending off flies or mosquitoes. After ten days of this combination, Mrs C. abruptly returned to her hallucinatory delirium; the onset of this precisely coincided with the cessation of her tics, which suggested that the latter might have served as 'lightning-conductors,' discharging her excitement in a relatively harmless way. The L-DOPA was immediately stopped again, but this did not diminish her excitement in the least. It became necessary to put side-rails on her bed and to have a nurse in constant attendance lest she injure herself in her extremity. On the night of 10 October, while her nurse had left the room for a minute, Mrs C. uttered a scream of terror, climbed over the side-rails, and fell heavily to the ground, breaking both hips and her pelvis.

The following months were months of great physical and mental torture for Mrs C.: she was in great pain from the injuries she had received; she developed a bedsore over the sacrum which had to be probed and washed several times a day; she lost 40

---

[86] It may be asked whether Gertie C. perhaps retained *unconscious* memories of this time, memories *repressed* from consciousness because of their deeply frightening and traumatic nature (such pseudo-amnesias, or inhibitions of memory, are not uncommon after frightful events – which include, of course, frightful psychoses). It is possible that there was some element of this, but it seems altogether more probable to me that Mrs C. – who was given neither to psychoses nor to crypto-amnesia – retained no memory whatever of the preceding three weeks, because these were filled with delirium, not psychosis.

pounds in weight; her dystonic rigidity and contractures grew more severe; and finally she was tormented by evil hallucinations which persisted without the least diminution for more than *five months* after the discontinuance of L-DOPA. By the summer of 1970 Mrs C. had come through the worst: her bedsore was healing, her rigidity and dystonia had become less extreme, and most important, her hallucinatory delirium was beginning to fade out.

As her periods of delirium diminished, and her intervals of lucidity increased, Mrs C. voiced a certain wistfulness: 'They're all disappearing now,' she said, 'the little people and *things* which have been keeping me company. Then I'll be my old plain self again.' But this was not to be. The day *after* delirium finally ceased, she had a strange experience while lying in bed. It started as an uncanny feeling – the sense that something extraordinary was about to happen; she felt herself compelled to look out of the window, and there to her amazement she saw a masked man climbing the fire-escape; when he drew level with her he brandished a stick and poked it in her direction, which filled her with terror; he then gave a 'devilish grin' and retreated down the fire-escape – *taking the fire-escape along with him.* It was this which indicated to Mrs C. that she had had 'a vision,' and that she had not only hallucinated a man but a fire-escape into the bargain. When Mrs C. described this to me the next day she shuddered all over, but also evinced, in her manner and choice of words, an unmistakable relish. The next evening the masked man on the fire-escape again appeared and this time came closer and flourished his stick in a fashion not only threatening but brazenly suggestive. On the third day Mrs C. decided to 'have it out' with me: 'You can't blame me,' she said. 'I haven't had anything for the last twenty years, and I'm not about to get anything *now,* you know . . . You surely wouldn't forbid a friendly hallucination to a frustrated old lady like me!' I replied that if her hallucinations had a pleasant and controllable character, they seemed rather a good idea under the circumstances. After this, the paranoid quality entirely dropped away, and her hallucinatory encounters became purely amicable and amorous. She developed a humour and tact and control – never allowing herself a hallucination before eight in the evening and keeping its duration to thirty or forty minutes at most. If her relatives stayed too late, she would explain firmly but pleasantly that she was expecting 'a gentleman visitor from out of town' in a few minutes' time and she felt he might take it amiss if he was kept waiting outside.

Mrs C. is alive and as well as she can be considering the severity of her illness. The deep peaceful look has returned to her eyes, and she seems to have regained her power for timeless contemplation of childhood scenes and moments. The only change in her from pre-DOPA days is that she now receives love, attention, and invisible presents from a hallucinatory gentleman who faithfully visits each evening.

MARTHA N.

℥ Miss N. was born in New York in 1908, the only daughter of devout Irish Catholic parents. She almost died from the flu in 1918, but did not suffer any clear-cut encephalitic symptoms then. After finishing high school, she started work with a telephone company; she was a thrice-elected 'Beauty Queen' at this time, and a valued companion at functions and dates. Parkinsonism presented itself when she was twenty-one years old, and caused such tremor that she ceased work that year. Concurrently she developed sleep-talking and sleep-walking. After this initial outburst of symptoms, her illness remained static for twenty-two years, during which time she lived at home with her parents, was able to walk, visit friends, play golf, and attend to all household and shopping duties.

With the death of her parents in 1951, Miss N.'s illness abruptly became worse, and in particular rigidity and dystonia developed, and overtook her, so that within two years she had become deeply disabled, losing the ability to walk or stand, and her voice and swallowing were also impaired. This precipitous deterioration in her status led to her institutionalization in 1954. Once admitted to hospital, her illness again seemed to come to a standstill, although the dystonia had led on to dystonic deformities.

I often saw Miss N. between 1966 and 1969 and found her intelligent and charming and pleasant to talk to. She showed at this time an immovable dystonic rigidity of both legs, a severe torticollis, a very soft voice, and extremely voluminous salivation. She was conspicuously sociable and affable in comparison with many other post-encephalitic patients. For fifty-one weeks in the year Miss N. was conspicuously 'together' and sane, but in the fifty-second week she had an 'Easter Psychosis.' This took the form of increasing rigidity, lessened ability to move or speak or swallow, depression, masking of the voice, and sometimes oculogyria. On Good Friday she would feel herself dying, and in a scarcely audible whisper request that we bring a priest to administer last rites. This done she would sink into a motionless, speechless 'swoon,' remaining this way till Easter Sunday, when she would rather suddenly 'come to' with a feeling of rebirth. Her voice, her movement, and all her abilities would be strikingly better than 'normal' for two or three weeks following this annual rebirth, and the diminution in her Parkinsonism and other problems was very remarkable during these weeks.

Miss N. was started on L-DOPA in June 1969. Her initial response to this was a retropulsion or insucking of the tongue, so severe that speech was impossible, and she was in continual danger of swallowing her tongue. In view of this her L-DOPA (2 gm. a day) was stopped. She was restarted on L-DOPA later, in the middle of July, and this time the tongue-pulsions and gaggings were not evoked at all, but, on the contrary, a striking improvement occurred. Her voice became much louder, her salivation virtually ceased, and her arms lost almost all their rigidity and akinesia; in effect Miss N. was 'normalized' except, of course, for the irreversible contractures of her feet and her neck. This superb therapeutic action showed itself with remarkable suddenness – in the course of an hour – and was induced by a mere 750 mg. of L-DOPA a day.

Her excellent state was maintained until 4 August – the day following my own departure for London. On this day Miss N. became extremely agitated, frightened, and depressed, showed intense tremor and rigidity alternating in her limbs, presented a fixed and corpse-like expression, and demanded last rites for her impending death. Her L-DOPA was stopped once again, and after a day she returned to her pre-DOPA self. On my return she asked me once more to try her on L-DOPA. 'It wasn't the drug which upset me,' she said. 'It was your going away. I couldn't be sure you would ever come back. I felt so afraid, I thought I would die.'

In September for the third time I gave her L-DOPA and her responses were *now* quite different from either of the first two times. She complained of rapid breathing and difficulty in catching her breath, and she had the beginnings of respiratory crises. She developed very rapid 'saluting' tics in both of her arms, her hands flying from her lap to her face three or four times every minute. She also developed palilalia, repeating her words innumerable times. Her reaction at this time was remarkably similar to that of her room-mate Miss D., so much so that I wondered if either was automatically 'imitating' the other. By the middle of September, Miss N. was ticcing 60 times to the minute, 60 minutes to the hour, and saying an incessant palilalic repetition of the following verse she had learned years before:

> I thought it said in every tick,
> I am so sick, so sick, so sick.
> Oh death, come quick, come quick, come quick!
> Come quick, come quick, come quick, come quick!

Since she was exhausting herself and maddening her fellow patients, I again found it necessary to stop L-DOPA.

Following this excited state Miss N. showed a severe 'rebound' when L-DOPA was stopped, becoming so rigid, tremulous, akinetic, and voiceless, and having so much difficulty in swallowing, that we had to tube-feed her. This 'withdrawal-reaction' continued for the remainder of September without any lessening in severity whatever.

In October I started Miss N. on L-DOPA for the fourth time and this time she again did well for some weeks, although she was more easily excited than usual, and when excited showed recurrence of her tics and palilalia. It was noted by the nursing staff, at this time, that she particularly showed tics when I was around. Miss N. knew that I was fascinated by tics, and that they would always attract my attention and interest.

In December, during a period of particularly grim weather, Miss N. again passed into a death-like stupor similar to that which she had shown on L-DOPA in August (and before L-DOPA, in her 'Easter Psychoses'). This time neither my presence nor anything I could do could alter her state: she lay motionless and frigid as if already a corpse. After three days of this state I stopped her L-DOPA, but this did not seem to make any difference. She continued in stupor for another ten days and during this time required total nursing care and tube-feeding once more. On Christmas day the sun came out and shone brilliantly for the first time in more than two weeks. Miss N. was taken in her chair onto the porch outside. Five minutes later she suddenly 'came to,' and within a few seconds was restored to herself. Her description of this was impressive and moving: 'I saw the sun,' she said. 'I saw the people all around me living and moving. I realized I was neither dead nor in Hell. I felt life stirring inside me. I felt something like a shell breaking inside me. And suddenly I could move and speak again.'

We gave Miss N. three months to recover from these experiences and to restore her physiological and psychological equilibrium. In March 1970, at her request, we started L-DOPA for the fifth time. Here, as before, there was a gratifying reduction of Parkinsonism and other symptoms for about three weeks. Then she started to develop singular hallucinations every evening, which always took essentially the same form. They would start with a feeling of *uncanniness,* a feeling that something unimaginably strange was about to happen, and the feeling that it had happened once before, in a dream or a past life, and that her coming experience would be a revisiting of the past. In this strange state, Miss N. would suddenly see two bearded men enter the room. They would walk to the window with an unhurried gait, and there light an old-fashioned lantern which they swung to and fro ('like a censer'). Miss N. would feel this swinging light was designed to capture her attention or 'bewitch' her, and she would feel intensely tempted to gaze at the light. At this point she would turn her head violently away and say, 'Get behind me, get behind me, you devils, you devils!' It was this sudden violent turning of the head and exclamation which drew the attention of Miss N.'s room-mate to the fact that she was having 'queer experiences' of some kind. Her equivocal visitors would then come to the head of her bed, would take pieces of shimmering gauze from their pockets, and wave these in circles in front of her eyes; she felt herself both shrinking and swooning as they did this before her, not knowing whether their activities were a curse or a blessing. Both men would bend over her face and kiss her, brushing her cheeks with the bristles of their beards. They would then walk gravely out of the room. With their departure Miss N. had an immense sense of regret and relief inseparably mixed. The feeling of 'strangeness' would disappear, and Miss N. would feel herself once again. These episodes would last ten or twelve minutes and would start on the stroke of eight every evening. When I asked Miss N. whether she thought her 'visitors' were real, she said: 'Yes and no. Not real like you, Dr Sacks, or the nurses, or this place. A different sort of reality, as if they had come from another world.' She later said, 'First I thought they were ghosts of patients who had died in this room, and then I realized they were supernatural. I could never decide whether they came from Heaven or Hell . . . it's funny – I am not usually superstitious, I don't normally believe in ghosts or spooks, but when the mood comes on me I *have* to believe.'

Since for two weeks the *status quo* was preserved, her apparitions coming at 8.00 and leaving sharp at 8.10, we continued Miss N. on her dose of L-DOPA; it was apparent, moreover, that she had started to derive a good deal of pleasure from the regular visits, for she would make herself up carefully 'in readiness' each evening. In her sixth week on L-DOPA, the visions assumed a more severe and ominous quality; the two bearded men were joined by a third and fourth and fifth and sixth, until the entire room was crowded with bearded men making supernatural gestures; moreover they would stay past their time, and continue their silent, sinister milling-around till 9.00 or 10.00 or 11.00 at night. At this stage Miss N. agreed that perhaps L-DOPA might be stopped. Her hallucinations continued for three weeks after the withdrawal of L-DOPA and then suddenly stopped: it was remarkably abrupt – one evening Miss N. failed to make herself up after supper and, when we asked why, said: 'There'll be no company this evening.' And, indeed, her 'company' never returned.

We gave Miss N. the remainder of the spring and the entire summer to recover her balance, and in October 1970 we started her on amantadine (an L-DOPA-like drug). And here, as with L-DOPA, there was an initial improvement in voice and movement and rigidity, etc. But after three weeks Miss N. complained of *pruritus vulvae.* We sent her to a gynaecologist, but he could find nothing the matter. Her pruritus then became a formication – a feeling that ants were crawling inside her; Miss N. would shudder all over as she described these symptoms, but would also exhibit unmistakable relish. Finally, the ants became tiny ant-sized men, crawling up her vagina, trying to get inside her. At this point Miss N. became violently agitated, and begged us to stop both the assault and the drug. We stopped the amantadine, but the hallucinatory assault persisted for more than six weeks before it disappeared, quite suddenly, without any warning or slow 'fading-out.'

Thus Miss N.–in her five trials on L-DOPA and her additional trial on an L-DOPA-like drug – showed remarkably different reactions on all six occasions. It was clear that the action of the drug was, in a sense, unpredictable, in that it might call forth a variety of behaviours: given the initial form of behaviour – whether tongue-pulsing, therapeutic, catatonic, ticcy-palilalic, formicatory, or hallucinatory – the rest of the reaction would follow this form. Miss N. showed strikingly little physiological constancy in her reactions to L-DOPA, but a striking dramatic unity in them once they were started. In view of her six so-strangely-mixed but ultimately uncontrollable reactions, we have not given Miss N.

L-DOPA or amantadine again. She has returned to her pleasant, easy-going, good-humoured, and prosaic self. She even 'skipped' her 'Easter Psychosis' in 1971 and 1972 – her first such omission in at least twenty years. She says, 'I have had enough visions and what-not to last me a lifetime.'

IDA T.

Mrs. T. was born in a village in Poland in 1901, had an uneventful childhood, and became a bride at sixteen and a mother at seventeen. In her twentieth year her life was cut across by a double tragedy: the death of her young husband, and the sudden onset of impatience, irritability, impetuosity, increased appetite, and a violent temper – a monstrous transformation of her previous character. The increasing violence and appetite of their bulky daughter was a source of great alarm to her peace-loving and penurious family, who found themselves wondering if a devil had possessed her. In her twenty-first year – when she had trebled her weight and terrorized the entire village – symptoms of a new kind appeared: increasing stiffness and slowness of movement, and other signs of a Parkinsonism which *held in* without diminishing her impulses to violence. At this juncture, her family took medical advice, and decided to ship off their now bomb-like daughter to the fabled doctors in the New World, who would doubtless know how to treat her.

By the end of her four-month transatlantic voyage 'Big Bertha' (as her shipmates had come to call her) had become completely motionless and speechless and stiff as a board, and on her arrival in the New World was at once moved into the newly opened 'Home for the Crippled and Dying.' For the next forty-eight years Mrs T. (or 'Big Bertha,' as the hospital staff too now called

her) continued to lie in Parkinsonian state, rigid, mute, motionless, and glaring, upon her specially reinforced catafalque of a
bed, attended by relays of diminutive nurses. She received no
communication whatever from her family, who had evidently
decided to 'dump' her and to retain possession of her effectively
orphaned, infant daughter. On rare occasions, if in pain or frustrated, Mrs T. would explode and chatter in fury like a maddened
machine-gun. She continued to display a voracious appetite,
which was soon joined by a voracious anality, her only demands
being for enemas or food. She was, however, sensible of attention and kindness, and would occasionally smile to her nurses, or
smackingly kiss them in a manner as explosive as her greeds and
rages. Indeed, all the nurses who came and went were fond of
'Big Bertha' and devotedly looked after her physical needs; she
would never have survived the 1920s without their devoted and
sedulous attentions.

When I first saw Mrs T. in 1966, she was a seal-shaped woman
weighing 400 pounds, entirely bald and covered with sebum.
The back of her head was totally flat, having been moulded from
a half-century of lying supine upon it. Her entire body was immovably rigid, and there were crippling dystonic-dystrophic,
flipper-like deformities of her hands and her feet. (These flipper-
like extremities, combined with her gigantic, greasy, streamlined
bulk, often gave one the curious impression of an enormous
Channel-swimmer 'frozen' miraculously, stroboscopically, in
mid-stroke.) Her eyes were as unblinking and hard and glower-
ing as a basilisk's. She was virtually without movement of any
kind, and even her breath was hardly perceptible. She greatly
resented my presence and questions, answering them with
grunts, expectorations, or spat-out monosyllables. Along with
Miss K., she was at once the most formidable and the most
pathetic human being I had ever seen.

This continued to be her state for the next three years, until
I brought her to our post-encephalitic 'community' and started
her on L-DOPA. I must confess that she refused the L-DOPA when
I asked her about it, and that I had it administered, at first, by
stealth, in her food. I did this after much inner conflict, in which
I was finally swayed by the nurses who had so long attended her,

who felt that there was 'a lovely person' beneath the formidable exterior of 'Big Bertha,' confined and longing to get out. She had no family or friends to say 'yea' or 'nay' for her.

The effects of L-DOPA were remarkably striking and sudden, and came on at a dose-level of 4 gm. a day. The frozen rigidity of her body suddenly 'cracked' and melted to a liquid, free-flowing motion, and her voice became much louder and more fluent, losing much of its explosive-obstructive sputtering-stuttering quality. I was summoned to the ward by an amazed and excited staff-nurse, and when I arrived I found Mrs T. smiling and gesturing and talking to the nurses nineteen-to-the-dozen; to me she said, 'Wonderful, wonderful! I'm moving inside – that dopey's a *Mitzphah* . . . Thank God you had sense to get it inside me!' To celebrate her 'awakening,' Mrs T. announced in a stentorian voice that she wanted a quart of chocolate ice-cream with each meal every day, and 'a big olive-oil enema – but *big!*' morning and evening. In the next three weeks, she talked a great deal to herself in Yiddish, or in guttural English with a strong Yiddish-Polish accent, chuckling and gurgling as she did so: all her talk was of the village where she had grown up as a child. At this time she also took to singing old Yiddish folk-songs and ballads in a sea-captain's rollicking bass – to the fury and amusement of everyone near her. The Sleeping Beauty had assuredly awoken, but as yet in a manner completely regressive and nostalgic; her mouth, her colon, and her past were the only things which mattered to her at the moment. She had yet to allow a *current* relationship.

At this stage I gave Mrs T. a small present, a token, a succulent cactus with a hideous yet beautiful spiny bulbosity. She was charmed with this plant and became immediately devoted to it, tending it and watching it for hours on end. I had the impression that it represented not only her first possession but her first *relation* in her forty-eight years 'underground' at Mount Carmel Hospital.

In the autumn of 1969, Mrs T. started to recognize and appreciate *as a person* a physiotherapist who was with us, who bathed and massaged her hands every day, and who designed special implements for them which she could hold in a pinch-grasp. Before this time, I think, Mrs T. had not clearly distinguished or

differentiated between the nurses who served her, but had regarded and treated them as identical – somewhat as a queen
termite treats her tiny workers. When not with her beloved plant
or physiotherapist, she was still implacably hostile, greedy, suspi-
cious, stubborn, negativistic, belligerent, querulous, and accus-
ing. But the plant and the physiotherapist brought out the best
in her.

The most moving event took place at the end of 1970 when
our social worker – after almost three years of persistent inquiry
– was able to locate her long-lost daughter; her daughter had, in
fact, come to America in the 1930s, but had never attempted to
seek out her mother because the rest of the family had said she
was dead. The reunion was not a simple one – it was a speechless
weighing-up and gazing on both sides, but it was a start; there
were months of disagreements, rages, silences, and quarrels, but
– somehow – by the middle of 1971, a deep mutual relation had
been forged, and each would greet the other with unmixed pleasure. One could see, in these intervening months, how Mrs T.
became humanized from week to week, as she emerged from her
pit of regression, desolation, and unreality. This one good relation was the thread which led the way from the maze of madness,
which drew her forth from the depths of Unbeing.

In the last year there have been some complications from the
continued use of L-DOPA – some return of her rigidity and stuttering, etc. But, all considered, she is still doing incredibly well
considering she was dead for forty-eight years.

FRANK G.

Mr G. was born in 1910, did reasonably at school, and seemed normal in all respects until the age of thirteen when he contracted the sleeping-sickness, and spent nine weeks in a state of deep stupor during which he was totally helpless and had to be tube-fed. When he recovered from this he showed a gross skewing of the right eye outwards and other signs of a third nerve palsy. He also seemed 'queer in the head,' 'sorta strange,' 'not himself any more.' He was unable to continue school, was considered mentally defective, and sent to work in a corrugated-box factory. For the next twenty years Mr G.'s life was monotonous and exemplary. He arrived at the factory on the dot each morning, worked at a steady unvarying rate, left the factory at five each evening, had supper and sat with his parents, went to bed at ten, and got up at six. His behaviour during these twenty years was conventional to the point of stereotypy: he would always greet the same people in the same words each day, make a comment about the weather, and subside into silence; he would read the headlines and a few sub-headings in the papers each day; he had no hobbies, no interests, no friends, and no social or sexual relations at all. He moved like a robot on his dull, undeviating, lifeless course – like a million 'chronic ambulatory schizophrenics' in the streets of America. Two or three times a year he would suddenly fly into a violent rage and attack someone, always an older man, whom he would allege to have been staring at him and trying to seduce him.

In his thirty-fifth year Mr G. found himself unable to maintain his rate of work, having developed a certain slowness of movement and speech. In his thirty-seventh year he was discharged from his job – to join the half-million population of out-of-work Parkinsonians. With the loss of his job Mr G. 'went to pieces,'

and became agitated, depressed, and unable to sleep. The monotonous structure of his life had been shattered, and he walked the
streets, unkempt and dirty, swearing and muttering to himself at
intervals. In this state Mr G. was admitted to a state mental
hospital where he gradually regained something of his former
equability and monotony, and in 1950 was transferred to Mount
Carmel Hospital.

During his twenty years at Mount Carmel Mr G. slowly 'deteriorated' in a number of ways: although he was physically quite
able to look after himself, wander around the hospital, or go out
in the streets, he became increasingly withdrawn and narrowed-
down in the range of his activities with each passing year. He
developed a multitude of fixed rituals and routines, but no real
relationships with anyone or anything. He became prone to stare
and hallucinate for several hours each day, but he kept his hallucinatory experiences to himself and kept them apart from his
behaviour and actions. His attacks of panic and rage became
somewhat commoner and would usually occur two or three times
a month: they were always connected with the feeling of being
slighted or seductively pressured.

In 1969, before he received L-DOPA, Mr G. showed 'flapping
tremor' of both arms, some rigidity and flexion of the neck,
profuse salivation, and bilateral ptosis, his eyelids so drooping
that his eyes were almost closed. His postural reflexes were considerably impaired. He showed mild akinesia, but no rigidity of
the arms. Additionally – quite unusual among the post-encephalitic patients I have seen – Mr G. showed bilateral signs of upper
motorneurone deficit and a mild mental dullness besides his
'queerness.' Finally Mr G. showed a 'humming tic' – a melodious
sound (mmmm ... mmmm ... mmmm ...) with each expiration.

Mr G. was placed on L-DOPA in May 1969, the dose being
gradually increased to 2 gm. a day. In these first three weeks Mr
G. showed exacerbation of his tremor and hurrying of gait as well
as sudden myoclonic jerks and spasms at times. He also showed
an increase of his expiratory humming tic and a tendency to toss,
grunt, and mutter during his sleep.

After a month these effects died away and Mr G. returned to
his previous state. Although continuing on 2 gm. of L-DOPA he

showed *no* reactions to this apparently for the ensuing three months. In October Mr G. developed violent out-thrustings ('propulsions') of the tongue, which was forced out to its roots 12 or 15 times a minute. When after two days of this we suggested stopping L-DOPA, Mr G. said, 'Don't – they'll stop by themselves.' An hour later the tongue pulsions *did* stop, and were never indeed to be seen again. For the ensuing six months Mr G. again reverted to his reactionless state, until in March 1970 he was carried away by a new wave of responses. He seemed to become irritable and touchy, and had a constant feeling that his right cheek was itching; he would scratch this impulsively and repeatedly in a tic-like way, and so violently that he continually caused it to bleed. He also showed an increased libido, spent many hours masturbating, and repeatedly exposed himself in the passage. During this distressed and agitated period Mr G.'s humming tic became a refrain *('tic d'incantation'),* a palilalic verbigeration of the phrase 'keep cool.' During the course of the day Mr G. would murmur 'keep cool, keep cool, keep cool . . .' hundreds if not thousands of times a day.

By May 1970 Mr G.'s exposures and assaults on other patients had become so frequent that the hospital administration threatened to transfer him to a state hospital – a threat which filled him with terror and impotent rage. The day after this threat Mr G. developed an oculogyric crisis combined with catatonia – the first he had ever had in his life: his eyes stared upwards, his neck was retracted with extraordinary violence, and the rest of his body showed statuesque immobility and cataleptic flexibility; he became completely inaccessible to all contact, and also, apparently, unable to swallow. This crisis or stupor lasted for ten days without interruption, during which time Mr G. required tube-feeding and nursing. When he 'came to' at last, he seemed a different man – as if he recognized defeat, and was broken inside. His impulsions and itching and tics and erotic and hostile excitement had all disappeared, and he now moved like a sleep-walker or a man in a dream. He was polite and pleasant and perfectly oriented, but his whole being seemed to be immured in a sort of 'sleep' or swoon; he gave an uncanny impression of being absent-as-a-person, and no longer in the world. He seemed almost disembodied – like a wraith or a ghost.

In August 1971 he died in his sleep. No cause of death was visible at *post mortem*.

MARIA G.

℃ Miss G. was born on a Sicilian farm in 1919, the younger daughter of strict and affectionate, if neurotic, Italian Catholic parents. She seemed intelligent as a child and did well at her school, although she had a reputation for being sprightly and 'fey.' In her eighth year she had a terrible nightmare which seemed to go on all night: she dreamt she had gone mad and been taken to Hell. This was the start of a month-long delirium with fever, hallucinations, and extraordinary movements; she scarcely slept at this time and could not be sedated. As the acute delirium faded away it became evident that a profound change had occurred in her character; for she was now intensely restless and violent and easily enraged, and lewd and impudent and always 'in trouble.' This behaviour was deeply shocking to her God-fearing parents and evoked from them hatred and threats and punishment. Indeed, her mother, speaking of all this to me more than forty years later, said: 'It was a punishment from Heaven because she was so evil. She was a naughty disobedient hateful child, and she deserved her sickness – she deserved all she got.'

By the age of twelve Miss G.'s behaviour had become constrained by a progressive stiffness and slowness of movement, and by the age of fifteen she was deeply Parkinsonian. For the next thirty years her parents – who in the meantime had moved to the United States – kept her in a back room where no one could see her; here she would lie face down on the carpet, sometimes biting it or chewing it with rage; her food would be thrown in like scraps to an animal, although a priest would be brought to see her every Sunday without fail.

In 1967, in view of her parents' increasing age and a heart ailment which was disabling her mother, Miss G. was admitted to Mount Carmel Hospital. At this time I found her profoundly Parkinsonian and catatonic: she showed a divergent squint and an internuclear paresis; salivation, which was exceedingly profuse and viscous; rigidity and akinesia of severe degree; violent 'flapping' tremor of her right hand at times; continual closing and clonus of the eyelids; and an impairment of postural reflexes so profound, that she would sit doubled over with her head on the ground. Her voice was very soft, but impulsive, and scarcely intelligible. She seemed quite intelligent and soon came to recognize everyone around her. Twice a month, she would have an oculogyric crisis, and on rare occasions a most violent rage; during her rages she would be able to rise to her feet and walk and yell and hit with great force; but for most of the time she was totally motionless. This was her state until given L-DOPA.

I started L-DOPA on 18 June 1969. Her response, which occurred at a dose-level of 1.2 gm. a day, was exceedingly swift and dramatic, occurring within hours on one particular day. She experienced a sudden surge of energy and strength, and a complete abolition of all her rigidity. She became able to walk the length of a passage, battling her stooping-tendency by the use of main force; her voice became loud and clear, though hurried, with a tendency to speak in short sentences or phrases; her salivation ceased almost completely; and her mood became joyous with a touch of elation. Her parents were summoned and visited her at once – their first such visit in her two years at hospital: her father embraced her with great gratitude and joy, and her mother exclaimed: 'A miracle from Heaven . . . a completely new person.' There followed a single wonderful week in which Miss G. was transformed in all possible ways. Her mother had bought her a wardrobe of dresses to celebrate her 'rebirth.' Dressed up in her finery, poised and made-up, Miss G. looked beautiful and much

Newspaper headlines from the 1920s indicating the magnitude of the epidemic, and public alarm and horror in response to it.

SLEEPY SICKNESS SPREADING.

FATAL CASES.

HUNT FOR ELUSIVE GERM.

Sleepy sickness continues to spread. New cases now reported as having occurred last week include:

BIRMINGHAM.—13; 5 deaths.

SHEFFIELD.—22; 1 death. Total cases March 10, 217; deaths 26.

d Walters Sinclair, 58, an engin-Greenock, died yesterday from use after a week's illness, and are reported at Donaghmore, far the only cases reported in reland outside Belfast, where 10 deaths have occurred in cases were reported during and one death.

of Mr. C. Bower Ismay, nd sportsman, of Hazel-rthamptonshire, con-grave anxiety. Mr. l 14 weeks ago while and was found un-

PERIL OF THE SLEEPY MICROBE.

EPIDEMIC WORST IN BRITAIN AND ITALY.

RECORD DEATH-ROLL

CHILDREN AMONG THE VICTIMS.

TRAGEDIES OF SLEEPY SICKNESS.

WARPED MINDS AND BROKEN BODIES.

PLEAS FROM VICTIMS

Since *The Daily Mail* published t letter of Mr. E. W. Hore, of Manchest concerning the pathetic case of daughter, who is a sufferer from after-effects of sleepy sickness, we ived a number of letters descri sequences of this dise art-broken

THE MYSTERY MALADY.

Alarming Spread of Sleepy Sickness.

WAR ON SLEEPY SICKNESS.

20,000 CASES LAST YEAR.

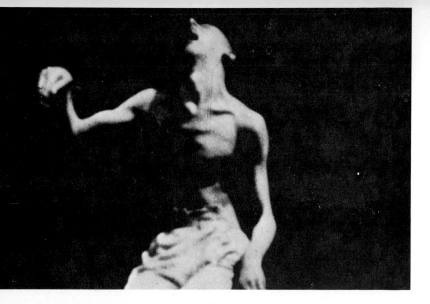

DEADLY AFTER-EFFECTS.

Sleepy sickness is without doubt the most devastating infective disease of modern times. The dreadful nature of this new disease is due not only to its high mortality but also to the very high percentage of victims who, even a year or two after the first attack, are visited with the most distressing after effects. A form of paralysis agitans known as "Parkinsonism" [Parkinson in 1817 first described paralysis agitans] is a common sequel, even in children as young as 10 years of age.

This disease is characterised by a rigidity of the musculature of the body, so that all voluntary movements can only be carried out slowly. The face becomes devoid of expression, and in severe cases even speech is affected. As the condition advances, the unfortunate person, owing to the muscular stiffness, is unable to feed or dress himself, and finally may become bedridden, unable to turn himself without assistance.

Neurasthenia, in its various forms, intractable insomnia, and disturbances in the respiratory mechanism are some of the other sequelæ of the disease, often incapacitating the patient for months or years.

MORAL DEGENERATION.

But even more tragic are the changes in moral character which often follow the disease.

Docile and well-behaved children undergo a mysterious transformation. They become spiteful, untruthful, and unmanageable. They often steal, or make themselves objectionable in a score of wanton and mischievous ways. Unresponsive to any appeal, they sometimes find themselves in court, and unless the nature of their trouble is recognised, may be set on the road to becoming life-long criminals.

Asleep For Three Years

IN THE WORLD AND YET OUT

From Our Own Correspondent

THE tragic case of a man being in the world and yet out of it was described to me yesterday.

This man, workless and homeless, more than three years ago walked into the West Highland Rest Home. He complained of being terribly tired, and it was obvious that his complaint was genuine. He simply could not keep awake.

When the doctor examined him he found the man was suffering from sleepy sickness, and he was put to bed right away. He is still sleeping.

Spoken to no one

"He has spoken to no one during the time," stated Mr. Peter MacDonald, the governor of the home, yesterday, "though in a subconscious way he has managed to take his food.

"In these brief intervals his hand just seems to drift from the bedclothes, as if being guided by some mystic form of propulsion.

"He does not recognise anyone, and after each meal he literally returns to the state of a living corpse. It is truly pitiful. There is no form of bodily decay about him. He is, in fact, putting on flesh.

"No one can tell," added Mr. MacDonald, "when, if ever, he will return to normal life. He is a problem and a vitally interesting one.

"I cannot, for sentimental reasons," said Mr. MacDonald, "allow the patient's name to be published, but the facts concerning him are accurate."

I was subsequently allowed to visit the ward where this strangely silent man is accommodated.

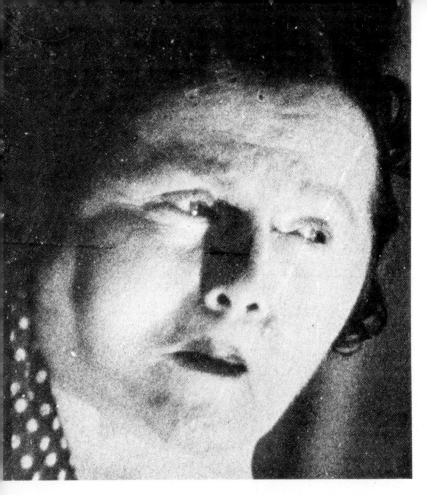

Following the great epidemic, numbers of patients passed into a strange, frozen 'sleep', in which they were transfixed in the endlessly prolonged first moment of their illness. This patient *(above)* had been transfixed in such a timeless entrancement since 1926; when 'awoken' briefly, in 1969, she felt that she was still in 1926 (see Rose R.).

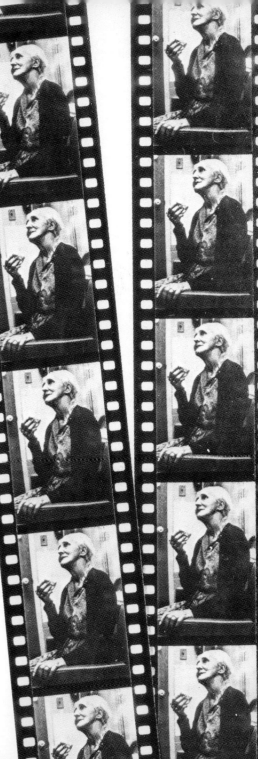

(Right) This patient (Frances M.), shown here, motionless, in a state of frozen expectation, was also 'asleep', although she was sometimes able to walk and talk in a bemused, 'sleep – walking' way. Her expression – unlike Rose R.'s – looked towards the future, in perpetual expectation of a possible awakening. Whereas Rose R. could not bear the modern world suddenly thrust on her by L-DOPA, Frances M. greeted her awakening with gratitude and delight, accepting with good humour the forty years that she had 'lost'.

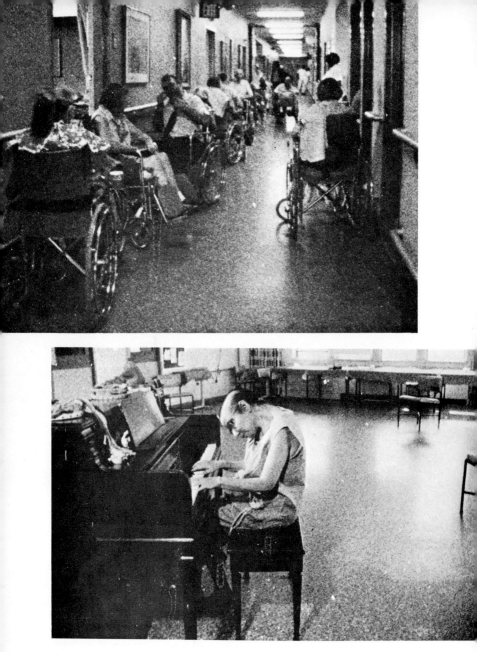

Unhappily, most large institutions are deficient in spaciousness and cosiness: their inmates tend to suffer from confinement and crowdedness, and from emptiness and loneliness.

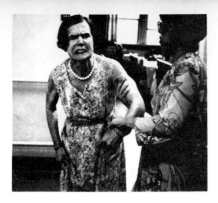

Institutions, insofar as they are *coercive*, aggravate the sickness of their inmates. Here we see one such patient, Margaret A., driven, by the combined effects of disease, L-DOPA and institutionalization, into a state of panic and rage, and into perpetual, compulsive water-drinking. In contrast, both her Parkinsonism and her neuroses all but disappear in more human conditions – for example, in the hospital garden and, above all, when visited by her much-loved sister.

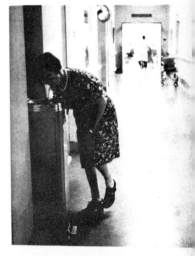

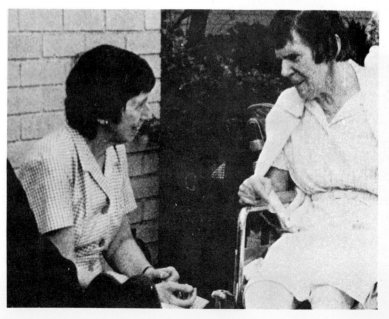

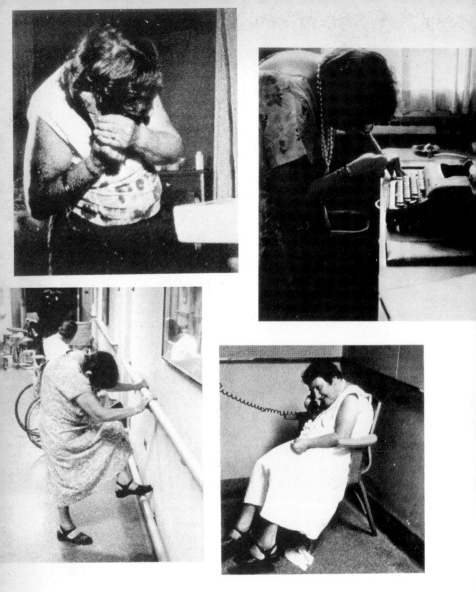

Some patients, however, despite disease, drug and institutionalization, manage to survive as vivid, individual, idiosyncratic people. Here we see one such patient, Hester Y., who had been in a state of virtual standstill for more than twenty years, 'awakened' by L-DOPA: now, alive to her appearance, she is seen doing her hair, despite the recurrence of a partial standstill (after many minutes entirely motionless, she is using her left hand to unlock her 'transfixed' right hand); we see her assiduously exercising her long-frozen limbs, typing her journal, and laughing as she speaks to her daughter on the phone. . .

younger than her age: the nurses now called her 'The Sicilian bombshell.'

In the first week of July various problems appeared. Miss G.'s high spirits turned to violence and mania, and she started to feel that she was being 'seduced' and 'teased'; she felt patients and staff were conspiring to 'get' her, and she was at once thrilled, terrified, and infuriated by the feelings this aroused. The merest glance would call forth a yell or the sudden violent flinging of whatever was to hand. She continually asked me how children were born and whether sex was 'natural' or punished by death. She became intensely anxious about her mother's health and made continual phone calls to home; the question she asked was always the same: 'You feeling OK, mother? You ain't going to die?' and she would weep and shudder after each of these phone calls. By the middle of July her days had become an ontological switch-back of 'ups and downs' – five furies a day followed by exhaustion and contrition. She was exceedingly formidable in these outbursts of fury, and would howl with great force like a maddened gorilla; she would rush down the corridors striking everyone round her, and if there was no one she would hit at the walls. Towards the end of each outburst she would bang her head on the walls and yell: 'Kill me, kill me! I'm bad, I must die!' Tiny doses of Thorazine (Largactil) – a mere 5 mg. – would 'break' these furies within a few minutes, but threw Miss G. into a deeply Parkinsonian, catatonic, and almost stuporous state.

On 16 July I reduced her L-DOPA from 1.2 gm. to 1.0 gm. a day. This immediately acted like a large dose of Thorazine, bringing Miss G. to a Parkinsonian-stuporous standstill. She spent four days in a profoundly disabled and depressed state, far more severe than her pre-DOPA state, and begged me repeatedly to increase her L-DOPA. On 20 July I increased it, infinitesimally, by 0.1 gm. a day. This immediately re-awakened the worst rage we had seen. Miss G. exploded into a murderous-catatonic fury with snarling, screaming, growling and roaring, clawing, scratching, smashing, and hurling; she scowled and glared in a bestial way, and looked like a great carnivore preparing to kill. In this state, she also showed violent out-thrustings of the tongue and a continual tonic protrusion of the lips *('schnauzkrampf')*. Since she seemed unable to speak, I gave her a pencil and paper, but she thrust these into her mouth and chewed them to pieces. After twenty-five hours of continuous fury – unmitigated by stopping her L-DOPA or injections – she collapsed into an exhausted, motionless sleep, curled up like a baby, with her thumb in her mouth. Feeling that Miss G. needed some weeks to 'cool off,' and since I myself was going away for a month, I did not re-start her L-DOPA till my return in September.

On my return, I found Miss G. was still intensely Parkinsonian-catatonic-depressed, immovably imploded in a physiological black hole – a state far worse than her pre-DOPA state, and one which necessitated near-total nursing care. She seemed scarcely alive now without her L-DOPA, but I feared she would become uncontrollably violent again if I re-started the drug. It seemed an impossible choice between impossible alternatives, but I could only try (and hope) for an intermediate state. I started Miss G. back on L-DOPA, therefore, using doses so small we had to make our own capsules. At 100 mg. a day, she showed no response; at 150 mg., 200 mg., and 250 mg. a day, she showed no response; at 300 mg. a day she suddenly 'exploded,' and went super-nova as she had done in the past.

This time her explosion went further than before, and caused her to shatter into behavioural fragments. In the ensuing two months her behaviour lost what unity it had shown before, and broke into innumerable 'sub-behaviours,' each perfectly organized and profoundly regressive – like a schizophrenic process, but deeper and more acute than any I had seen. I felt we had opened a Pandora's box, or disclosed a nest of ontological snakes. And yet it was impossible to stop the L-DOPA, or even to reduce it by the minutest fraction, for her response to this was immediate coma, with depressed respiration and signs of anoxia. I tried this twice, both times with results which could have been fatal. She had lost any state between death and madness; she had lost the *possibility* of any intermediate state once she started over-reacting to L-DOPA.

In these two months, Miss G. became very sensitive, and would shield her food and her possessions with her hands, fearfully and angrily scowling at 'stealers.' She developed an insatiable hoard-

ing urge, and surrounded herself with a miscellany of objects –
torn papers, gnawed candies, and pencils and fruit, the contents
of her handbag, bits of bread, and occasionally faeces – all gathered together in her chair and her bed. She showed lightning-
quick tics and impulsions of gaze, her eyes darting around with
extraordinary speed; frequently her gaze would be 'captured' or
captivated by some object or other which had chanced to enter
its field; flies, in particular, compelled her attention; when her
gaze was caught she would have to make a violent effort of her
entire body to 'release' it. She was continually 'bewitched' by
objects around her, and forced to watch them, or touch them, or
lick them, though at times she could countermand these entice-
ments with 'block.' She showed insatiable appetite and uncontrollable voracity, and after eating would have an irresistible urge to
lick her plate, and to stuff her fingers and the utensils into her
still-chewing mouth. When drinking, her tongue would be violently extended, or she would *lap* with an incredible cat-like
celerity.

She repeatedly complained that she was filthy and shameful,
and was continually picking and brushing her person, her hands
moving separately as if independently controlled. Occasionally,
she would pick at or brush the people around her. At times she
felt the whole world like a goad, or a horde of pestering, picking
impingements, and she would shrink down in her chair and cover
her face, or lie on the floor in a foetal position. Increasingly she
lived in a world of her own, battling with or surrendering to her
own apparitions. Each day she became more narcissistic and regressive, and less prone to react to anything round her. She
developed innumerable strange habits and mannerisms, some of
them so strange as to defeat interpretation, and others which
were plain tokens of self-destruction – biting and kicking herself,
choking and scratching herself, putting her head in an invisible
noose, or laying it flat on an invisible block, pantomimes and
evocations of violence and death. Only in the evenings would her
torments diminish, and a calm would descend on this distracted
woman: at such times she would go back to weaving a basket,
which she had been engaged on for several months, and which

– alone – had been exempt from her rabid destructions. I last saw
Miss G. on the evening of 21 December, calmly weaving her
basket in bed. She was found dead and cold in her bed the next
morning, her rigid arms still clutching her favourite basket.

RACHEL I.

&. Following an attack of *encephalitis lethargica,* Mrs I. developed a progressive Parkinsonian disability which by 1964 had
completely immobilized her with intense rigidity and dystonia of
her trunk and extremities. Her speech, curiously, was an aspect
of function scarcely touched by her otherwise so-engulfing Parkinsonism, and showed that she retained her intelligence, memory, and humour despite having been so long 'walled up' in her
immobilizing syndrome. Twice a month, usually on Sundays, her
condition would be transformed by peculiar attacks in which she
would feel herself flooded by wave upon wave of unlocalizable
pain and anguish which compelled her to scream out in a high
perseverative voice. These attacks, which began and ended quite
suddenly, and had occurred for twenty or more years, had never
been demonstrably associated with any physical disease and were
therefore presumed to be *crises* or 'thalamic attacks' of an unusual
sort. They demonstrated a potential for affective and catatonic
excitement which was inapparent or disguised at all other times.

In the latter part of 1967 Mrs I. started to show a slight senile
deterioration of recent memory although her general intellectual
organization remained quite intact and above normal in quality.
I had several times approached her about the use of L-DOPA, but
she was very fearful regarding its use and would say, 'No, I won't
try it – it'll blow me to pieces.' In September 1970, she changed

her mind, saying, 'I suppose at this stage I have nothing to lose.'

Her reaction to L-DOPA was catastrophic from the start. Ten days after beginning the drug and on a dose of 1 gm. daily, without any therapeutic effect or warning signs whatever Mrs I. *did* 'blow up.' She became intensely excited, deliriously hallucinated, seeing tiny figures and faces all around her, and hearing voices, which suddenly appeared and disappeared in all parts of the room; she also became uncontrollably echolalic, repeating anything one said to her in a shrill screaming voice hundreds or thousands of times in succession. Haunted by hallucinations and echoing indefinitely to external stimuli, Mrs I. gave the impression of a hollow, untenanted, ghost-filled house, as if *she herself* had been 'dispossessed' by echoes and ghosts. Despite stopping L-DOPA immediately, and despite the heaviest possible use of sedatives and tranquillizers, it proved impossible to stop this monstrous excitement. It continued unabated for three weeks, and almost twenty-four hours a day, during which time she had no rest except for short-lived exhausted stupors. During this period she showed a sharp decline in her intellectual status, becoming visibly less able to recognize familiar figures, and less able to create complex hallucinations, with each passing day; it was impossible to avoid the impression that she was being combusted or 'burnt out' by the uninterrupted intensity of her cerebral excitement. In the fourth week the excitement suddenly came to an end and was replaced by a state of coma. This continued for a month, during which time she required total nursing care, tube-feeding, etc. When Mrs I. awoke from her coma she had lost the power to recognize anyone or anything, could make only non-verbal noises, and showed no recognizable signs of mental 'presence' at all. She seemed to have become a complete mental blank, wiped clean of all structure like a terminal dement. She lingered in this mindless and functionally decorticate state for seven weeks before expiring in an attack of pneumonia.

AARON E.[87]

  Mr E. was born in 1907, the elder of fraternal twins. His parents had immigrated to the States a few years before, and at the time of Mr E.'s birth had established a flourishing delicatessen in the right part of Brooklyn. Mr E.'s early life was one of work, seriousness, and laborious self-improvement, delivering newspapers and half a dozen other jobs as a boy and adolescent, and supplementing his education with night classes, public lectures, and long hours spent in the Brooklyn public library. By the age of twenty-three Mr E. had established himself as an up-and-coming accountant, was able to marry and take out a mortgage.

Over the next thirty years Mr E. showed exceptional vigour and enterprise, and was able to expand into a six-man corporation. During these intervening years he enjoyed excellent health and never lost a day's work through illness or 'indisposition.' He was a freemason, a prominent member of the local synagogue, a vice-president of the local school board, and actively interested in civic affairs. He had a large circle of friends and business acquaintants, went to the theatre every Thursday, played golf every Sunday, and went on a camping trip with his wife and five children to the Adirondacks every summer. He was the epitome of the self-made man and the American success story.

It is probable, in retrospect, that his first symptom of Parkinson's disease might have showed itself in his trips to the mountains in situations of unusual exertion or stress. At such times he would occasionally show a tendency to stutter, and an unusual

---

[87] Aaron E. and the following patient (George W.) did *not* have post-encephalitic disorders, but 'ordinary' Parkinson's disease – in Aaron's case sufficiently severe to demand hospitalization, in George's case mild enough to permit a full and independent life outside. Though they differ, radically, from the other patients whose stories I relate, I felt I should include them to show L-DOPA may have profound and complex effects, and even (as in Aaron's case) an absolutely decisive effect, in patients with 'ordinary' Parkinson's disease.

impatience, restlessness, and alacrity of movement; he would also get abnormally tired and find particular difficulty in 'getting going' once he had 'settled down' in his chair. But if these were Parkinsonian symptoms they were unrecognized at the time, and it was only in 1962, in his fifty-sixth year, that Mr E. developed an unmistakably Parkinsonian tremor of the hands and an increasing rigidity of his arms and back. His symptoms were considerably helped by Artane and similar drugs, and he fought them off with his usual vigour, continuing to do a full day's work, maintain his social life, and play golf until 1965.

In 1965, Mr E. felt that everything was becoming too much for him; these feelings had been brewing for more than a year, and had been fought down by him again and again; when they finally broke through, they did so suddenly and explosively. With no warning, and with none of his usual deliberation, Mr E. precipitately announced his retirement from work, his resignation from the local school and synagogue boards, and a great reduction of all his other activities and commitments. He 'renounced' his life as an active man, and almost as a member of society. He now spent the greater part of his time at home, looking at the newspapers and television, and pottering in the garden at the back of the house. He continued to follow the market and keep in touch with his broker, but to a smaller and smaller degree with each passing month, ceasing altogether in 1966. Prematurely retired, and no longer the bread-winner, Mr E.'s status at home very sharply declined; he partly fell from, and partly resigned, his position as paterfamilias and master of the house, letting all major decisions be undertaken by his wife and his sons. He started to show signs of depression, anxiety, dependence, passivity, self-pity, and querulousness – incredible to those who had known him as an active, driving, powerful, and resourceful man only a few years before. His loss of status and general autonomy, and his Parkinsonian symptoms, seemed to play upon and reinforce one another; and by 1967 Mr E. had not only become a complete invalid, but had developed the personality and traits of one.[88]

---

[88] Life changes, powerful emotions, can not only exacerbate, but can *precipitate* Parkinsonism (at least in predisposed individuals; see n. 115, p. 238). When I

In view of his severe disability and depression and dependence, Mr E. was admitted to Mount Carmel Hospital as a private
patient in the summer of 1967. This greatly increased all his
symptoms, Parkinsonian and otherwise; he saw his hospitalization
not as 'a new start' and 'a form of therapy' – as his family and the
hospital brochures suggested – but as a 'putting-away' and a sign
that 'everything was finished' as far as he was concerned. When
I saw him at this time, he showed a picture of Parkinson's disease
which was severe, but could not possibly be mistaken for a post-
encephalitic picture. He exhibited very little spontaneous speech

---

saw Mr E., and heard his story, I was strongly reminded of another patient,
Edward J. Mr J. had been employed in a government office since the age of 21,
was very attached (perhaps without realising it) to his work, and greatly distressed when, at 55, he had to retire (this being the mandatory retirement age
in his office). As he walked back, sadly and for the last time, from his office, he
found that his right arm had lost its swing, and that his right leg was dragging.
His immediate thought was that he had had a stroke, but when he consulted a
neurologist he was told no, that he had Parkinson's disease on this side. 'But
that's impossible!' he cried. 'How can I have Parkinson's? I was playing tennis
with my son last weekend!'

The neurologist seemed surprised, but reiterated, 'Well, you have Parkinson's
now,' and advised that he consult Irving Cooper, the neurosurgeon, regarding
a thalamotomy (the treatment of choice for hemi-Parkinsonism in the early '60s).
Dr Cooper confirmed the diagnosis, and being busy, scheduled surgery for a
date two months ahead. The day before surgery, Mr J. strode into his office,
waved his arms around, skipped, and said, 'My Parkinson's is gone now!'

'Nonsense!' said Dr Cooper, 'You're on my list for tomorrow.'

'Examine me,' said Mr J. 'Decide for yourself.'

Dr Cooper examined him (Mr J.'s story was confirmed by Cooper himself),
could no longer find a trace of Parkinsonism, and took him off the operating list
for the next day.

Mr J. then remained in apparently good health for three years, returning to
part-time employment, and to playing tennis with his son on weekends. Until,
in 1965, an appalling tragedy happened: his wife was killed by a hit-and-run
driver as she returned home, during the great black-out, that autumn. Mr J.
seemed to take the news very well, but the next morning when he woke up he
was drooling, shaking in both arms, and grossly Parkinsonian – and in this state
was admitted to Mount Carmel a month later. He was severely depressed, as well
as Parkinsonian on both sides, when I saw him, and I immediately started him
on antidepressants. With these, and support, and time, his depression lifted, and
with this his Parkinsonism lifted a certain amount too, but it did not disappear
completely, as it had three years previously. (Still later, in 1969, I put him on
L-DOPA.)

This is the most striking case I know of a patient who must be presumed to
have had a latent (or subclinical) Parkinsonism – suddenly pushed into clinical

or movement, although when spoken to he would liven up and talk with a touch of his old animation. He was unable to rise without aid from his chair, to initiate gait, or to walk stably once started, having strong tendencies to 'freezing,' festination, and pulsion. He was thin and haggard, and looked older than his age. His posture was listless and stooped, and his face had a hopeless look under its Parkinsonian mask. He showed moderately severe rigidity in all his limbs, and much shaking of the hands when tired or distressed. He presented the picture of a man who was both severely disabled and broken in spirit, and I could scarcely believe that he had been in full command of a vigorous and varied life only two years before. Mr E. continued in this disabled and defeated state, until he was given L-DOPA.

He was started on L-DOPA in March 1969. The dose was slowly raised to 4.0 gm. a day over a period of three weeks without *apparently* producing any effect. I first discovered that Mr E. was responding to L-DOPA by accident, chancing to go past his room at an unaccustomed time and hearing regular footsteps inside the room. I went in and found Mr E., who had been chairbound since 1966, walking up and down his room, swinging his arms with considerable vigour, and showing an erectness of posture and a brightness of expression completely new to him. When I asked him about these effects he said with some embarrassment: 'Yes! I felt the L-DOPA beginning to work three days ago – it was like a wave of energy and strength sweeping through me. I found I could stand and walk by myself, and that I could do everything I needed for myself – but I was afraid that you would see how well I was and discharge me from hospital . . . you see, I've gotten so used to depending on people and having them take care of my

---

Parkinsonism, first reversibly, by great emotional stress. Such cases are seen, occasionally, by all neurologists, and remained a great puzzle until the advent of PET scanning in the mid-1980s. This is able to directly visualise dopamine levels in the midbrain and basal ganglia, and it has shown that dopamine levels may be reduced in the brain by 30–50% without producing any clinical symptoms; but that if it is reduced still further, to less than 20% of normal, Parkinsonian symptoms promptly appear. Probably Mr J. was in such a borderline situation, with a markedly (but not yet critically) reduced level of brain dopamine, and was pushed 'over the border' by situations of great stress, which led to depletion past the critical point of his already-reduced dopamine.

needs, I've lost all confidence in myself . . . I've got to unlearn the habit of depending, I suppose . . . you'll have to give me time for this, you know.' I reassured Mr E. that I understood his position, and would in no sense hurry him or force him beyond his wishes or capacities.

The requisite dose of L-DOPA (5.5 gm. a day) was achieved after another two weeks and brought about a virtual 'normalization' in every way. Mr E. now talked and walked with perfect facility, and could do everything he wanted: he was no longer detectably Parkinsonian in any way. But he remained very fearful of expanding his so-constricted life, and did much less than his capacities allowed. It took a month before Mr E. plucked up courage to leave his room and walk freely around the hospital; it took four months before Mr E. ventured outside the hospital to walk round the block and look at the world 'outside'; and it was nine months before Mr E. said he felt sufficiently well and confident to return to his home and former style of life. During those nine months he presented a picture of health; he had filled out again, had a good colour, and no longer looked older than his age. Thus, to overcome Mr E.'s Parkinsonism was a matter of days; but to overcome his invalidism and fear and pessimism took all of nine months.

Mr E.'s leaving the hospital and return to his home had a moving and triumphal quality about it; half the hospital turned out to see him off, and the *New York Times* itself published a picture (August 26, 1969); it was the first time in fifty years that a Parkinsonian patient who had entered Mount Carmel had ever left it to return to his home. There followed three pleasant and full months during which Mr E. – still taking 5.0 gm. of L-DOPA a day – resumed a fairly active domestic and social life, seeing friends and neighbours he had turned away from in 1965, gardening a little, playing golf on Sunday, and even discussing the market a bit with his broker. He appeared increasingly confident and tranquil during these first three months at home.

In his thirteenth month on L-DOPA, however, some problems arose, affecting his movements and emotional reactions. He developed sudden flickering movements (chorea), especially severe about the mouth and face, and tending to dance from one muscle

group to another;[89] his actions became rather abrupt and precipitate, and he now started to gesticulate a great deal with his arms
and body when he was speaking (he was not formerly given to
such gestural exuberance). He became impatient and restless; he
became somewhat irritable and inclined to quarrel; he developed
a hectoring and bullying manner, with apprehension and anxiety
beneath. In short, he was now showing a progressive psychomotor excitement induced by L-DOPA. Mr E. tended at this time to
minimize all his symptoms: 'They're nothing,' he would say,
'nothing to speak of . . . I don't mind them, why should anyone
else mind?' And indeed, the choreic and urgent quality of Mr E.'s
behaviour was not in itself a real disability; it prevented him from
nothing that he wished to do; it was far more obvious to others

---

[89] Chorea (literally 'a dance') was rather rare before the advent of L-DOPA,
usually being seen only in the hereditary Huntington's chorea, and the chorea
which sometimes occurred with rheumatic fever ('St Vitus's Dance'). Now
chorea is extremely common, since virtually every patient with Parkinson's
disease placed on L-DOPA develops chorea sooner or later – so much so that some
neurologists have spoken of chorea as 'anti-Parkinsonism.' It is certainly very
striking and convincing to see, in such patients, the interconversions of the two:
the massive hardness and tension of Parkinsonian rigidity transformed to the
softness and fluttering of (anti-Parkinsonian) chorea; particularly dramatic, in
patients with *dystonia musculorum deformans,* is to see a heavy, sluggish, rolling
wave of dystonia break into a fine, sparkling spray or spume of chorea . . . Chorea
is a sort of physiological confetti, and gives the impression of being weightless
and forceless; choreic movements occur 'spontaneously,' requiring neither deliberate effort, nor the convulsive tension which eventuates in tics; they 'happen,'
suddenly, without effort or warning, in a way which suggests a complete absence
of resistance, indeed a complete absence of inertia. One can treat chorea stochas-
tically or statistically, and say that such-and-such an amount is likely to occur in
such-and-such a time; but it is impossible to treat its movements *individually* –
to say *when* or *where* the next movement will occur. Nor is experience of any
use here: one realizes, after a while, that choreic movements are *inherently*
unpredictable in individual terms – one can no more say when and where they
will occur than one can predict this of bubbles in a boiling liquid, or of the
disintegration of atoms in a radioactive substance . . . or other *essentially quantal*
phenomena which can only be quantized in probabilistic terms. We have spoken
earlier of the need for relativistic and quantal models in neurology, and we see
that we do not have to go as 'far out' as the peculiar standstills (considered on
pp. 111–112) to find biological 'macro-quantal' phenomena. Seeing chorea as
a sparkling emission, and Parkinsonism or dystonia as strongly constrained travelling waves; seeing, above all, their interconversions, one enjoys a sort of
double vision, the contrast and complementarity of two basic modes – the
discrete and the continuous, the quantal and the relativistic.

than it was to himself; and it was obviously a state far preferable to his previous Parkinsonian-depressive state. These movements could be reduced only partially by reducing the L-DOPA: thus I found Mr E. best on 4.0 gm. a day; on 4.5 gm. he was far too choreic, and at 3.5 gm. a day he showed reversion to his Parkinsonism. At this stage, therefore, Mr E. had begun to walk a tight-rope of 'normality' with chasms of 'side-effects' to either side.

In the sixteenth month on L-DOPA Mr E. started to develop spontaneous reversions to Parkinsonism, tiredness and depression which were at first infrequent and brief. Within two weeks of their onset these fluctuations had become abrupt, severe, and frequent, and Mr E. started swinging, several times a day, between states of driven excitable chorea and states of intense weariness and Parkinsonism. Finally, the excited choreic states ceased altogether, and Mr E. found himself clenched, without any intermission at all, in an intolerably severe Parkinsonian state – *much* more severe than his pre-DOPA state. Attempts to alter his state by increasing his L-DOPA – the recommended treatment – were entirely useless. Motionless, almost speechless, salivating, intensely rigid, Mr E. was brought back to Mount Carmel Hospital. His return in this state was not only intensely humiliating to himself, but caused a wave of apprehension among the seventy other Parkinsonian patients receiving L-DOPA. They had seen Mr E. leave in triumph, and now they saw his tragic return. I frequently overheard such comments as, 'He was the star patient – he did better than anybody. If *he* gets into such trouble, what'll happen to *us?*'

With Mr E.'s readmission to hospital I stopped his L-DOPA – a withdrawal which caused great weakness and lassitude and apathetic depression, as well as a violent resurgence of Parkinsonian tremor. This acute 'withdrawal syndrome' lessened after two weeks, and Mr E. seemed to return to his pre-DOPA status. With his state apparently stable once more, I restarted him on L-DOPA, hoping for a renewal of his original reaction. This, however, did not occur: Mr E. now showed himself to have become unusually and pathologically sensitive to L-DOPA, so that on a dose of no more than 1.5 gm. a day he immediately redeveloped chorea and swung into the up-and-down cycle which he had shown before, culminating once again in an intense contracted Parkinsonian akinesia. It was therefore necessary to withdraw his L-DOPA again, and I decided to let two months elapse without L-DOPA in the hope of restoring his original reactivity. In October 1970 I started him on L-DOPA for the third time, using the smallest possible doses, and increasing these extremely slowly. This time Mr E. showed a still more inordinate sensitivity to the drug, becoming violently choreic on a dose no greater than 250 mg. a day – less than a twentieth of the dose that he had originally been taking – and for the third time L-DOPA had to be stopped. I therefore decided that six months had to elapse before we tried L-DOPA again.

During these six months Mr E. fell into a peculiar state, completely unlike anything he had ever shown before. He would sit motionless in his wheelchair in the corridor all day with his eyes open but curiously blank; he seemed wholly indifferent to everything around him, and also to his own fate as a person. When I asked him how he felt he would reply, *'Comme ci, comme ça,'* or 'That's the way it goes,' without any expression. He showed no active attention to anything around him, although he registered its happening in a mechanical way. I tried hard to elicit some feeling from Mr E. and failed completely; and he himself said: 'I have no feelings – I've gone dead inside.' During these months Mr E. looked somehow dead, like a ghost or a ghoul or a zombie. He had ceased to convey any feeling of living presence, and had become a mere absence seated in a wheelchair. During this time (March 1971) I tried L-DOPA for the fourth time, and now Mr E. showed no reaction whatever: where he had reacted so intensely six months before to 250 mg. a day, he now showed not a trace of any reaction to 5,000 mg. a day. He said: 'I knew this would happen – I'm burnt out inside. Nothing you can do will make any difference.' I could not help wondering whether he was right, and whether we had indeed in some way totally destroyed his potential for reacting to L-DOPA or to anything else.

In the summer of 1971 Mr E. – who had not been taking L-DOPA or other drugs since the spring – started to look and feel more *alive*, and to show a return of reactions and feelings which had been in abeyance for the previous nine months. In October 1971 I started him on L-DOPA for the fifth time, and his reactions to this have been substantially and moderately successful up to the present time (September 1972). Mr E. has shown nothing to match the marvellous effect seen in 1969; there is never a time when he could be mistaken for 'normal'; he has bouts of chorea and Parkinsonism and depression and occasional festination, and a new symptom – dystonic spasms affecting his neck; but, despite these problems, his overall mobility and mood are obviously much better than they were in the days before L-DOPA. He is able to get around the hospital and look after his own physical needs, for most of the time, and once a month or so he feels up to a weekend at home. He reads the papers and gossips, and takes a very real interest in everything about him. Although his life is constricted and monotonous – as is unfortunately true of so many patients in such institutions – he nevertheless seems to have achieved a real and useful equilibrium over the last ten months, and perhaps he will continue to hold this indefinitely in the future.

GEORGE W.[90]

Mr W. was born in the Bronx in 1913, left school at fourteen, and joined his father in the family laundry business. He married in his early twenties and combined his daily slogging in the laundry with a full family and social life.

In his fiftieth year Mr W. noticed a tendency for his right hand

---

[90] See n. 87, p. 190.

to tremble if he became over-excited or over-tired – a symptom which was initially dismissed by his doctor as a 'nervous tremor.' Two years later, he started to experience some difficulty with quick or fine movements in his hand and found that his handwriting was becoming smaller. Subsequently he developed an overall stiffness of the entire right side of his body.

These and other symptoms were so slowly progressive that when I first saw Mr W. as a private patient – eight years after the onset of his tremor – he was still able to do a full day's work in his sweltering laundry, to drive his car, to walk several blocks, and to look after himself in every way. He did, it was true, show considerable rigidity and akinesia of his right side, and when he walked showed no swing of the right arm and a tendency to drag his right foot; his voice was virtually normal; his face was moderately masked. The only change which had been necessitated by his illness was that Mr W. had had to learn to write with his left hand – he had always, fortunately, been 'ambidextrous.' Although there was no sign of Parkinsonism on the left side of his body, I had the impression that his left arm was a trifle hyperactive, because he seemed to gesticulate a good deal with his arm and showed a tic-like or manneristic tendency to adjust his spectacles every two or three minutes. (When I first saw Mr W., I was uncertain as to whether this over-activity of the left arm was pathological, or whether it was simply a 'compensation' for the deficiency of activity on his right side: his subsequent reactions to L-DOPA showed that its activity was in fact pathological.)

Mr W. had found Artane and similar drugs quite useful since 1965, and was in two minds about the use of L-DOPA when he first came to see me in 1970. 'I hear it's a wonderful drug,' he said. 'They keep calling it a "miracle drug" in the papers. I've often talked with Mrs W. about taking it, but we can't make up our minds. I can still do a full day's work, and almost everything else I want, but things are getting more difficult from one year to another. Maybe I could carry on for another few years . . . Of course, it would be wonderful if I could get back the full use of my right side. But then there are all of these "side-effects" I keep hearing about.'

There was no urgency in the matter, and Mr W. and I postponed any decision about the use of L-DOPA until the summer of 1971. We finally decided to try it after he had shown an excellent reaction to amantadine during April and May of that year. Mr W.'s initial reaction to L-DOPA was rather strange, and consisted of the development of manifest Parkinsonism in his 'normal' left side. This negative reaction disappeared after a few days and was replaced by a remarkable loosening-up and mobilization of his right side – to such an extent, indeed, that Mr W. seemed and felt absolutely normal in all ways in his third week on the drug. In his fourth week on L-DOPA (he was taking at this time 3.5 gm. a day) he developed a distressing restlessness and alacrity which drove him to walk much too fast: 'I'm sort of scared by all this *drive,'* he said at the time. 'I hurry so much I'm practically running – I'm scared I'll get a heart-attack or something. I keep having to tell myself to walk more slowly.' At this time he also developed some chorea, grimacing, irregularity of breathing, stuttering, and periods of exhaustion and rigidity in the middle of each day. At this time we discussed stopping L-DOPA but Mr W. said, 'Let's wait a bit longer – maybe things will settle down and I'll adjust to the stuff.'

Things did settle down and Mr W. did adjust to his L-DOPA. His 'side-effects' disappeared within a month – his dose of L-DOPA remaining unchanged – and he returned once more to a state of complete or apparently complete 'normality.' He is still maintaining this now – more than a year later. But it is normality with a catch to it, as Mr W. and those who know him are fully aware. I have recently (September 1972) had a letter from Mr W. in which he says: '. . . I've been on L-DOPA for fifteen months now. It's amazing stuff but there is a "but" . . . At best I feel completely normal and I can do everything I want. At these times nobody would know there was anything the matter with me . . . but I've become very over-sensitive, and the moment I over-exert myself or over-excite myself, or if

I am worried, or get tired, all the side-effects immediately come back. If anyone even talks about "side-effects," or if I think about them, they also come back. Before I took L-DOPA I had Parkinson's all the time. It was always there and never changed too much. Now I'm OK. I'm *perfect* when everything is going smoothly, but I feel like I'm on a tight-rope, or like a pin trying to balance on its point.[91] If you ask whether L-DOPA is good or bad for me, I'd say it was *both.* It has wonderful effects but there is a hell of a "but" . . .'

---

[91] Many other patients besides George W. use such images to express their sense of an extremely fined-down and precarious balance, an ever-diminishing fulcrum or base, an ever-increasing liability to upset. Such patients, although they appear perfectly normal *when* they are normal, have lost the latitude, the broad base, of true health or stability, and have entered the knife-edged state of *metastability:* they have lost the 'give,' the resilience, the *suppleness* of health, and are now in a state essentially *brittle* – a 'rigid-labile state,' in Goldstein's term. One feels of such patients – and this too is an image frequently voiced by them – that they no longer dwell in a world of gentle slopes and gradients, a secure and familiar terrestrial landscape, but that they have been transported to a sort of nightmare world, a moonscape of fearful pinnacles and precipices, a (literally) *horrid* realm of points and edges . . . We have seen, again and again, how the morbid comes to resemble the mechanical in its lack of intrinsic stability and control. Thus the horrid, punctate, acicular state of metastable patients is extraordinarily evocative of the world which Newton devised, and precisely shares its character, its improbability, and its peculiar perils: '. . . To suppose that all the Particles in an infinite Space should be so accurate poised one among another,' Newton writes, '. . . [were] as hard as to make not one Needle only, but an infinite number of them . . . stand accurately poised upon their Points . . . the Principle . . . is a precarious one' (Newton: second letter to Bentley).

Given this mountainous, precarious landscape, where there is no safe point of equilibrium and stability, it is inevitable that these DOPA-inflamed Parkinsonian patients should be liable to violent crashes and falls. Images of exciting heights and terrible falls (metaphorical perceptions of their precarious states) may haunt or obsess such endangered patients, and be vividly conveyed to all those around them. Thus Lucy K.: 'Look at me, look at me! I can fly like a bird!' and Margaret A.'s 'wonderful flying floating feeling'; but these elevated states are accompanied by indefinable yet intense anxieties – thus Rose R., her jubilation darkened by a shadow from the future, exclaims: 'Things can't last. Something awful is coming!' No patient depicted this more vividly and memorably than Frances D.: 'I'd done a vertical take-off,' she said. 'I'd gone higher and higher on L-DOPA – to an impossible height. I felt I was on a pinnacle a million miles high . . . And then . . . I *crashed* . . . I was buried a million miles deep in the ground.'

CECIL M.[92]

༆ Cecil M. was born in London in 1905, developed the sleep-ing-sickness during the great epidemic, but appeared to have made a complete recovery from this until the onset of Parkin-sonian and other symptoms twenty years later (1940). His initial symptom was megaphonia – a tendency to bellow and raise his voice – which was followed by the development of grunting, and a tendency to clench and grind the teeth. Within a few months of their onset these presenting symptoms disappeared, and were replaced by a Parkinsonian syndrome with impairment of bal-ance, a tendency to backwards-falling, festination, freezing, and predominantly left-sided rigidity and tremor. By 1942, the clini-cal picture had stabilized and was to show no significant changes for the next quarter of a century. Mr M., who was an intelligent and resourceful man, found that he could lead a full life despite his symptoms: he continued to drive to business each day, to lead an active family and social life, and to maintain his many interests, hobbies, and physical activities – especially swimming, of which he was particularly fond, and which allowed a far more fluid and fluent motion than walking.

Mr M. was placed on L-DOPA in 1970. His initial responses may be described in his own words: 'In the early stages it seemed to have given me a new lease of life. I felt exhilarated and rejuvenated. The stiffness went out of my left arm and leg. I could use my left arm to shave and also to type. I could bend down with

---

[92] Cecil M. was *not* an inmate of Mount Carmel, but an outpatient in London. Thus his 'situation' was quite unlike that of the profoundly ill patients who had been 'asleep' at Mount Carmel for decades; on the other hand, it was essentially similar to that of the many thousand post-encephalitic patients all over the world who, despite a certain degree of disability, have been able to lead full, indepen-dent, and essentially normal lives.

ease to do my shoe up. And of course I could walk with complete freedom and enjoy moving about, which is something I dreaded doing before. And the tremor in my left arm almost disappeared.'

On the sixteenth day of taking L-DOPA, when Mr M. was enjoying his new-found mobility and feelings of energy, he started to suffer from a recrudescence of the 'lock-jaw' or *trismus* he had briefly experienced in 1940. Over the next week Mr M.'s trismus became intense and continual, so that he could no longer open his mouth to eat or speak. Concurrently with this he experienced a return and indeed an exacerbation of his Parkinsonian freezing, rigidity, and tremor. At this point he indicated that he wished the L-DOPA to be stopped.

Mr M. has declined any subsequent trials of L-DOPA. He says: 'I have had this condition for more than thirty years and I have learnt to live with it. I know exactly where I am, what I can do, and what I can't do. Things don't change from day to day – or at least they didn't change till I was given L-DOPA. Its effect was very pleasant at first, but then it turned out more trouble than it was worth. I can get along perfectly well without it – why should I try L-DOPA again?'

LEONARD L.

☙ I first saw Leonard L. in the spring of 1966. At this time Mr L. was in his forty-sixth year, completely speechless and completely without voluntary motion except for minute movements of the right hand. With these he could spell out messages on a small letter-board – this had been his only mode of communication for fifteen years and continued to be his only mode of communication until he was given L-DOPA in the spring of 1969.

Despite his almost incredible degree of immobility and disability, Mr L. was an avid reader (the pages had to be turned by someone else), the librarian at the hospital, and the producer of a stream of brilliant book reviews which appeared in the hospital magazine every month. It was obvious to me, from my first meeting with Mr L. – and this impression was reinforced by all my subsequent meetings with him – that this was a man of most unusual intelligence, cultivation, and sophistication; a man who seemed to have an almost total recall for whatever he had read, thought, or experienced; and, not least, a man with an introspective and investigative passion which exceeded that of almost any patient I had ever seen. This combination of the profoundest disease with the acutest investigative intelligence made Mr L. an 'ideal' patient, so to speak, and in the six and a half years I have known him he has taught me more about Parkinsonism, post-encephalitic illness, suffering, and human nature than all the rest of my patients combined. Mr L. deserves a book to himself, but I must here confine myself to the barest and most inadequate outline of his state, before, during, and after the use of L-DOPA.

The picture which Mr L. presented in 1966 had not changed since his admission to the hospital, and indeed he himself – like so many other 'mummified' post-encephalitic patients – seemed a good deal younger than his chronological age: in particular he had the unlined face of a man in his twenties. He showed extreme rigidity of his neck, trunk, and limbs and marked dystrophic changes in his hands, which were no larger than those of a child; his face was profoundly masked, but when it broke into a smile the smile remained for minutes or hours – like the smile of the Cheshire Cat; he was totally voiceless except at times of unusual excitement when he could yell or bellow with considerable force. He suffered from frequent 'micro-crises' – upturnings of the eyeballs, associated with transient inability to move or respond; these lasted a few seconds only, and occurred dozens, and sometimes hundreds, of times a day. His eye movements, as he read, or glanced about his surroundings, were rapid and sure, and gave the only external clue to the alert and attentive intelligence imprisoned within his motionless body.

At the end of my first meeting with Leonard L. I said to him:

'What's it like being the way you are? What would you compare it to?' He spelt out the following answer: 'Caged. Deprived. Like Rilke's "Panther."'[93] And then he swept his eyes around the ward and spelt out: 'This is a human zoo.' Again and again, with his penetrating descriptions, his imaginative metaphors, or his great stock of poetic images, Mr L. would try to evoke the nature of his own being and experience. 'There's an awful presence,' he once tapped out, 'and an awful absence. The presence is a mixture of nagging and pushing and pressure, with being held back and constrained and stopped – I often call it "the goad and halter." The absence is a terrible isolation and coldness and shrinking – more than you can imagine, Dr Sacks, much more than anybody who isn't this way can possibly imagine – a bottomless darkness and unreality.' Mr L. was fond of tapping out, or voicelessly murmuring – in a sort of soliloquy – passages from Dante or T. S. Eliot, especially the lines:

> Descend lower, descend only
> Into the world of perpetual solitude,
> World not world, but that which is not world,
> Internal darkness, deprivation
> And destitution of all property,
> Desiccation of the world of sense,
> Inoperancy of the world of spirit . . .

'At other times,' Mr L. would tap out, 'there's none of this sense of pushing or active taking-away, but a sort of total calmless, a nothingness, which is by no means unpleasant. It's a let-up from the torture. On the other hand, it's something like death. At these times I feel I've been castrated by my illness, and relieved from all the longings other people have.' And when he was in *these*

---

93   Sein Blick ist vom Vorübergehn der Stäbe
          So müd geworden, dass er nichts mehr hält.
          Ihm ist, als ob es tausend Stäbe gäbe
          Und hinter tausend Stäben keine Welt.

(His gaze from going through the bars has grown so weary that it can take in nothing more. For him it is as though there were a thousand bars, and behind the thousand bars no world.)

moods Mr L. would think of Abelard, and would tap out or murmur:

> For thee the fates, severely kind, ordain
> A cool suspense from pleasure and from pain,
> Thy life a long, dead calm of fix'd repose;
> No pulse that riots, and no blood that glows.
> Still as the sea, 'ere winds were taught to blow,
> Or moving spirit bade the waters flow.

At other times, Mr L. would describe for me states of perception and being to which he was frequently prone, both in his waking and his dreaming states – states which I have elsewhere called dynamic vision, and kinematic-mosaic vision.[94] My knowledge of such states, as they occur in post-encephalitic patients, has been especially derived from Mr L., who is so articulate, and from other patients (particularly Hester Y. and Rose R. as well as other patients whose histories are not given here), who frequently experienced such states without having Mr L.'s passion and power to describe them.

It was only very gradually, over the following years, with Mr L.'s help and that of his devoted mother – who was continually with him – that I was able to form any adequate picture of his state of mind and being, and the way in which this had developed in the preceding years. Mr L. had shown precocity and withdrawal from his earliest years, and these had become much accentuated with the death of his father when he was six. By the age of ten he would often say: 'I want to spend my life reading and writing. I want to bury myself among books. One can't trust human beings in the least.' In his early adolescent years Leonard L. was indeed continually buried in books, and had few or no friends, and indulged in none of the sexual, social, or other activities common to boys of his age. At the age of fifteen his right hand started to become stiff, weak, pale, and shrunken: these symp-

---

[94] Such states may also occur in other intoxications induced by belladonna, LSD, etc., in psychoses, and especially during migraine attacks: see Ch. 3 in my book *Migraine*.

toms – which were the first signs of his post-encephalitic disease – were interpreted by him as a punishment for masturbation and for blasphemous thoughts; he would often murmur to himself the words of the 137th psalm ('If I forget thee, O Jerusalem, let my right hand forget its cunning') and 'If thy right hand offend thee cut it off.' He was reinforced in these morbid phantasies by the attitude of his mother who also saw his illness as a punishment for sin (compare Maria G.). Despite the gradual spread and progression of his disability, Leonard L. was able to go to Harvard and to graduate with honours, and had almost finished a thesis for his Ph.D. – in his twenty-seventh year – when his disability become so severe as to bring his studies and activities to a total halt. After leaving Harvard, he spent three years at home; and at the age of thirty, almost totally petrified, he was admitted to Mount Carmel Hospital. On his admission he was at once given charge of the hospital library. He could do little but read, and he *did* nothing but read. He indeed became buried in books from this time on, and thus, in a sense, achieved a dreadful fulfilment of his childhood wish.

In the years before I gave him L-DOPA I had many conversations with Leonard L., conversations which were necessarily somewhat one-sided and cursory since he could only answer my questions by painfully tapping out answers on his spelling-board – and his answers tended to assume an abbreviated, telegraphic, and sometimes cryptic form. When I asked him how he felt he would usually tap out 'meek,' but he would also intimate that he sometimes had a sense of intense violence and power which was 'locked up' inside him, and which he experienced only in dreams. 'I have no exit,' he would tap out. 'I am trapped in myself. This stupid body is a prison with windows but no doors.' Although for much of the time, and in many ways, Mr L. hated himself, his disease, and the world, he also had a great and unusual capacity for love. This was especially apparent in his reading and his reviewing, which showed a vital, humorous, and at times Rabelaisian relish for the world. And it was sometimes evident in his reaction to himself when he would spell out: 'I am what I am. I am part of the world. My disease and deformity are part of the world. They are beautiful in a way like a dwarf or a toad. It's my destiny to be a sort of grotesque.'

There existed an intense and mutual dependence between Mr L. and his mother, who came to the hospital to look after him for ten hours a day – a looking-after which included attention to his most intimate physical needs. One could see, when his mother was changing his nappies or bib, a look of blissful baby-like contentment on Mr L.'s face, admixed with impotent resentment at his degraded, infantilized, and dependent state. His mother, similarly, showed and expressed a mixture of pleasure with her life-giving, loving, and mothering role, admixed with intense resentment at the way in which her life was being 'sacrificed' to her grown-up but helpless 'parasite' of a son. (Compare the relationship of Lucy K. and her mother.) Both Mr L. and his mother expressed uncertainty and ambivalence about the use of L-DOPA; both of them had read about it, but neither had actually seen its effects. Mr L. was the first patient in Mount Carmel whom I put on L-DOPA.

Course on L-DOPA

L-DOPA was started in early March 1969 and raised by degrees to 5.0 gm. a day. Little effect was seen for two weeks, and then a sudden 'conversion' took place. The rigidity vanished from all his limbs, and he felt filled with an access of energy and power; he became able to write and type once again, to rise from his chair, to walk with some assistance, and to speak in a loud and clear voice – none of which had been possible since his twenty-fifth year. In the latter part of March, Mr L. enjoyed a mobility, a health, and a happiness which he had not known in thirty years. Everything about him filled him with delight: he was like a man who had awoken from a nightmare or a serious illness, or a man released from entombment or prison, who is suddenly intoxicated with the sense and beauty of everything round him. During these two weeks, Mr L. was drunk on reality – on sensations and feelings and relations which had been cut off from him, or distorted, for many decades. He loved going out in the hospital garden: he would touch the flowers and leaves with astonished delight, and sometimes kiss them or press them to his lips. He suddenly desired to see the night-city of New York, which (although so close to) he had not seen, or wanted to see, in twenty years: and on his return from these night-drives he was almost breathless with delight, as if New York were a jewel or the New Jerusalem. He read the 'Paradiso' now – during the previous twenty years he had never got beyond 'Inferno' or 'Purgatorio' – with tears of joy on his face: 'I feel saved,' he would say, 'resurrected, re-born. I feel a sense of health amounting to Grace . . . I feel like a man in love. I have broken through the barriers which cut me off from love.' The predominant feelings at this time were feelings of freedom, openness, and exchange with the world; of a lyrical appreciation of a real world, undistorted by phantasy, and suddenly revealed; of delight and satiety with self and the world – 'I have been hungry and yearning all my life,' said Mr L., 'and now I am full. Appeased. Satisfied. I want nothing more.' He experienced a vanishing of hostility, anxiety, tensions, and meanness – and in their place felt a sense of ease, of harmony and safety, of friendship and kinship with everything and everyone which he had never in his life experienced before – 'not even before the Parkinsonism,' as he was the first to admit. The diary which he started to keep at this time was full of expressions of amazement and gratitude. *'Exaltavit humiles!'* he wrote on each page: and other exclamations like 'For *this* it was worth it, my life of disease,' 'L-DOPA is a *blessed* drug, it has given me back the possibility of life. It has opened me out where I was clammed tight-shut before,' and 'If everyone felt as good as I do, nobody would think of quarrelling or wars. Nobody would think of domination or possession. They would simply enjoy themselves and each other. They would realize that Heaven was right here down on earth.'

In April, intimations of trouble appeared. Mr L.'s abundance of health and energy – of 'grace' as he called it – became *too* abundant and started to assume an extravagant, maniacal and grandiose form; at the same time a variety of odd movements and other phenomena made their initial appearance. His sense of harmony and ease and effortless control was replaced by a sense of *too-muchness,* of force and pressure, and a pulling-apart – a pathological driving and fragmentation which increased, obviously and visibly, with each passing day. Mr L. passed from his sense of delight with existing reality, to a peremptory sense of mission and fate: he started to feel himself a Messiah, or the Son of God; he now 'saw' that the world was 'polluted' with innumerable devils, and that he – Leonard L. – had been 'called on' to do battle with them. He wrote in his diary: 'I have Risen. I am still Rising. From the Ashes of Defeat to the Glory of Greatness. *Now* I must Go Out and Speak to the World.' He started to address groups of patients in the corridors of the hospital; to write a flood of letters to newspapers, congressmen, and the White House itself;[95] and he implored us to set up a sort of evangelical lecture-tour, so that he could exhibit himself all over the States, and proclaim the Gospel of Life according to L-DOPA.

Where, in April, he had had a marvellous sense of ease and satisfaction he now became uneasy and dissatisfied, and increasingly filled with painful, unsatisfiable appetites and desires. His hungers became transmogrified into insatiable passions and greeds. He ascended to heights of longing and phantasy which no reality could have met – least of all the grim and confining reality of a Total Institution, an asylum for the dilapidated and dying,[96] or – as he himself had described it three years earlier – a 'human zoo.' The most intense and the most thwarted of these yearnings were of a sexual nature, allied with desires for power and possession. No longer satisfied with the pastoral and innocent kissing of flowers, he wanted to touch and kiss all the nurses on the ward – and in his attempts to do so was rebuffed, at first with smiles and jokes and good humour, and then with increasing asperity and anger. Very rapidly, in May, relationships became strained, and Mr L. passed from a gentle amorousness to an

---

[95] Mr L. never actually sent out any of these letters, and spoke with irony of himself as 'a Parkinsonian Herzog.'

[96] The hospital was, in fact, originally called 'The Mount Carmel Home for the Crippled and Dying,' and despite having changed its lugubrious name, necessarily retained some of its original character.

enraged and thwarted erotomania.[97] Early in May he asked me if I could arrange for various nurses and nursing aides to 'service' him at night, and suggested – as an alternative – that a brothel-service be set up to meet the needs and the hungers of DOPA-charged patients.

By mid-May, Mr L. had become thoroughly 'charged up,' in his own words, 'charged and super-charged' with a great surplus, a great *pressure,* of libidinous and aggressive feelings, with an avidity and voracity which could take many forms. In his phantasies, in his notebooks, and in his dreams, his image of himself was no longer that of the meek and mild and melancholy one, but of a burly caveman equipped with an invincible club and an invincible phallus; a Dionysiac god packed with virility and power; a wild, wonderful, ravening man-beast who combined kingly, artistic, and genital omnipotence. 'With L-DOPA in my blood,' he wrote at this time, 'there's nothing in the world I can't do if I want. L-DOPA is power and irresistible force. L-DOPA is wanton, egotistical power. L-DOPA has given me the power I craved. I have been waiting for L-DOPA for the

---

[97] Such a suppression of sexuality, indeed, is all too common in asylums and institutions, and could have serious repercussions even in patients who were in a less extreme position than Leonard L. Two post-encephalitic patients, Maurice P. and Ed M., were both admitted in the same week in 1971. Both were relatively young, still in their forties, both had been married, both had recently been divorced by their wives. Both were overwhelmed by the calamity of events, and – like Miron V. – immediately became psychotic on admission. Both were placed on L-DOPA, and went through the spectacular drama of 'awakening' and 'tribulation.' But here their stories diverged completely. Ed achieved a clean separation, marked by affectionate understanding and lack of neurosis; liberated by this, remobilized and re-energized by L-DOPA, he found a happy sexual relationship outside the hospital, and a subsequent happy marriage inside the hospital. Finding love, finding work (he discovered a talent for drawing, and soon became the hospital artist), finding *himself,* he found 'accommodation' of a most spacious kind, and has held it now for more than eight years, despite the severest post-encephalitic disease. Maurice, unhappily, though also a man of charm and parts, never achieved a clean separation from his wife; the two remain linked in obsessive mutual torture. Neither has he found work or friends. He is not 'permitted' any 'accommodation,' any freedom, and remains trapped in a torturing sexual neurosis, punctuated by bouts of violent masturbation and near-rape. At such times, like Leonard, he cries, 'Take away the DOPA – I'd sooner be dead than tortured like this.'

past thirty years.'[98] Driven at this time by libidinal force, he started to masturbate – fiercely, freely, and with little concealment – for hours each day. At times his voracity took other forms – hunger and thirst, and licking and lapping, biting and chewing, and sucking his tongue – all of which stimulated him and yielded something very similar to sexual pleasure (compare Margaret A., Rolando P., Maria G., *et al.*).

Coinciding with this surge of general excitement, Mr L. showed innumerable 'awakenings' and specific excitements – particular forms of urge and push, repetition, compulsion, suggestion, and perseveration. He started to talk with great speed, and to repeat words and phrases again and again (palilalia). He continually seized and held different objects with his eyes, and would be unable to relinquish his gaze voluntarily. He showed urges to pant and to clap his hands, and once he had started to do either of these he was unable to stop, but proceeded with continually increasing violence and speed until a sort of clench or freezing set in: these frenzied crescendos – a catatonic equivalent of Parkinsonian hurry and festination – yielded 'a surge of excitement, just like an orgasm.' In the latter half of May, reading became difficult because of uncontrollable hurry and perseveration: once he had started to read he would read faster and faster without regard for the sense or syntax, and unable to stop this festinant reading he would have to shut the book with a snap after each sentence or paragraph, so that he could digest its sense before rushing ahead. Tics appeared at this time, and grew more numerous daily: sudden impulsions and tics of the eyes, grimaces, cluckings, and lightning-quick scratchings. Finding himself distracted and decomposed by this increasing furor and fragmentation, Mr L. made his final effort at control, and decided – at the start of June – on an act of supreme coherence and catharsis – the writing of an autobiography: 'It'll bring me together,' he said; 'it'll cast out the devils. It'll bring everything into the full light of day.'

Using his shrunken, dystrophic index-fingers, Mr L. typed out an autobiography 50,000 words in length, in the first three weeks

---

[98] Compare the sentiments expressed by Freud about cocaine quoted in the Appendix: 'Miracle' Drugs: Freud, William James, and Havelock Ellis, p. 323.

of June.[99] He typed almost ceaselessly – twelve or fifteen hours a day, and *when* he typed he indeed 'came together,' and found himself free from his tics and distractions, from the pressures which were driving and shivering his being; when he left the typewriter, the frantic, driven, ticcing palilalia would immediately assert its hegemony again.

During this writing, Mr L. felt a returning sense of strength and freedom, and a need of absolute solitude and concentration. He said to his mother at this time: 'Why don't you take off for a week or a month, go to Florida maybe – you could do with a rest. I'm independent now – I won't need you so much. I can do everything I want for myself right now.' His mother was greatly disturbed by these sentiments, and now showed how much *she* was in need of their relationship of symbiosis and dependence. She became greatly agitated, and came to me and to others several times at this period, saying that we had 'taken away' her son, and that she couldn't go on unless he were 'restored' to her: 'I can't bear Len, the way he is at the moment,' she said, 'the way he's so active and full of decision. He has pushed me away. He only thinks of himself. I need to be needed – it's the main need I have. Len's been my baby for the last thirty years, and you've taken him away with your darned El-Dopey!'[100]

In the last week of June, and throughout July, Mr L. returned

---

[99] Mr L.'s autobiography is a remarkable document, unique of its kind. Its style and content clearly show the conflicts which were raging in Mr L. at this time. For the most part, he shows an extraordinary humour, detachment, and passion for accuracy, and provides penetrating and moving descriptions of his early years, the development of his illness, and his reactions to this, his fellow patients at the home they all shared, his reactions to L-DOPA, his feeling towards the drug, towards me, and towards others. It is *also* interlarded with waves and floods of sexual phantasy, jokes, pseudo-reminiscences, etc., which would rise up and engulf him from time to time; some of these are conflated with carnivorous and cannibalistic phantasies, with thoughts of raw meat to satisfy his needs.

[100] Mrs L.'s attitude was not uncommon among relatives of our invalid patients. The restoration of activity and independence was by no means always welcomed by some of these relatives, and was sometimes passively or actively opposed. Some of these relatives had built their own lives around the illnesses of the patients, and – unconsciously, at least – did everything they could to reinforce the illness and dependence ensuing. One sees such social and familial reinforcement of illness in neurotic and schizophrenic families, of course, and quite commonly also in migrainous families.

to his violently frenzied and fragmented state, and now this passed beyond all bounds of control, and brought into action ultimate physiological safeguards which in themselves were highly distressing or disabling.

His sexual and hostile phantasies now assumed hallucinatory form, and he had frequent voluptuous and demoniac visions, and erotic dreams and nightmares each night.

At first, Mr L. ingeniously controlled these hallucinations by confining them to the blank screen of his television set or a picture which hung on the wall opposite his bed. The latter – an old picture of a Western shanty-town – would 'come to life' when Mr L. gazed at it; cowboys on horses would gallop through the streets, and voluptuous whores would emerge from the bars. The screen of the television set was 'reserved' for the production of grinning and leering demoniac faces. Later in July, this 'controlled' hallucinosis (which had some analogies to that of Martha N. and Gertie C.) broke down, and his hallucinations 'escaped' from the picture and screen, and spread irresistibly in his whole mind and being.[101] His tics, his palilalia, his frenzies increased.

---

[101] Leonard L. had, in fact, been hallucinating for years – long before he ever received L-DOPA (although he was unable or unwilling to admit this to me until 1969). Being particularly fond of 'Western' scenes and films, Leonard L. had, indeed, ordered the old painting of the shanty-town as long ago as 1955 *for the sole and express purpose of hallucinating with it* – and it was his custom to 'animate' it for a hallucinatory matinée after lunch every day. It was only when he was maddened by L-DOPA that this chronic (and comic) and benign hallucinosis escaped from his will and imaginative control, and assumed a frankly psychotic character.

Those who hallucinate are, not unnaturally, usually reticent about their 'visions' and 'voices,' etc., for fear that they will be regarded as eccentric or mad; and this was equally true of the large population of post-encephalitic patients resident at Mount Carmel. Moreover these patients also had, of course, very great physical difficulties in communication. It has taken many years for these patients to trust me, to *entrust* me with some of their most intimate experiences and feelings; and thus it is only *now* (in 1974), after we have known each other for almost a decade, that I find myself in a position to make a double observation: first, that at least a third, and possibly a majority, of the deeply disabled and longest-institutionalized patients are 'chronic hallucinators'; and secondly, that in most cases it would be quite incorrect to use the term 'schizophrenic' of either the patients or their hallucinations. My reasons for saying this are, in essence, as follows: that most of the patients' hallucinations lack the ambivalent, often paranoiac, and in general uncontrollable nature of schizophrenic hallucinations; but that they are, in con-

His speech became broken by sudden intrusions and cross-associations of thought, and by repeated punning and clanging and rhyming. He started to experience forms of motor and thought 'blocking' very similar to those of Rose R. and Margaret A.: at such times he would suddenly call out, 'Dr Sacks! Dr Sacks! I want . . .', but be unable to complete what he wished to say; the same block was also manifest in his letters to me, which were full of violent, exclamatory starts (usually my name, followed by two or three words – in one such letter, impotently repeated twenty-three times) followed by sudden haltings and blocks. And in his walking and movements such blocks were apparent, which suddenly arrested him in mid-motor stream: he seemed, at such times, to be in collision with an invisible wall.

This period also saw the onset and progress of rapid exhaustions or reversals of response – an up-or-down or 'yo-yo' reaction essentially similar to those shown by Hester Y., Margaret A., Maria G., Rolando P., and many of our other most severely affected patients. At such times, Mr L. would pass within minutes (and as his oscillations grew more severe, within seconds) from an intensely aroused and excited state to one of profound exhaustion, associated with severe recrudescence of Parkinsonian and catatonic immobility and rigidity. These switches (of reaction between agitated-manic-ticcy-akathisia and exhausted-depressed-Parkinsonian-akinesia) took place with continually increasing frequency and suddenness – at first related to the times of L-DOPA administration, and controllable to some extent by the times and

---

trast, very like scenes of normal life, very much like that healthy reality from which these pathetic patients have been cut off for years (by illness, institutionalization, isolation, etc.). The function (and form) of schizophrenic hallucinations, in general, has to do with the *denial of reality;* whereas the function (and form) of the benign hallucinations seen in Mount Carmel has to do with *creating reality,* imagining a full and happy and healthy life of a sort which has been cruelly denied to them through Fate. Thus I regard it as a sign of these patients' health, of their enduring wish to live, and live fully – if only in the realms of imagination and hallucination, which are the only realms where they still enjoy freedom – that they hallucinate all the richness and drama and fullness of life. They hallucinate to *survive* – as do subjects exposed to extreme sensory, motor, or social isolation; and for this reason, whenever I learn from such a patient that he constructs a rich and benign hallucinatory 'life,' I encourage him to the full, as I encourage all creative endeavours which reach out to life.

the dosage: but then 'spontaneously,' without any reference to dosage or times. During this period his total daily intake of L-DOPA was reduced from 5 gm. to 0.75 gm. a day, without making the least difference to his pattern of reaction; at this time also we followed the Cotzias schedule of giving him his L-DOPA in small frequent doses – we even tried him on hourly doses of the drug; but this also made no difference to his rapid and violent oscillations of response. All his reactions had become all-or-none. The 'middle-ground' of health, temper, harmony, moderation had almost entirely disappeared at this time, and Mr L. became completely 'decomposed' into pathological immoderations of every sort.

We could only guess at the relative importance of various determinants in this catastrophic reaction – the possibility of L-DOPA accumulating within him; a 'functional' conflagration, whereby one form of excitement led to another; the inevitability of exhaustions or 'crashes' given such stimulation; the lack of real absorbing occupation, or effective catharsis, with the finishing of his book; the deteriorating relationship between him and the nursing staff; or the implicit (if not explicit) demand by his mother for him to be sick and dependent, and her disapproval or 'veto' of any improvement. It seemed likely that *all* of these factors – as well as others which we could not formulate – were playing some part in determining his reactions.

The closing scene of this so-mixed summer was precipitated by institutional disapproval of Mr L.'s ravening libido, the threats and condemnations which this brought down on him, and his final, cruel removal to a 'punishment cell' – a tiny three-bedded room containing two dying and dilapidated terminal dements. Deprived of his own room and all his belongings, deprived of his identity and status in our post-encephalitic community, degraded to the physical and moral depths of the hospital, Mr L. fell into suicidal depression and infernal psychosis.[102]

---

[102] I thought at this time, and still think, that among the important non-pharmacological determinants of the reactions of these patients to L-DOPA – and especially the form and severity of their 'side-effects' after a period of enormous improvement – the repressive and censorious character of the institution they found themselves in played a considerable part. In particular, the hospital admin-

During this dreadful period at the close of July, Mr L. became obsessed with notions of torture, death, and castration. He felt the room was a network of 'snares'; that there were 'ropes' in his belly which were trying to strangle him; that a gibbet had been set up, outside his room, for his impending and deserved execution for 'sin.' He felt that he was going to burst open, and that the world was coming to an end. He twice injured his penis, and once tried to suffocate himself by burying his head in his pillow.

We stopped his L-DOPA towards the end of July. His psychoses and tics continued for another three days, of their own momentum, and then suddenly came to a stop. Mr L. reverted during August to his original motionless state.

During August he scarcely moved or spoke at all – he had been returned to his original room – but reflected deeply on the preceding few weeks. In September he 'opened up' again to me, tapping his thoughts on his original letter-board. 'The summer was great and extraordinary,' he said (paraphrasing, as he was prone to, a poem of Rilke's),[103] 'but whatever happened then will not happen again. I thought I could make a life and a place for myself. I failed, and now I am content to be as I am; a *little*

---

istration frowned upon any manifestations of sexuality among the inmates and often treated this with an irrational and cruel severity. Leonard L., Rolando P., Frank G. and many other patients were, I think, driven at times into depressive or paranoid psychoses by the combination of a DOPA-induced libidinous arousal and its frustration or punishment by the conditions and policies of institutional life. If, as Mr L. suggested, some mode of sexual release had been provided or permitted, the effects of L-DOPA might – perhaps – have been less malignant.

A further factor, which doubtless added to Mr L.'s sexual drives and their guilty moral recoil, was the too-close relation between him and his mother. His mother – who, in a sense, was herself in love with her son, as he was with her – became indignant and jealous of Mr L.'s new thoughts: 'It's ridiculous,' she spluttered. 'A grown man like him! He was so *nice minded* before – never spoke about sex, never looked at girls, never seemed to think about the matter at all . . . I have sacrificed my life for Len: I am the one he should constantly think of; but now all he thinks of is those *girls!*' On two occasions, Mr L.'s thwarted sexuality became incestuous in direction, which outraged (but also titillated) his ambivalent mother. Once she confided to me that 'Len was trying to *paw* me today; he made the most horrible suggestions. *He said the worst thing in the world* – Bless him,' and she blushed and giggled as she said this to me.

[103] Der Sommer war sehr gros.
Wer jetzt kein Haus hat, baut sich keines mehr.

better perhaps, but no more of – all that.' At his request, then, I restarted Mr L. on L-DOPA in September 1969. He now showed the most extraordinary sensitivity to it – reacting strongly to a total dose of 50 mg. a day, where he had originally required 5,000 mg. a day. His response now was *entirely* pathological; he showed not a trace of therapeutic response, simply tics and tension and blocking of thought. 'You see,' he said afterwards, 'I told you so. You will never see anything like April again.'

In the past three years I have, in place of L-DOPA, repeatedly tried the use of amantadine, a drug with effects somewhat similar to, but milder than those of L-DOPA. I have given him amantadine eleven times in all. His reaction to this initially was very favourable, though lacking the intensity of the effects of L-DOPA. For almost ten weeks in the autumn of 1969 Mr L. was able to speak and move with some facility on amantadine without too much in the way of 'side-effects'; but towards the end of the year his reactions to amantadine became more pathological, the therapeutic reaction being displaced by a return to Parkinsonism and 'block,' on the one hand, and an accession of tics and restlessness, on the other. With each succeeding use of amantadine the therapeutic effects became less marked and shorter in duration, and the pathological effects more marked. On his eleventh and final trial of amantadine in March 1972, Mr L. showed only pathological reactions to this. He said at this time, 'This is the end of the line. I have *had* it with drugs. There is no more you can do with me.'

Since this final, futile trial of amantadine, Mr L. has recovered his 'cool' and composure. He has, apparently, conquered his hopes and regrets, the violent feeling of promise and threat, which drugs thrust on him for more than three years. He has, finally, assimilated the entire mixed experience, and used his strength and intelligence to accommodate to it. 'At first, Dr Sacks,' he recently said, 'I thought L-DOPA was the most wonderful thing in the world, and I blessed you for giving me the Elixir of Life. Then, when everything went bad, I thought it was the worst thing in the world, a deathly poison, a drug which sent one down to the depths of hell; and I cursed you for giving it to me. I was terribly mixed in my feelings between fear and hope, and hatred and love . . . Now I accept the whole situation. It was wonderful, terrible, dramatic, and comic. It is finally – *sad,* and that's all there is to it. I'm best left alone – no more drugs. I've learned a great deal in the last three years. I've broken through barriers which I had all my life. And now, I'll stay myself, and you can keep your L-DOPA.'

Perspectives

PERSPECTIVES

ᕲ The terrors of suffering, sickness, and death, of losing ourselves and losing the world, are the most elemental and intense
we know; and so too are our dreams of recovery and rebirth, of
being wonderfully restored to ourselves and the world.

Our sense that there is *something the matter,* that we are ill or
in error, that we have departed from health, that we are possessed
by disorder and no longer ourselves – this is basic and intuitive
in us; and so too is the sense of *coming to* or awakening, of
resipiscence or recovery, being restored to ourselves and the
world: the sense of health, of being well, fully alive, in-the-world.

Scarcely less basic are our *perversions* of being. Given certain
conditions, we create our own sickness; we imagine and construct
innumerable diseases, whole worlds of morbidity which can defend or destroy:

> . . . As the other *world* produces *Serpents,* and *Vipers,* malignant
> and venimous creatures, and *Wormes,* and *Caterpillars,* that en-
> deavour to devour that world that produces them . . . so this
> world, ourselves, produces all these in us, in producing *diseases,*
> and *sicknesses,* of all these sorts; venimous and infectious diseases,
> feeding and consuming diseases, and manifold and entangled
> diseases, made up of several ones . . . O miserable abundance, O
> beggarly riches!
>
> DONNE

And as we allow diseases, so we can collude with them, and
connive at them, greedily embracing sickness and suffering, plotting our own ruin, in a horrible peccancy of body and mind:

. . . We are not onely *passive,* but *active,* in our owne *ruine;* we do not onely stand under a *falling house,* but *pull* it downe upon us; and wee are not onely *executed,* but wee are *executioners,* and *executioners of our selves.*

DONNE

But, by the same token, we can resist and combat our own diseases, employing not only the remedies which physicians and others provide, but resources and strengths of our own which are inborn or acquired. We would never survive without these powers of health, so deep and far-reaching, which are, finally, the deepest and strongest we have. Yet we know so much of the devices of disease, and so little of the powers of health that are in us:

To well manage our affections, and wild horses of *Plato,* are the highest Circenses; and the noblest Digladiation is in the Theater of ourselves; for therein our inward Antagonists, with ordinary Weapons and down right Blows make at us, but also like Retiary and Laqueary Combatants, with Nets, Frauds and Entanglements fall upon us. Weapons for such combats are not to be forged at *Lipara;* Vulcan's Art doth nothing in this Internal Militia . . .

SIR THOMAS BROWNE

These are the terms in which we experience health and disease, and which we naturally use in speaking of them. They neither require nor admit definition; they are understood at once, but defy explanation; they are at once exact, intuitive, obvious, mysterious, irreducible, and indefinable. They are *metaphysical* terms – the terms we use for infinite things. They are common to colloquial, poetic, and philosophical discourse. And they are indispensable terms in medical discourse, which unites all of these. 'How are you?', 'How are things?', are metaphysical questions, infinitely simple and infinitely complex.

The whole of this book is concerned with these questions – 'How are you?', 'How are things?' – as they apply to certain patients in an extraordinary situation. There are many legitimate answers to this question: 'Fine!', 'So-so', 'Terrible!', 'Bearing up',

'Not myself', etc.; evocative gestures; or simply *showing* how one is, how things stand, without use or need of special gestures or words. All of these are intuitively understood, and *picture* for one the state of the patient. But it is not legitimate to answer this metaphysical question with a list of 'data' or measurements regarding one's vital signs, blood chemistry, urinalysis, etc. A thousand such data don't begin to answer the essential question; they are irrelevant and, additionally, very crude in comparison with the delicacy of one's senses and intuitions:

> The *pulse,* the *urine,* the *sweat,* all have sworn to say nothing, to give no Indication, of any dangerous *sicknesse* . . . And yet . . . I feele, that insensibly the *Disease* prevailes.

> DONNE

The dialogue about how one is can only be couched in human terms, familiar terms, which come easily and naturally to all of us; and it can only be held if there is a direct and human confrontation, an 'I-Thou' relation, between the discoursing worlds of physicians and patients.[104]

---

[104] In *The Revised Confessions* de Quincey tells us how much he suffered from 'the pressure on the heart from the incommunicable.' This pressure, no doubt, is known to all of us; but it may approach the most agonizing level in patients whose sufferings are not only intense, but so strange as to seem, at first, beyond the possibilities of communication. Such difficulties in communication, clearly, can arise from the very strangeness, the extraordinary quality, of patients' problems, their experience; but an equal, if not greater, difficulty may be created by physicians themselves who, in effect, decline to listen to their patients, to treat them as equals, and who are prone to adopt – from force of habit, or from a less excusable sense of professional apartness and superiority – an approach and language which effectively prevent any real communication between themselves and their patients. Thus patients may be subjected to forms of interrogation and examination which smack of the schoolroom and the courtroom – questions of the form: 'Do you have *this* . . . do you have *that* . . .?' which by their categorical nature demand categorical answers (yes and no answers, answers in terms of *this* and *that*). Such an approach forecloses the possibility of learning anything new, and prevents the possibility of forming a picture, or pictures, of what it is like to be as one is. The fundamental questions – 'How are you?' and 'What is it *like?*' – can only be answered analogically, allusively, in terms of 'as if' and likeness, by images, similitudes, models, metaphors, that is, by *evocations* of one sort and another. There can be no reaching out into the realm of the incommunicable (or the scarcely communicable) unless the physician becomes a fellow traveller, a fellow explorer, continually moving *with* his patients, discovering

The situation is radically different with regard to the subject matter and discourse of logic, mathematics, mechanics, statistics, etc. For here the terms of reference – quantities, locations, durations, classes, functions, etc. – are clear-cut and finite, and thus admit of precise definition, enumeration, estimation, and measurement. Moreover, one's attitude in such matters is radically different: one is no longer 'a man in his wholeness wholly attending'; one de-personalizes one's self and the object under survey, making of both an 'It.'[105] Here, then, the basic question is: 'What

---

with them a vivid, exact, and figurative language which will reach out towards the incommunicable. *Together* they must create languages which bridge the gulf between physician and patient, the gulf which separates one man from another.

Such an approach is neither 'subjective' nor 'objective'; it is (in Rosenstock-Huessy's term) *'trajective.'* Neither seeing the patient as an impersonal object nor subjecting him to identifications and projections of himself, the physician must proceed by sympathy or empathy, proceeding in company with the patient, *sharing* his experiences and feelings and thoughts, the inner conceptions which shape his behaviour.. He must feel (or imagine) how his patient is feeling, without ever losing the sense of himself; he must inhabit, simultaneously, two frames of reference, and make it possible for the patient to do likewise.

[105] I should make it clear that my purpose is to distinguish two modes of clinical approach, and to indicate their complementarity – not to advocate either as against the other. We are faced, as physicians, with two sorts of problem, each requiring its own approach and language: one is the problem of *identification,* the other is the problem of *understanding.* Identification, in this sense, is essentially legal in nature – the same term ('case') is used in medicine and law. Faced with a 'case' of something or other, we seek for 'evidence' which will enable us to arrive at a diagnostic decision. This evidence may take various forms – *symptoms* which form the grounds of complaint; *signs* which are regarded as specific to specific disorders; *tests* to confirm or refute our suspicions. When we have gathered the requisite testimony we say, 'This is a case of such-and-such' and 'The requisite treatment is such-and-such': the case has been 'considered' and is now ready to be 'disposed of' or 'closed.' Our sole concern in this judicial process is the treatment of diagnostically relevant criteria, and the search for data which meet these criteria. The business of 'understanding' is nowhere relevant, nor is the question of 'care' for the patient: diagnostic medicine could be entirely carried out by the rote application of rules and techniques, which a computer could undertake as well as a doctor.

Such a mechanical and technological medicine is ethically neutral and epistemologically sound – it advances continually, it has saved countless lives. It only becomes unsound and wrong if it excludes non-mechanical or non-technological approaches, if it displaces clinical dialogue and an existential approach. 'Cases' are abstract; patients are people, people who are suffering, perplexed, and fearful. Patients need proper diagnosis and treatment, but they also need understanding and care; they need human relationship and existential encounter, which cannot be provided by any technology.

exactly is the case with regard to *this* at this particular time and place?' And the answer is couched in terms of when, where, and how much: the world is reduced to pointing and points.[106]

Both types of discourse are complete in themselves; they can neither include nor exclude one another; they are complementary; and both are vital in understanding the world. Thus Leibniz, comparing metaphysical and mechanical approaches, writes:

> I find indeed that many of the effects of nature can be accounted for in a two-fold way, that is to say by a consideration of efficient causes and again independently by a consideration of final causes . . . Both explanations are good, not only for the admiring of the work of a great artificer, but also for the discovery of useful facts in Physics and Medicine. And writers who take these diverse routes should not speak ill of each other . . . The best plan would be to join the two ways of thinking.

Leibniz stresses, however, that metaphysics comes first: that although the workings of the world never contravene mechanical considerations, they only make sense, and become fully intelligible, in the light of metaphysical considerations; that the world's mechanics subserve its design.[107]

Thus our theme and plea relates to the *complementarity* of both approaches – the development of the technical without any forfeit of the human: what Buber has called 'the humanization of technology, before it dehumanizes us.' Such a complementarity is bound to be present if the physician stands in a proper relation to his patients – a relation which is neither sentimental nor mechanical – but one which is based on deep *consideration,* on an inseparable combination of wisdom and care. Thus Leibniz, who amongst so much else was one of the greatest of jurists, regarded legalisms and mechanisms as purely secondary, and defined law and judgement in fundamentally ethical and existential terms – as *'caritas sapientis.'* If we care, and care wisely for our patients, everything else will fall into place.

[106] The entire body of the *Philosophical Investigations* is, in a sense, concerned with the distinction between *pointing language* (a language in which 'every word has a meaning. The meaning is correlated with the word. It is the object for which the word stands.') and *evocative language.* Wittgenstein here shows, with extreme penetration and clearness, how a pointing-language (or calculus) is always inadequate to describe the real world, how its use is confined to what is abstract and 'unreal.'

[107] These quotations and paraphrases of Leibniz are taken from his *Discourse on Metaphysics* and his *Correspondence with Arnauld,* which, though written in the

If this were clearly understood, no trouble would arise. Folly enters when we try to 'reduce' metaphysical terms and matters to mechanical ones: worlds to systems, particulars to categories, impressions to analyses, and realities to abstractions. This is the madness of the last three centuries, the madness which so many of us – as individuals – go through, and by which all of us are tempted. It is this Newtonian-Lockean-Cartesian view – variously paraphrased in medicine, biology, politics, industry, etc. – which reduces men to machines, automata, puppets, dolls, blank tablets, formulae, ciphers, systems, and reflexes. It is this, in particular, which has rendered so much of our recent and current medical literature unfruitful, unreadable, inhuman, and unreal.

There is nothing alive which is not individual: our health is *ours;* our diseases are *ours;* our reactions are *ours* – no less than our minds or our faces. Our health, diseases, and reactions cannot be understood *in vitro,* in themselves; they can only be understood with reference to *us,* as expressions of our nature, our living, our being-here *(da-sein)* in the world. Yet modern medicine, increasingly, dismisses our existence, either reducing us to identical replicas reacting to fixed 'stimuli' in equally fixed ways, or seeing our diseases as purely *alien* and bad, without organic relation to the person who is ill. The therapeutic correlate of such notions, of course, is the idea that one must attack the disease with all the weapons one has, and that one can launch the attack with total impunity, without a thought for the *person* who is ill. Such notions, which increasingly dominate the entire landscape of medicine, are as mystical and Manichean as they are mechanical and inhuman, and are the more pernicious because they are not explicitly realized, declared, and avowed. The notion that disease-causing agents and therapeutic agents are things-in-themselves is often ascribed to Pasteur, and it is therefore salutary to remember Pasteur's death-bed words:

Bernard is right; the pathogen is nothing; the *terrain* is everything.

1680s, were only published in the 1840s, subsequent to the death of Locke, Hume, and Kant.

Diseases have a character of their own, but they also partake of our character; we have a character of our own, but we also partake of the world's character: character is monadic or microcosmic, worlds within worlds within worlds, worlds which express worlds. The disease-the man-the world go together, and cannot be considered separately as things-in-themselves. An adequate concept or characterization of a man (Adam, in Leibniz's example) would embrace all that happened to him, all that affected him, and all that he affected; and its terms would combine contingency with necessity, allowing the perpetual possibility of 'alternative Adams.' Leibniz's ideal is thus a perfectly shaped and detailed *history,* (or disclosure), or *biography,* an integral combination of science and art.[108]

In our own time, the most perfect examples of such biography (or 'pathography') are the matchless case-histories of Freud. Freud here shows, with absolute clarity, that the on-going nature of neurotic illness and its treatment cannot be displayed *except* by biography.

But the history of neurology has nothing, or almost nothing, of this sort to offer.[109] It is as if some absolute and categorical

---

[108] In the case of illness, one's confinement, one's surroundings, one's hopes and one's fears, what one hears, or believes, one's physician, *his* behaviour, are all coalesced in a single picture or drama. Thus Donne, on his sick-bed, writes: 'I observe the Phisician, with the same diligence, as hee the disease; I see he feares, and I feare with him: I overtake him, I overrun him in his feare, and I go the faster, because he makes his pace slow; I feare the more, because he disguises his fear, and I see it with the more sharpnesse, because hee would not have me see it . . . he knows that my fear may disorder the effect, and working of his practice.'

[109] Among the few exceptions may be mentioned the fascinating and witty 'Confessions of a Ticqueur,' at the start of Meige and Feindel's 1902 book *Tics,* and the very fine psychoanalytically oriented case-histories of post-encephalitic syndromes given in Jelliffe's two books on the subject (Jelliffe, 1927; Jelliffe, 1932). The finest recent examples of such biographical case-histories have been provided by A. R. Luria (*The Mind of a Mnemonist* and *The Man with a Shattered World* both rev., 1987). In our own, technological age, there has often been a downgrading of case-history as being 'unscientific' or 'mere description,' though in the last twenty years, most especially through the writing and example of Luria, there has been a reconsideration of narrative as an indispensable scientific tool – Luria writes, in this regard, of 'Romantic Science,' and of science as 'the ascent to the concrete.' A new respect is being accorded now to case-histories, these being seen not just as histories of disease ('pathographies'), but histories

distinction had been made between the nature of neurotic and neurological illness, the latter being seen as arrays of 'facts' without design or connection. Everything real and concrete, in a sense, has a history and a life: did not Faraday provide a charming example of this in his 'History of a Candle'? Why should diseases be exceptions? And why especially such extraordinary illnesses as Parkinsonism and post-encephalitic 'syndromes,' which have such profound (if generally unregarded) analogies to neurotic illness? If ever an illness and a 'cure' called out for a dramatic and biographic presentation, the story of Parkinsonism and L-DOPA does so. If we seek a 'curt epitome' of the human condition – of long-standing sickness, suffering, and sadness; of a sudden, complete, almost preternatural 'awakening'; and, alas! of entanglements which may follow this 'cure' – there is no better one than the story of these patients.

Not that there is any dearth of writing on the subject: a vast flood of papers, articles, reports, reviews, editorials, proceedings of conferences, etc., has poured forth since Cotzias's pioneer paper in February 1967, to say nothing of rhapsodic (and often unscrupulous) advertisements and newspaper articles. But there is, I believe, something quite fundamental which is missing in these. One mulls over whole libraries of papers, couched in the 'objective,' styleless style *de rigueur* in neurology; one's head buzzes with 'facts,' figures, lists, schedules, inventories, calculations, ratings, quotients, indices, statistics, formulae, graphs, and whatnot; everything 'calculated, cast-up, balanced, and proved' in a manner which would have delighted the heart of Thomas Gradgrind.[110] And nowhere, *nowhere,* does one find any colour, reality, or warmth; nowhere any residue of the living experience;

---

of people, histories of *life.* (See Luria, 1977; Sacks, 1986; Sacks, 1987; Sacks, 1990a) A similar revaluation of historical description, when describing complex, unrepeatable, unique events in palaeontology and biology, has been given new force recently, by the writings of Stephen Jay Gould (see especially Gould, 1989).

[110] 'Thomas Gradgrind, Sir – peremptorily Thomas – Thomas Gradgrind. With a rule and a pair of scales, and the multiplication tables always in his pocket, sir, ready to weigh and measure any parcel of human nature, and tell you exactly what it comes to. It is a mere question of figures, a case of simple arithmetic.' – *Hard Times*

nowhere any impression or picture of what it *feels* like to have Parkinsonism, to receive L-DOPA, and to be totally transformed. If ever there were a subject which needed a non-mechanical treatment, it is this one; but one looks in vain for life in these papers; they are the ugliest exemplars of assembly-line medicine: everything human, everything living, pounded, pulverized, atomized, quantized, and otherwise 'processed' out of existence.

And yet – it is the most enchanting of subjects, as dramatic, and tragic, and comic as any. My own feelings, when I first saw the effects of L-DOPA, were of amazement and wonder, and almost of awe. Each passing day increased my amazement, disclosing new phenomena, novelties, strangenesses, whole worlds of being whose possibility I had never dreamt of – I felt like a slum-child suddenly transplanted to Africa or Peru.

This sense of worlds upon worlds, of a landscape continually extending, reaching beyond my sight or imagination, is one which has always been with me, since I first encountered my post-encephalitic patients in 1966, and first gave them L-DOPA in 1969. It is a very mixed landscape, partly familiar, partly uncanny, with sunlit uplands, bottomless chasms, volcanoes, geysers, meadows, marshes; something like Yellowstone – archaic, prehuman, almost prehistoric, with a sense of vast forces simmering all round one. Freud once spoke of neurosis as akin to a prehistoric, Jurassic landscape, and this image is still truer of post-encephalitic disease, which seems to conduct one to the dark heart of being.[111]

---

[111] The use of this Conradian phrase (though Conrad was not in my conscious thoughts as I wrote!) epitomizes a certain *doubleness* of attitude, a complexity of feeling which I cannot wholly resolve.

Thus I note of Hester Y. that her sudden awakening filled me, and all those around her, with 'awe,' and that we found her awakening 'just like a miracle.' I quote the words of Ida T.: 'wonderful, wonderful! . . . that dopey's a *Mitzphah!*' and of Maria G.'s parents: 'A miracle from Heaven . . . a completely new person.' On the other hand, I note the 'dark' side of patients' awakenings; that Frances D. (who called L-DOPA *'Hell-* DOPA') found herself face to face with 'very deep and ancient parts of herself, monstrous creatures from her unconscious, and from unimaginable physiological depths below the unconscious . . . prehistoric and pre-human landscapes . . .'; and that even in a patient as prosaic and good-humoured as Lillian W. there was a sense of the anarchic, the absurd, the grotesque, of crises and symptoms so surrealistic and strange as to seem lacking

Wittgenstein once remarked that a book – like the world – could convey its subject-matter by *examples,* anything further being redundant. My prime intention, in this book, has been to provide examples.

Hitherto we have travelled, in imagination, *with* our patients, tracing with them the course of their lives, their illness, and their reactions to L-DOPA. Now, we can remove ourselves from this itinerary, from history and happening, and gaze more fully at certain aspects of the landscape, at patterns-of-reaction which have special importance.

We have no need to look farther afield – above or below or behind or beyond anything which we have seen so far. We have no need to chase after 'causes,' or theories and explanations – anything which lies *outside* our observations:

> Everything factual is, in a sense, theory . . . There is no sense in looking for something behind phenomena: they *are* theory.

GOETHE

---

not only in moral nature, but in any intelligible nature at all. I was forced to use terms which I had never previously allowed into scientific descriptions.

I was forced, too, to wonder if my previous world-views had not been too pallid, too superficial, and altogether too 'rational' – mere skimmings or skatings on the surface of reality; if I had not been denying the fierce complexity of Nature, profoundly important determinants of being – forces below the surface of the conscious, forces below the surface of the world, powers beyond powers, depths beneath depths, extending into the infinite depths of our world-home, the cosmos. On the surface there was Apollonian light and calm, everything 'rational and reconciled'; beneath – I knew not what chthonic or Dionysiac depths. The extraordinary phenomena presented by my patients hinted at unseen, unsuspected, and almost *wanton* human depths, innumerable 'Ids' below the lowest level of which Freud spoke – or perhaps one vast 'Id,' like the primordial energy of the cosmos itself. This deepest 'Id' of all – neither 'good' nor 'evil,' moral nor immoral, rational nor irrational, orderly nor unruly (unless all of these at once, complected together); this endlessly resourceful, creative force seemed to be the very spirit of Nature itself, the urge *to be* (and to persist and grow in self-being), that ever-living, ever-struggling, self-realizing *conatus* of which Spinoza and Leibniz spoke in identical terms.

Thus, when I speak of being led to 'the dark heart of Being,' I imply nothing base, Manichean, or arcane, nothing diabolic or morally dark. I imply altitude, depth, the abyss, the heights – a vision of the numinous centre of things, the radiant spirit of the phenomenal world.

We have no need to go beyond the evidence of our senses. But what we need is an approach, a language, which is adequate for the subject. The terms of existing neurology, for example, cannot begin to indicate what is happening with the patient; we are concerned not simply with a handful of 'symptoms,' but with a *person,* and his changing relation to the world. Moreover, the language we need must be both particular and general, combining reference to the patient and *his* nature, and to the world and *its* nature. Such terms – at once personal and universal, concrete and metaphorical, simple and deep – are the terms of metaphysics, or colloquial speech. These terms, of course, are those of 'health' and 'disease,' the simplest and deepest terms we know. Our task – in the context of patients' reactions to L-DOPA – is to explore the meaning of these terms, to avoid superficial definitions and dichotomies, and to *feel* (beyond the range of formulations) the intimate, essential nature of each.

The quantitative welfare statistics of existing studies of L-DOPA are really a paradigm of the Benthamite felicific calculus ('the greatest good of the greatest number'), or of F. Y. Edgeworth's 'Hedonical Calculus.' The brevity and use of such an actuarial approach can be conceded at once, whereas its limitations (and cruelties) are covert and implicit, and need exposure to the full light of day. The utilitarian approach is not couched in terms of particulars and universals, and its terms necessarily hide both from sight; it gives us no insight whatever into the general design of behaviour, or into the ways in which this is exemplified in particular patients; it positively stands in the way of such insight.

If we are to learn anything *new* from our study, we must pay attention to the precise forms and relationships of all phenomena seen, to 'health' and 'disease' in terms of design. We need infinite terms for infinite states (worlds), and must go to Leibniz, not Bentham, for appropriate concepts. The Leibnizian 'optimum' – health – is not a numerical quotient, but an allusion to the greatest fullness of relationship possible in a total world-manifold, the organization with the greatest richness and reality. Diseases, in this sense, depart from the optimum, for their organization or design is impoverished and rigid (although they have frightening strengths of their own). Health is infinite and expansive in mode, and reaches out to be filled with the fullness of the world; whereas disease is finite and reductive in mode, and endeavours to reduce the world to itself.

Health and disease are alive and dynamic, with powers and propensities and 'wills' of their own. Their modes of being are inherently antithetical: they confront one another in perpetual hostility – our 'Internal Militia,' in Sir Thomas Browne's words. Yet the outcome of their struggle cannot be pre-determined or pre-judged, any more than the outcome of a chess game or tournament. The rules are fixed but the strategy is not, and one can learn to outplay one's antagonist, Sickness. In default of health, we manage, by *care,* and control, and cunning, and skill, and luck.

Health, disease, care – these are the most elemental concepts we have, the only ones adequate to bear the discussion. When we give L-DOPA to patients, we see first an emergence from sickness – an AWAKENING; then a relapse, and a multiplication of problems and troubles – TRIBULATION; finally, perhaps, the patient reaches a sort of 'understanding' or balance with his problems – this we can call ACCOMMODATION. It is in terms of this sequence – Awakening . . . Tribulation . . . Accommodation – that we can best discuss the consequences of L-DOPA.

AWAKENING

Virtually all patients with true Parkinsonism show some sort of 'awakening' when given L-DOPA.[112] This is true of all but three (Robert O., Frank G., Rachel I.) of the patients described in this book, and of all but a score of the two hundred Parkinsonian patients to whom I have given L-DOPA.[113] In general –

---

[112] Patients with 'pseudo-Parkinsonism' (e.g. Parkinsonian-like pictures associated with disease of the cortex – a not uncommon situation in elderly patients) show virtually no awakening at all. I drew attention to this in 1969 (see Sacks, 1969) and suggested at this time that trial with L-DOPA might thus be useful in distinguishing such patients from true Parkinsonians.

The aetiology of the Parkinsonism, in itself, is not of significance in modifying reactions to L-DOPA: thus toxic Parkinsonism, associated with manganese or carbon monoxide poisoning, may respond well to L-DOPA. Among my own patients who have done well when given L-DOPA have been three who suffered from syphilitic Parkinsonism (Wilson's 'syphilitic mesencephalitis') associated with tabes.

[113] A few patients may fail to show awakening on L-DOPA and instead be thrust into deeper illness; moreover, the response may be quite different at different times in a single patient. Thus, among post-encephalitic patients at Mount Carmel not described in this book, one initially became comatose with the administration of L-DOPA, but when given it a year later showed a dramatic awakening. Another (Seymour L.), when first given L-DOPA in April 1969, showed a dramatic but very short-lived awakening, which was compromised within a month by respiratory crises, side-to-side lunging movements of the neck and trunk, hallucinations, tics, etc., necessitating discontinuance of the drug; when given a *minute* dose of L-DOPA (100 mg. daily) twenty months later, he showed a disastrous reaction, being immediately precipitated into a state of greatly exacerbated Parkinsonism and catalepsy, followed by coma; but when placed on L-DOPA for the *third* time, in October 1972, he not only did well, but has maintained this excellent reaction up to the time of writing (October 1974). I have seen similar sequences with other patients, for example Gertie C., who was put on L-DOPA again early in the summer of 1974, after a gap of almost four years, and has since maintained a stable, happy, and tranquil reaction and a renewed ability for speech. I cannot judge whether such unexpectedly auspicious responses to renewed administration of L-DOPA have some simple physiological

though this is not always the case – awakening is most profound and most rapid in patients with the severest disease, and may be virtually instantaneous in patients with 'imploded' (or 'black hole') types of Parkinsonism-catatonia (e.g. Hester Y.). In patients with ordinary Parkinson's disease, awakening may be extended over a matter of days, although it usually reaches its zenith within two weeks or so. In post-encephalitic patients, as our case-histories have shown, awakening tends to be much prompter and more dramatic; moreover, post-encephalitic patients, in general, are much more sensitive to L-DOPA, and may be awakened by a fifth or less of the doses required for 'ordinary' patients.

An 'ordinary' patient may be in excellent (behavioural) health apart from his Parkinsonism, and this itself may be mild, and of relatively short duration; for such a patient, therefore, getting well or awakening chiefly consists in a reduction or apparent abolition of his Parkinsonism; there are other aspects to awakening, even in such patients, but these are much more readily studied in profoundly and chronically disabled post-encephalitic patients, who suffer from a great number of disabilities in addition to Parkinsonism. These patients, we have seen, may show profound reductions not only of their Parkinsonism, but of innumerable other problems – torsion-spasms, athetosis, chorea, tics, catatonia, depression, apathy, torpor, etc., etc. – from which they concurrently suffered. Such patients recover, not from one malady, but from a multitude of illnesses, and in extremely short order. All manner of disorders, which are not usually taken to have a dopamine-substrate or to be amenable to L-DOPA, may nevertheless vanish as the Parkinsonism vanishes. Such patients, in short, may experience a virtually total return to health, a recovery which is over and above anything one could predict from our knowledge of the location and functions of L-DOPA, etc., or from our currently accepted physiological picture of the brain. That such virtually simulta-

---

explanation, or whether they have occurred in consequence of a great inner act of psychophysiological *'accommodation'* (as described in the section on this).

neous-instantaneous awakenings occur is not only of profound therapeutic interest, but of momentous physiological and epistemological interest.[114]

Certain feelings are invariably experienced during a profound awakening, and are described by patients in figurative terms very similar to those which an 'outside' observer would invoke. The sudden relief of Parkinsonism, catatonia, tensions, torsions, etc., is experienced as a deflation or detumescence, a sudden relief of an internal pressure; patients often compare it to passing flatus, eructation, or emptying of the bladder. And this is exactly how it looks to an external observer: the stiffness or spasm or swelling disappears, and suddenly the patient is 'relaxed,' and at ease. Patients who comment on the 'pressure' or 'force' of their Parkinsonism, etc., are clearly not speaking in physical terms, but in ontological or metaphysical terms which correspond to their experience. The terms of 'pressure' or 'force' indicate something about the *organisation* of illness, and give a first inkling of the nature of ontological or 'inner' space in these patients; and in all of us.

This return-to-oneself, resipiscence, 'rebirth,' is an infinitely dramatic and moving event, especially in a patient with a rich and full self, who has been *dispossessed* by disease for years or decades (e.g. Hester Y.). Furthermore, it shows us, with wonderful clarity, the dynamic relation of sickness to health, of a 'false self' to the real self, of a disease-world to an optimum-world. The automatic return of real being and health, *pari passu* with the drainage of disease, shows that disease is not a thing-in-itself, but parasitic on health and life and reality: an ontological ghoul, living on and

[114] Such a 'global' awakening was indeed unintelligible in relation to the prevailing notions of neuroanatomy in 1969 – notions which saw the 'motor,' the 'perceptual,' the 'affective,' and the 'cognitive' as residing in separate and non-communicating compartments of the brain. But anatomy has been revolutionised in the past twenty years, most especially by Walle Nauta, who has shown that all these supposedly-separate compartments of brain function are richly interconnected and in continual communication; only with this new neuroanatomy does one understand how the motor, the sensory, the affective, the cognitive, can – and indeed must – go together (see Nauta, 1989; Sacks, 1989).

consuming the grounds of the real self. It shows the dynamic and implacable nature of our 'internal militia'; how opposed forms of being fight to possess us, to dispossess each other, and to perpetuate themselves.[115]

That a return to health or resipiscence is possible, in these patients with half a century of the profoundest illness, must fill one with a sense of amazement – that the potential for health and self can survive, after so much of the life and structure of the person has been lost, and after so long and exclusive an immersion in sickness. This also is of major importance, not only therapeutically, but theoretically as well.[116]

---

[115] This reciprocity between health and sickness is quite apparent even in the absence of L-DOPA. One sees, in practice, again and again, how Parkinsonism may suddenly burst into apparency – from a previously inapparent, latent or virtual condition – if a person becomes ill, profoundly exhausted, shocked, depressed, etc., how it takes over and flourishes with the ebbing of health; one sees, equally clearly, how it may then 'go away' again – retreat into inapparency, latency, virtuality – with the return of strength and abounding health. Thus, two years ago, I had occasion to see an old lady who, the day before falling and breaking her hip, had been 'full of life,' and had shown not the least sign of Parkinsonism (or none that was recognized); the following day, when I saw her, she was in some pain, but – more significantly – had suffered, and showed, an existential collapse, a sense that she was 'finished' and that death was near, a draining away of her vitality and *da-sein;* now, in addition to looking half-dead, she was deeply Parkinsonian; three days later, she 'was herself' once again – she felt full of life and no longer showed the least trace of Parkinsonism. She has continued in excellent health since this time, and has not again shown any manifest Parkinsonism. I have no doubts, however, that it is *there* (in potential, in propensity, latent, dormant, *in posse*), and will again come to the forefront if her health, her real-being, is injured or lost.

[116] Such awakenings may be compared to so-called *'lucid intervals.'* At such times – despite the presence of massive functional or structural disturbances to the brain – the patient is suddenly and completely *restored to himself.* One observes this, again and again, at the height of toxic, febrile, or other deliria: sometimes the person may be recalled to himself by the calling of his name; then, for a moment or a few minutes, he *is* himself, before he is carried off by delirium again. In patients with advanced senile dementias, or pre-senile dementias (e.g. Alzheimer's disease), where there is abundant evidence of all types regarding the massive loss of brain structure and function, one may also – very suddenly and movingly – see vivid, momentary recalls of the original, lost person. (There may be brief, sudden normalisations of an otherwise profoundly abnormal EEG in these tantalisingly lucid moments: compare figure 1, p. 328.)

Again, there is described, and I have seen, the sudden 'sobering' effect of illness, tragedy, bereavement, etc., on profoundly deteriorated, 'burnt-out,'

If we are to understand the *quality* of awakening, and of the awakened state – health – we must depart from the physiological and neurological terms which are generally used, and heed the terms which patients themselves tend to use. Currently used neurological and neuro-physiological terms have reference to alterations of energy-level and energy-distribution in the brain; we must also use energetic and economic concepts, but in a radically different way from the way in which they are generally used.

We have already spoken (n. 31, p. 30) of the two schools in classical neurology – the holists and topists, or, in their own vernacular – the 'lumpers' and 'splitters.' Holists refer to the

---

hebephrenic schizophrenics; such patients – who may have been 'decomposed' into a swarm of mannerisms, impulsions, automatisms, and mocking 'selflets' for decades – may *come together* in a moment faced with an overwhelming reality.

But one need not look for such far-out examples. All of us have experienced sudden composures, at times of profound distraction and disorganization; sudden sobriety, when intoxicated; and – especially as we grow older – sudden total recalls of our past or our childhood, recalls so complete as to be a re-being. All of these indicate that one's self, one's style, one's *persona* exists as such, in its infinitely complex and particular being; that it is not a question of this system or that, but of a total organisation which must be described as a self. Style, in short, is the deepest thing in one's being. An extraordinary example of this is provided by a number of letters which I once saw, written by Henry James when he was in a terminal, extremely febrile, pneumonia delirium: these letters show clear evidences of delirium, but their *style* is unmistakably and uniquely that of Henry James, and indeed, of 'late' Henry James.

Many neuropsychologists, pre-eminently Lashley, have spent their lives 'in search of the Engram': the work of Lashley, in particular, has conclusively shown how individual skills and memories may survive massive and varied extirpations of the brain. Such experimental observations, like careful and thoughtful clinical observations (most notably those of Luria, as set out in *The Man with a Shattered World*), indicate that one's *persona* is in no way 'localisable' in the classical sense, that it cannot be equated with any given 'centre,' 'system,' 'nexus,' etc., but only with the intricate totality of the whole organism, in its ever-changing, continuously modulated, afferent-efferent relation with the world. They show, instead, that one's ontological organisation, one's entire being – for all its multiplicity, all its shimmering, ever-shifting succession of patterns (Hume's 'bundle of perceptions,' Proust's 'collection of moments') – is nevertheless a coherent and continuing entity, with a historical, stylistic, and imaginative continuity, with the unity of a life-long symphony or poem.

Note (1990): Such a dynamic, biological concept of consciousness as reflecting ever-shifting 'global mappings' in the brain, ceaseless relatings of current perceptions to past mappings, has been articulated with great force recently, by Gerald Edelman.

'total energy' of the brain as if this were something uniform, undifferentiated, and quantifiable. They speak, for example, of arousal and activation, of increased activity in an activating-system – an increase which can be defined and (in principle) measured by counting the total number of impulses which pass up this system. In more idiomatic terms, it is said that patients are 'turned on' or 'switched on' by L-DOPA. The limitation, and finally, the unreality, of such terms is that they are purely quantitative, and that they speak of magnitudes without reference to qualities. In reality, one *cannot* have magnitudes destitute of quality. Although patients do speak of feeling more energy, more 'pep,' more 'go,' etc., they clearly distinguish the qualities of pathology and health: in the words of one patient awakened by L-DOPA – 'Before I was *galvanized,* but now I am *vivified.'*

Topists, by contrast, envisage a mosaic of different 'centres' or 'systems,' each imbued with a different kind of energy; they see energy as parcelled or partitioned in innumerable packages, all of which are 'correlated' in some mysterious way. Thus, patients on L-DOPA may be given a 'vigilance-rating,' a 'motility-rating,' an 'emotivity-rating,' etc., and correlation-coefficients established between these. Such notions are completely alien to the experience of the patient, or to that of a sympathetic observer who *feels with* his patients. For *nobody* is conscious of their 'emotivity,' for example, as distinct from their 'vigilance': one is conscious only of feeling alive, attentive, aware – and of the total, infinite character of one's attention and awareness. To break up this unity into isolated components is to commit an epistemological solecism of the first order, as well as to be blind to the feelings of one's patients.

Awakening consists of a change in awareness, of one's total relation to one's self and the world. All post-encephalitic patients (all *patients*), in their individual degrees and ways, suffer from defects and distortions of attention: they feel, on the one hand, cut-off or withdrawn from the world, on the other hand immersed, or *engrossed,* in their illness. This pathological in-turning of attention on itself is particularly marked in cataleptic forms of illness, and is beautifully illustrated by a cataleptic patient who once said to me: 'My posture continually yields to itself. My posture continually enforces itself. My posture is continually suggesting itself. I am totally absorbed in an absorption of posture.'

Awakening, basically, is a reversal of this: the patient ceases to feel the presence of illness and the absence of the world, and comes to feel the absence of his illness and the full presence of the world.[117] He becomes (in D. H. Lawrence's words) 'a man in his wholeness wholly attending.'

Thus the awakened patient *turns* to the world, no longer occupied and preoccupied by his sickness. He turns an eager and ardent attention on the world, a loving and joyous and innocent attention, the more so because he has been so long cut-off, or 'asleep.' The world becomes wonderfully vivid again. He finds grounds of interest and amazement and amusement all round him – as if he were a child again, or released from gaol. He falls in love with reality itself.

Reunited with the world and himself, the entire being and bearing of the patient now changes. Where, previously, he felt ill at ease, uncomfortable, unnatural, and strained, he now feels at ease, and at-one with the world. All aspects of his being – his movements, his perceptions, his thoughts, and his feelings – testify simultaneously to the fact of awakening. The stream of being, no longer clogged or congealed, flows with an effortless, unforced ease: there is no longer the sense of *'ça ne marche pas,'* or stoppage inside.[118] There is a great sense of spaciousness, of

---

[117] Instinctively and intuitively all patients use certain metaphors again and again. Thus, there are the universal images of rising and falling, which come naturally and automatically to every patient: one *ascends* to health and happiness and grace, and one *descends* to depths of sickness and misery. But a dangerous confusion can also arise: there are enticing ascensions and 'fraudulent heights' of mania, greed, and pathological excitement; and although these are quite different from the solid elevation of health, yet they may be confused with and 'compensate' for it. Another universal metaphor is that of *light* and *darkness:* one emerges from the darkness and dimness of disease, into the clear light of health. But sickness has brilliance and false lights of its own.

[118] This partly mechanical, partly infernal, sense of inner stoppage, or of a senseless, maddening going-which-goes-nowhere, so typical of Parkinsonism and neurosis, is nowhere better expressed than in D. H. Lawrence's last poems and letters.

freedom of being. The instabilities and knife-edges of disease disappear, and are replaced by poise, resilience, and ease.

These feelings, variously coloured by individual disposition and taste, are experienced, with greater or less intensity, by every patient who becomes fully awakened from the use of L-DOPA. They show us the full quality – the zenith of real being (so rarely experienced by most 'healthy' people); they show us what we have known – and almost forgotten; what all of us once had – and have subsequently lost.

This sense of a return to something primal, to the deepest and simplest thing in the world, was conveyed to me, most vividly, by my patient Leonard L. 'It's a very sweet feeling,' he said (during his own so-brief awakening), 'very sweet and easy and peaceful. I am grateful to each moment for being itself . . . I feel so contented, like I'm at home at last after a long hard journey. Just as warm and peaceful as a cat by the fire.' And this was exactly how he *looked* at that moment –

> . . . Like a cat asleep on a chair, at peace, in peace,
> and at one with the master of the house, with the mistress,
> at home, at home in the house of the living,
> sleeping on the hearth, and yawning before the fire.

> Sleeping on the hearth of the living world
> yawning at home before the fire of life
> feeling the presence of the living God
> like a great reassurance
> a deep calm in the heart

> Men that sit in machines
> among spinning wheels, in an apotheosis of wheels,
> sit in the grey mist of movement which moves not,
> and going which goes not,
> and being which is not.

> . . . going, yet never wandering, fixed yet in motion,
> the kind of hell that is real, grey and awful
> the kind of hell grey Dante never saw . . .

a presence
as of the master sitting at the board
in his own and greater being,
in the house of life.

D. H. LAWRENCE

TRIBULATION

Thanne schal be greet tribulacionn.

WYCLIF BIBLE

For Fortune lays the Plot of our Adversities in the founda-
tion of our Felicities, blessing us in the first quadrate, to blast
us more sharply in the last.

SIR THOMAS BROWNE

⮑ For a certain time, in almost every patient who is given
L-DOPA, there is a beautiful, unclouded return to health; but
sooner or later, in one way or another, almost every patient is
plunged into problems and troubles.[119] Some patients have quite

---

[119] But there is not always a halcyon period before 'tribulations' set in. Thus
Hester Y. 'went critical' on a particular day, within seconds, and without any
'warning' whatsoever (n. 65, p. 100). Moreover, there was a quality of too-
muchness *from the start* – she seemed excessively aroused, exuberant, and showed
a strange motor pressure and perseveration almost at once. Hester was a patient
with a particularly severe, all-or-none type of post-encephalitic disorder – but
similar explosive reactions were sometimes seen even in some patients with
'ordinary' Parkinson's disease. One such patient, a schizophrenic, Bert E., whom
I started on L-DOPA in 1986, showed a mild, dose-related activation as I gradually increased the dosage; but then, suddenly, with a further small (5%) increase,

mild troubles, after months or years of good response; others are uplifted for a matter of days – no more than a moment compared to a life-span – before being cast back into the depths of affliction.

No simple statement can be made as to which patients get into most trouble first, nor can any firm prediction be made as to how and when trouble will present itself. But it is reasonable to say that patients who were in the greatest trouble originally – whether their troubles were neurological, emotional, socio-economic, or whatever – *tend* (other things being equal) to get into the greatest trouble on L-DOPA.[120]

'went critical,' and within the course of an hour went into a state of 'hypernormality' – of striking, almost frenetic activity of mind and body. He had been 'as usual' – with some lessening of rigidity and tremor, but still almost speechless, and needing help to get out of bed, etc. – on Sunday morning, but then, suddenly, in the middle of the day, he 'flipped' (as the nurses put it): leapt out of his chair, ran down the corridor, started shadow-boxing, and then started talking 'a mile a minute,' all his talk being about sports and games of various kinds (football, baseball, mathematical games, etc.). What first appeared as a normal if dramatic 'awakening' or 'release' showed clearly manic qualities within a day or two. At this point I made a small (5%) decrease of his L-DOPA; but this, instead of damping down his hyperactivity a little, caused an instant return to severe, tremulous, and almost helpless Parkinsonism. It is clear that Bert's reactions had already escaped from a simple, linear dose/response equivalence by the time he went critical, had already moved into some complex, non-linear realm of suddenness and unpredictability.

[120] So general a statement requires addition and qualification. By and large, patients with ordinary Parkinson's disease – who constitute the vast majority of our present Parkinsonian population – can expect the longest periods of unclouded response, and the mildest 'side-effects' when these finally come; whereas patients with post-encephalitic Parkinsonism appear much more prone to early and drastic adverse responses. But there are exceptions, and important ones, to any such 'rule': *no* Parkinsonian patient, however favourable his 'starting-situation,' can be *guaranteed* a long period of favourable response; conversely, one sees profoundly disabled post-encephalitic patients – like Magda B., and others whose histories are not given in this book – who astonish themselves and everyone by doing famously on L-DOPA, and *continuing* to do so. The incalculable nature of individual responses (which is hidden by the statistical presentations usually used) indicates how numerous and complex must be the determinants of response, and how many of them must be *latent (in posse),* strengths and weaknesses unexpected because unseen.

There is, however, one group of patients who are almost invariably tipped into disaster by the use of L-DOPA: these are patients with supervening dementia; they are the most vulnerable of all to L-DOPA, and not only to L-DOPA but to stresses of all kinds. The story of Rachel I. exemplifies the special dangers which attend the giving of L-DOPA to such patients. (See Sacks et al., 1970b; and Sacks et al., 1972.)

There has been a widespread, indeed universal, tendency to lump all these troubles into the category of 'side-effects,' a term which is at once dismissive and reassuring. Sometimes the term is used for convenience, without carrying any particular implications; more commonly, following the precedent of Cotzias, and a widely accepted medical practice, the term is used to denote some essential distinction from effects which are desired or expected – a distinction which allows them to be *excised,* if one wishes. Nothing is pleasanter than such an assumption, and nothing so requires dispassionate inquiry. This is very well realized by clear-minded patients, often better than by the physicians who treat them.[121]

The term 'side-effects' is objectionable, and to my mind untenable, on three sets of grounds: practical, physiological, philosophical. First, the vast majority of what are now called 'side-effects' had long ago been observed as characteristic responses of 'normal' animals given L-DOPA; in this situation, where there were no therapeutic assumptions, intentions, or insistences, there was no thought of introducing such categorical distinctions. Secondly, the use of such a term hides the actual structure and interrelation of 'side-effects,' and therefore prevents any study of this. The enormous number and complexity of 'side-effects' from L-DOPA, though an affliction to patients, is uniquely instructive if we wish to learn more of the nature of disease, and of being; but the possibility of such learning is foreclosed if we take the term 'side-effects' to be the end of the matter. Thirdly, to speak of 'side-effects' here (or in the context of technology, economics, or anything whatever) is to divide the world into arbitrary bits, and deny the reality of an organized *plenum.*

The therapeutic corollary of all this is that we may commit ourselves (and our patients) to chimerical hopes and searches for 'abolishing side-effects,' while excluding from our attention the very real ways in which they *can* be modified, or be made more bearable. Nobody has ever commented more pungently on the

---

[121] One such patient, Lillian T., now in Mount Carmel, when admitted to a large neurological hospital in New York, for the ninth time, for the 'treatment of side-effects' – in her case, a violent head-thrusting from side to side – said to her physician: 'These are *my* head-movements. They are no more a "side-effect" than my head is a "side-effect." You won't cut them out unless you cut off my head!'

futility of chopping down 'side-effects,' as opposed to the necessity of looking at the 'whole complexion and constitution' of what is actually happening, than our metaphysical poet as he lay on his sickbed:

> Neither is our *labour* at an end, when wee have cut downe some *weed,* as soone as it sprung up, corrected some *violent* and dangerous *accident* of a *disease,* which would have destroied *speedily;* nor when wee have pulled up that *weed,* from the very root, recovered *entirely,* and *soundly,* from that *particular disease;* but the whole *ground* is of an *ill nature,* the whole soile *ill disposed;* there are inclinations, there is a propensenesse to *diseases* in the *body,* out of which without any other *disorder, diseases* will grow, and so wee are put to a *continuall* labour upon this *farme,* to a continuall studie of the whole *complexion* and *constitution* of our *body.*

> DONNE

All patients, then, move into trouble on L-DOPA; not into 'side-effects,' but into *radical trouble:* they develop, once more, their 'propensenesse to diseases,' which can sprout and flower in innumerable forms. Why should this be so, we are compelled to wonder? Is it something to do with L-DOPA *per se?* Is it a reflection of the individual reactivity of each patient – of a universal reactivity all organisms show, when exposed to continued stimulation or stress? Does it depend on the expectations and motives of patients, and of physicians and others who are significant at this time? Are the overall life-style and life-circumstances relevant? All of these questions are real and important; all must be asked, and tested if possible; all of them overlap and dovetail to form the total *plenum* of patients' being-in-the-world.

We see, in Donne, a great variety of words relating to the nature of disease: disposition, inclination, propensity, complexion, constitution, etc., a richness of language which both distinguishes and unites two aspects of disease – its *structure* and *strategy.* Freud reminds us repeatedly that we must clearly distinguish the *liability to illness* from the *need for illness:* it is one thing, for example, to be migraine-prone, and another to want an attack as

an excuse for breaking an unpleasant appointment. Schopenhauer's thesis is that the world presents itself to us under two
aspects – as Will and Idea – and that these two aspects are always
distinct and always conjoined; that they totally embrace, or *in-
form,* one another. To speak in terms of either alone is to lay
oneself open to a destructive duality, to the impossibility of con-
structing a meaningful world: this is exemplified in the epistemological inadequacy of such statements as 'He did badly on
L-DOPA out of sheer spite,' or 'He did badly on L-DOPA because
he had too much (too little) dopamine in the brain.' The spite
may indeed have been there, and the alteration of dopamine may
indeed have been there, both significant, both crucial, both aspects of the way he was doing. But neither consideration alone
can afford us an adequate picture, or the possibility of an adequate picture, of the total situation. Perhaps the patient's spite
was the 'final cause,' and his dopamine the 'efficient cause'; both
considerations, both ways of thinking, as Leibniz reminds us, are
useful, and both *need to be joined.* But how shall we unite the 'final
cause' with the 'efficient cause,' the will with the matter, the
motive with the molecule, when they seem so remote, and dispar-
ate, from each other? Here again – as always – we are rescued
from the wastes of mechanism and vitalism by common sense,
common language, metaphysics: by terms which unite in their
two-facedness the concepts of structure and intention – words
like *plan* and *design,* and by the innumerable exemplifications of
such words which colloquial speech presents to us, and which we
– as scientists – so often feel impelled to reject and ignore.

For a brief time, then, the patient on L-DOPA enjoys a perfection of being, an ease of movement and feeling and thought, a
harmony of relation within and without. Then his happy state –
his world – starts to crack, slip, break down, and crumble; he
lapses from his happy state, and moves towards perversion and
decay.[122] We are forced to use words of this nature, however

---

[122] Awakening is characterized by perfect satisfaction, a perfect filling of the
organism's needs. At such a time the patient says (as did Leonard L., in effect):
'I have what I need, I need no more. I have *enough,* and all is well'; *he* says this,
and (we may imagine) all his starved cells are saying this as well. Being-well is
'enoughness' – satisfaction, contentment, fulfilment, assuagement. To the ques-

unexpected they may seem in this context, if we are to gain any
dynamic understanding of the development of those dissolutions
and departures and perversions which constitute the essence of
downfall, of disease. What we need so much – and not only in

---

tion, 'How much?' of a drug should be given, there is only one correct answer,
and that is 'Enough!'

But, alas! this happy state, this state of 'enoughness,' never endures. After a
time 'enoughness' is lost, and thereafter there is *no longer* any correct dose to
give: 'enoughness' is replaced by 'not-enoughness' and 'too-muchness,' and it is
no longer possible to 'balance' the patient. Nothing is sadder than this insidious
loss of balance, the steady attrition of therapeutic latitude, of health; nevertheless
it occurs – and seemingly inevitably, in every patient who is given L-DOPA. One's
wish, the temptation, is to deny it occurs, and to promise the patient that the
'right' dose, the 'right' response, has only been temporarily or fortuitously lost,
and can be found once again by ingenious manipulations and 'titrations' of
dosage. To do so is to lie, or at least to delude – to raise expectations which
cannot be met.

The problem of 'titration' – giving so much of a substance to obtain so much
of a response – which is so easy and straightforward in chemistry (where one has
simple stoichiometric equivalence) sooner or later becomes *the* problem with the
continued administration of L-DOPA (or with the administration of any drug
designed to alter behaviour). Let us review the sequence of responses we have
seen in all our patients – the sequence of responses which occurs in *any* patient
maintained on L-DOPA. To begin with, we see a simple, solid, beneficial response
– the patient *gets better,* after he has been given so much of the drug; and it seems,
for a while, that his new-found improvement can be maintained on a fixed
'maintenance-dose' of L-DOPA: *at this stage,* therefore, the notion of 'titration,'
of a simple stoichiometric balancing or commensuration between dose and response, seems to have been achieved, and to be perfectly feasible. But *then,*
invariably, 'complications' occur, and these have the following general pattern:
First, patients become more and more 'sensitive' to the effects of L-DOPA, sometimes to a quite extraordinary degree (as with Leonard L., who initially required
5,000 mg. a day, but later responded to a hundredth of this dose). Secondly, we
see qualitative alterations in response to L-DOPA, so that reactions which were
originally simple and straightforward now become increasingly complex, variable, unstable, and paradoxical – they may become, indeed, *impossible to predict* (at
which point infinitesimal alterations of dosage may precipitate responses *incalculable* in magnitude or kind) – a sort of 'macro-quantal' situation analogous to the
'Curie point' in heating ferromagnetic materials. At such a time we can no longer
converge on any correct or appropriate dose of L-DOPA (we see this very clearly
in the case of Frances D.) – there is no longer any such thing as a correct dose,
as 'enough' – the therapeutic window has closed. We are now in a veritable
double-bind – there is no longer any evidently right thing to do, and whatever
we do is the wrong thing to do. At this stage, then, there is no mid-point of
response any longer; the patient is no longer titrable with L-DOPA; there is no
longer any equivalence between dose and response; there has ceased to be any
commensurability between stimulus and response.

medicine – is an anatomy of wretchedness, an epistemology of disease, which will follow Burton, Schopenhauer, Freud, etc., and extend their considerations to all other (monadic) 'levels': one must see, for example, that Galen's *circulus vitiosus,* the vicious circle, is a universal of pathology at all possible levels; and that this is equally true of exorbitance and extravagance, and of all self-augmenting deviations from the ease, the harmony, the unforcedness of health. So Donne, in his relapse into sickness, continually asks himself, What went wrong? And why? Might it have been avoided? etc., and by inexorable stages is driven to the most universal concept of disease and 'propensenesse' to this.

The first symptom of returning disease, of going wrong, is *the sense* that something is going wrong. This so-obvious point cannot be emphasized too strongly. The patient does not experience a precisely formulated and neatly tabulated list of symptoms, but an intuitive, unmistakable sense that 'there is something the matter.' It is not reasonable to expect him to be able to define exactly what is the matter, for it is the indefinable sense of 'wrongness' that indicates to him, and to us, the *general* nature of his malaise: the sense of wrongness which he experiences is, so to speak, his first glimpse of a *wrong world.* [123] This sense of wrongness carries with it a precursory quality, of a perfectly precise kind: whatever is experienced conveys or intimates what will or may be experienced in the future, the expansion and evolution of an already-present character. [124]

---

[123] Of interest, in this connection, is a case of epilepsy described by Gowers. The affected patient invariably suffered from an abrupt and authentic sense of *wrongness* ('whatever was taking place before the patient would suddenly appear to be *wrong* – i.e. morally wrong . . .') immediately before convulsion and unconsciousness.

[124] An interesting and perhaps essential formal model of this quality is to be found in Cantor's concepts of infinite sets and transfinite cardinals. The laws of ordinary, inductive mathematics do not apply to these, for the 'least part' of such transfinites are equal to the whole, and convey their infinite (i.e. world-like) quality. All of us have perhaps thought of this reflexive quality with regard to an infinite series of maps: the map which contains a map of the map, which contains a map of the map of the map, etc. Indeed, this image has been specifically mentioned to me by a number of patients who find themselves embedded in interminable reflexive states of precisely this type. (See, for example, Rose R., n. 54, pp. 75–76.)

Thus, Donne, experiencing the first 'grudging' of his illness, writes:

> In the same instant that I feele the first attempt of the disease, I feele the victory.

Unease and discord – in the most general of senses – are the sign and source of returning disease. The forms and transforms are infinitely varied, and never the same in any two patients. Individuality is inherent in disease, as in everything; diseases are 'perverse' individual creations – worlds, base worlds, simpler and starker than the worlds of health.

Common to all worlds of disease is the sense of pressure, coercion, and force; the loss of real spaciousness and freedom and ease; the loss of poise, of infinite readiness, and the contractions, contortions, and postures of illness: the development of pathological rigidity and insistence.

In patients with ordinary Parkinson's disease, the first 'side-effects' of L-DOPA are most easily seen in movement and action: in a certain haste, alacrity, and precipitancy of movement, in the exaggerated force and extent of movements ('synkinesis') and in the development of various 'involuntary' movements (choreatic, athetotic, dystonic, etc.). In post-encephalitic patients, for various reasons, excesses of 'temperament' are particularly prominent, and these perhaps indicate more clearly the general form of disease. One sees this particularly clearly in such patients as Rolando P., Margaret A., Leonard L., etc., but one also sees it in patients with common Parkinson's disease, like Aaron E.

Paradoxically, deceptively, such exaggerations first appear as excesses of health, as exorbitant, extravagant, inordinate well-being; patients such as Leonard L. slip by degrees, almost insensibly, from supreme well-being to pathological euphorias and ominous ectasies. They 'take off,' they exorb, beyond reasonable limits, and in so doing sow the seeds of their subsequent breakdowns. Indeed, exorbitance is *already* a first sign of breakdown: it indicates the presence of an unmeetable need. Defect, dissatisfaction, underlie exorbitance: a 'not-enoughness' somewhere leads to greed and 'too-muchness,' to a voracity and avidity which *cannot* be met.[125]

If we ask, Where is the defect, the dissatisfaction, the avidity?, we must recognize that it may be anywhere, in the *plenum* of being: that it may be in their molecules, their motives, or their relations with the world. Unsatisfied need, insatiable greed, defines the eventual position of *all* patients on L-DOPA. This leads us to an inexorable economic conclusion – that there is a lacuna somewhere, an unassuageable gap, to be found in the situation of every single patient. Such a gap may be of any type – a chemical or structural hiatus in the midbrain itself; a wound or lacuna in emotional being; an isolation approaching Limbo in relation to the world: one way or another, there is a gulf which cannot be filled *and stay filled;* not, at least, through the agency of L-DOPA alone. A chasm develops between supply and demand, between need and capacity; an inner division of being takes place, so that there is a simultaneous suffering from surfeit and starvation – 'one halfe lackes meat, and the other stomacke' – in the metaphor which Donne applies to his sickness.

We see from their responses to the continued and continual administration of L-DOPA – if we did not see it before – that these patients have needs over and above their need for L-DOPA (or brain-dopamine); and that beyond a certain point or period no mere *substance* – however 'miraculous' – can compensate, indemnify, or cover up these other needs. These patients not only lack meat, but stomach as well: what will happen if we stuff a man who lacks some of his stomach? These considerations are passed over in the current insistence that patients can be 'titrated' with L-DOPA indefinitely, in a perfect commensuration of supply and demand. They can be 'titrated' with L-DOPA *at first,* as eroded ground can be watered, or a depressed area given money; but sooner or later, complications occur; and they occur because there is complex trouble in the first place – not merely a parching

---

[125] A sense of 'not enough!'; a craving for 'more!'; an avidity for 'still more!'; surely the pattern is all too familiar! We are compelled to recognize a precise formal analogy between the concept of pathological propensity and that of addiction or sin. The concept of this analogy is a notion we can neither dismiss nor dispense with.

or depletion of one substance, but a defect or disorder of *organisation* itself, invariably in the brain, and elsewhere as well.

This danger, this dilemma, was quite clearly recognized by Kinnier Wilson, forty years ago: he says, in effect, that there is just so much we can do, by restoring to pathological cells their missing 'pabulum,' but that beyond this there is futility and danger if we try to 'whip up' the patient's impoverished and decaying cells. Whether we try to stuff cells beyond their capacity, or whether the cells themselves show an incontinent 'avidity,' and 'try' to assimilate or function beyond their capacity, the end-result will be the same. Moreover, a static metaphor – like stuffing a man who lacks half his stomach – is not adequate to describe what actually occurs; the image of 'whipping up' decayed and flagging cells, and of their accelerated breakdown under this stress, is much more germane to the eventual consequences of L-DOPA. For what we see, in every patient maintained on L-DOPA, is that his tolerance for the drug becomes less and less, while his need for the drug becomes greater and greater: in short, that he gets caught in the irresoluble vicious circle of 'addiction.'[126]

---

[126] Such dangers and dilemmas are in no sense peculiar to the use of L-DOPA. They tend to occur, one way or another, with the prolonged use of *all* cerebral stimulants and depressants, with *all* drugs which have supposedly specific effects on behavioural disorders. Perhaps the closest analogy is the use of stimulants (amphetamines) to combat the intense sleep and drowsiness of narcoleptic patients – who, in the severest cases, may tend to sleep twenty-four hours a day, to sleep away the whole of their lives; such sleepers may be brilliantly awakened by the use of amphetamines, and be able to resume normal life for weeks or months; but, sooner or later – as with patients on L-DOPA – they tend to show both a waning and a spreading of effect, the advent of psychoses, and other 'side-effects' of amphetamines, along with a recurrence of their original sleep. Similar considerations apply to the use of amphetamines, cocaine, or other stimulants to combat 'neurasthenia' and neurotic depressions.

Especially similar patterns of response occur with the prolonged use of tranquillizers to combat emotional and motor excitements. Thus the phenothiazide or butyrophenone tranquillizers are often superbly effective in the *short-term* treatment of neuroses and psychoses, and may restore the patient to a merciful calm, but *thereafter* there comes an ever-increasing likeliness of drug-induced Parkinsonism, dyskinesia, and other 'side-effects,' along with a recurrence of the original neurosis. Such effects are especially germane with regard to the extraordinary effects of haloperidol (so-called anti-DOPA) on Gilles de la Tourette or multiple-tic syndrome (a disorder associated with an excess of brain-dopamine).

Let us now plot the steps by which this occurs, the successive positions of the patient as he plays the losing game he cannot stop.[127] He becomes over-stimulated, over-reactive, over-excited – exorbitant; but underlying all this is an increasing need or deficit; he is, so to speak, striving to gain by illegitimate means what he is no longer attaining by legitimate means. Or, to return to our economic metaphor: he is no longer 'earning his keep'; his real assets and reserves are continually dwindling; he is subsisting on a loan, on borrowed time and money, and this – while it preserves appearances – further depletes his own reserves and earning-power, and brings nearer the day of reckoning, of repayment; he is experiencing a transitory 'boom,' but sooner or later the 'crash' must come.[128]

Our patients, then, ascend higher and higher into the heights of exorbitance, becoming more active, excited, impatient, increasingly restless, choreic, akathisic, more driven by tics and urges and itches, continually more hectic, fervid, and ardent, flaming into manias, passions, and greeds, into climactic voracities, surges, and frenzies . . . until the crash comes at last.[129]

Almost all such patients at first show a 'miraculous' reduction or abolition of their tics; but many of them, sooner or later, run into a series of 'tribulations' – Parkinsonism, apathy, and similar 'side-effects' – along with a recurrence of their original tics; the most fortunate, the toughest – like patients on L-DOPA – finally achieve a more or less acceptable 'accommodation' or *modus vivendi.*

[127] The process of sickening, going-down, deteriorating, etc., has always been visualized as a circular process, with a peculiarly terrible force and shape of its own. Morbid process and propensity were classically identified with sin and peccability – hence Galen's vicious circle: the fundamental image of Dante's 'Inferno.' But the best image, the image the patient feels, is that of a spiral, a whirlpool, a vortex – being sucked down, irresistibly, and with ever-increasing velocity, in the orbits of an accelerating and deteriorating spiral. There is a swirling violence, a sort of deadly attraction, as these patients are sucked into the depths.

[128] This pattern – of a single supreme moment, which once attained can never be attained again – is all too familiar with regard to alcohol, opium, stimulants, and other 'addictive' drugs. De Quincey writes: '. . . the movement is always along a kind of arch; the Drinker rises through continual ascents to a summit or apex, from which he descends through corresponding steps of declension. There is a crowning point in the movement upwards, which once attained cannot be renewed.'

[129] I have emphasized, in this and preceding descriptions, what I take to be a

The form and tempo of 'crashing' are immensely variable in Parkinsonian patients; and in many of the stabler, more fortunate patients, there is more the feeling of gentle subsidence and detumescence, than of a sudden violent crash. But whatever the form and tempo it takes, there is descent from the dangerous heights of pathology – a descent which is at once protective, yet also destructive.[130] Patients do not descend to the ground, as a punc-

---

generic tendency ('exorbitance') common to all excitations in this phase of reaction. This mode of description departs from that of classical neurology, which describes excitations as localizations; in either holistic or topistic terms. If one speaks in these terms, one will speak of the following items in response to L-DOPA: an increase in the magnitude of each excitation, a spread of excitation to other areas of the brain, and a continuous proliferation of 'new' excitations *(de novo)*, until the brain is *lit up* with innumerable excitations. Pavlov – who is both holist and topistic in approach – ascribes each widening distribution of excitations partly to the centrifugal spread of charge in a homogeneous brain-conductor ('irradiation'), and partly to the sequential stimulation of anatomically or functionally contiguous systems ('chain-reaction').

Allied to the images of illumination (Sherrington's 'myriad of twinkling lights' and Pavlov's 'bright halo with wavering borders' – both images of awakening and consciousness) are those of conflagration: flares being lit in the cerebral city, until it finally goes up in flames; a fire being lit in the cold house of being, which first warms, then consumes, the whole of the house.

Addendum (1990): In this spreading, irradiating process, more and more cerebral functions, more and more 'neuronal groups' (as Edelman would call them) are activated or 'turned on'; and once this has occurred, apparently, a permanent change may take place, these neuronal groups becoming sensitised or kindled – so that, even if L-DOPA is stopped and restarted, in any future trials of L-DOPA, they will be promptly reactivated. The brain, apparently, *learns* these 'side effects,' incorporates them as part of a new (and malignant) repertoire.

The reactions to L-DOPA become more and more complex, and in a way which is individual and unique to each patient. Each wave of excitement kindles new responses, which are thereafter facilitated and become part of the excitement. Something of this, indeed, seemed to occur *before* L-DOPA, in those patients who were prone to crises (pp. 18–19): such crises tended to *evolve,* adding new features, becoming more complex, with each repetition.

[130] Generically similar reactions have been described by Pavlov, in experimental animals submitted to 'supra-maximal' stress. Such animals, after a time, show diminutions or reversals of response, entering into 'paradoxical' and 'ultra-paradoxical' phases. Pavlov speaks, in such cases, of 'transmarginal inhibition consequent upon supra-maximal excitation,' and regards this inhibition as protective in type. Goldstein, working with patients, describes essentially similar phenomena, and regards them as basic biological reactions; Goldstein speaks here of an 'excitation-course' rising to a peak, with reversal of responses, or 'equalization,' after this peak. One sees too, at the level of single neurons, how response to continued massive stimulation is always bi-phasic, the neuron adapting to, or resisting, further stress.

tured balloon would sink to the ground. They sink or crash below the ground, into the subterranean depths of exhaustion and depression, or the equivalents of these in Parkinsonian patients.

In patients with ordinary Parkinson's disease (Aaron E., for example), these crashes may not occur for a year or more, and may be relatively mild when they *do* occur. Their 'akinetic episodes' (as the crashes are usually called) tend, at first, to be short and slight, and to come on two or three hours after each dose of L-DOPA. Gradually they become more severe and longer, increasingly abrupt in onset and offset, usually losing their relation to times of giving L-DOPA.

The qualities of these states are varied and complex, more so than is usually described in the literature: among these qualities are lassitude, fatigue, somnolence, torpor, depression, neurotic tension, and – specifically – a recrudescence of Parkinsonism itself. Such states vary from mildly unpleasant and disabling to intensely distressing and disabling; in Aaron E. for example, they were far more disabling and unpleasant than his original (pre-DOPA) state, the more so because they occurred with such suddenness, and so unpredictably.

In post-encephalitic patients, these crashes tend to be far more severe, and may occur within seconds, and scores of times daily (as in Hester Y., for example). But their complexity and severity are highly instructive, and show us more clearly what goes on at such times. One sees from the reactions of such patients that one is not dealing with any mere exhaustion of response – an assumption which is rather generally made, and taken as the basis of hopefully therapeutic 'titration' of drug-dosage.[131] There is, no doubt, an element of exhaustion in these variations of response; but their instantaneity, profundity, and complexity show us that other transformations – of a fundamentally different nature – are

---

[131] Thus, in the summer of 1970, Cotzias *et al.* published a table with recommended alterations of drug-dosage for different clinical states. If akinetic episodes occurred, the dosage of L-DOPA was to be increased by 10%; if they *still* occurred, by another 10%. Such recommendations, to my mind, can be dangerously misleading in the management of patients; moreover, they lack any sound theoretical basis. It is only fair to add that Cotzias, and many other neurologists, are now readier to relinquish such fixed rotas and tables and rules-of-thumb, and to play each patient 'by ear,' with a full appreciation of the *individual* nature of all responses, and their real complexity.

also occurring. Thus, in Leonard L., Rolando P., Hester Y., etc., we see virtually instantaneous changes from violently explosive, 'expanded' states to intensely contracted, 'imploded' states – or, in the astronomical image suggested by Leonard L., from 'super-nova' states to 'black holes,' and back again. The two states we see – which at various times have been called 'up' states and 'down' states – show a precise formal analogy of structure; they represent different phases, or transforms, of each other; they depict for us, as for our patients, the opposite 'poles' of an ontological continuum.[132]

The 'down' states, then, do not represent simple and – so to speak – 'normal' exhaustions, with the protective and recuperative capacities of such exhaustions; nor can they be adequately represented as 'protective inhibitions' (in Pavlov's term) or protective 'equalizations' (in Goldstein's term). They are much less benign, for they consist of total *recoils* or rebounds or reversals of response, which fling patients, in an almost uncontrollable trajectory, from pole to pole of their being or 'space.'[133] The opposite of each exorbitance is a counter-exorbitance, and patients may be bounced between these as in a frictionless space:

---

[132] These deeply pathological states seem to lead us towards exceedingly strange yet possible images of 'inner space' in such patients; and such images, it must be stressed, occur spontaneously to imaginative patients. Thus the 'shape' of behaviour, when reduced to exorbitances, becomes that of an *hour-glass,* with a 'waist' fined down to almost-zero proportions; or, putting the matter less concretely, of an infinite yet closed ontological space, everywhere hyperbolic, and negatively curved: a space, moreover, which allows *no exit,* for it runs into itself like a Möbius strip. And *this* image, too, may be expressed by some patients: thus Leonard L., when most torturingly enclosed, compared himself to a fly trapped in a Klein bottle. Such images – of an essentially relativistic 'ontological space' – require a detailed and formal elaboration, if they are to be anything more than intriguing and suggestive.

[133] Pavlov – speaking of similar switch-backs in experimental animals, and in manic-depressive patients – talks of 'waves of excitation followed by troughs of inhibition.' Many patients, similarly, speak of waves running through them, or of being tossed up and down like a boat in heavy seas. These undulant images seem entirely appropriate, if one departs from the notion of simple, sinusoidal waves, and instead visualizes torrential excitements which *surge hyperbolically,* getting steeper and steeper, as they get higher and higher, and thus have the potential of infinite height. Such waves – fortunately – do not occur in terrestrial seas; they reflect forces and spaces of an extraordinary type; they only occur in a non-linear space, which we must endeavour to imagine as best we can.

their extremities and excursions tend to *increase,* in a frightening paradigm of positive feed-back or 'anti-control'; and 'between-states' (control-states) tend to *decrease* towards zero. Thus, once such ontological oscillations or reverberations have started, the possibilities of 'normality' become smaller and smaller, and 'in-between' states are less and less seen. Almost all of my patients who have found themselves in such situations use the image of a tight-rope to express how they feel: and this, indeed, is almost literally true, for they have become ontological funambulists above a pit of disease; or, in an allied metaphor, they seek a vanishing still-point amid total exorbitance – thus Leonard L.'s tortured wish: 'If only I could find the eye of my hurricane!'

With the continuation of such states – which may be highly persistent despite withdrawal of L-DOPA (see Rachel I., for example) – further splits or decompositions may occur, exorbitances splitting into facets or aspects, sharply differentiated 'equivalents' of being; Hester Y., for example, showed this 'crystalline' split-ting and was able to describe it particularly clearly. This further schism leads to an ontological delirium, with behaviour refracted into innumerable facets, and instantaneous jumps between these facets or aspects.[134]

These considerations, to my mind, depict the *general* form or design of reactions to L-DOPA. They have not departed from the general ground of physiological energetics or economics. They have outlined, in the sparest detail, various energetic-economic positions, or phases, of brain-state, and their interrelations, some-thing which would be susceptible, in principle, to a precise math-ematical exposition.

The administration of L-DOPA is a *general* treatment, which one hopes to match with brain-reactions or phases. One would sus-pect on theoretical grounds, as one finds in practice, that it be-comes increasingly less possible to match dose-level and brain-

---

[134] Consideration of these sparkling effervescent deliria, and of the kinematic vision and 'standstills' with which they may be associated (see Hester Y.), leads us to an aspect of 'inner space' even stranger and more difficult to imagine than the curved spaces we have looked at; kinematic phenomena show us a dimen-sionless 'space' where there is a succession without extension, moments without time, and change without transit: in short, the world of quantum mechanics.

phase. For dose-level has only a single dimension or parameter: we can increase or decrease the dose – nothing else (altered spacing of doses can be subsumed under this); whereas brain-reaction and behaviour flower into many dimensions, which cease to become describable or determinable in linear terms. To insist or suppose that responses can always be 'titrated' by dose-level is to pretend that the brain is a sort of barometer, to make a reduction of its real complexity. 'Biological organisation cannot be reduced to physico-chemical organisation,' Needham reminds us, 'because nothing can ever be reduced to anything.' And one finds, in practice, that once patients have entered complex states of perturbation and turbulence, their reactions to L-DOPA become singularly difficult to predict – if not, at times, inherently unpredictable. Once akinetic episodes have started to occur, for example, their severity may sometimes be modified by increasing L-DOPA, sometimes by decreasing L-DOPA, and sometimes by neither – all depending. Depending on two or ten or fifty variables, themselves interdependent, and complexly linked. Jevons used to compare complex economic situations to *weather,* and we must use the same image here: the brain-weather or ontological weather of these patients becomes singularly complex, full of inordinate sensitivities and sudden changes, no longer susceptible to an item-by-item analysis, but requiring to be seen as a whole, as a *map.*

To imagine that such a meteorological situation can be 'played' by the application of fixed formulae and rules of the most simplistic type is to play blind-man's-buff in the world of reality;[135] to be an alchemist or an astrologer – a purveyor of 'secrets'; to be 'a mathematical chimaera bombinating in a biological vacuum' (to borrow Huxley's paraphrase of the original Rabelais). The therapeutic game cannot be played this way, whatever our

---

[135] It is, of course, not fortuitous that those who are most apt to speak of L-DOPA as 'a miracle drug' are also most prone to publish complicated tables and formulae and rules for proper dispensing of the 'magical stuff.' Such mystical and mechanistic attitudes can not only endanger patients, but are deeply unscientific in that they go with an improper attitude to Nature – the arrogant feeling that Nature exists to be commanded and *ruled,* instead of the humble feeling that we need to understand her.

wishes; but – to the extent that it can be played at all – it can be played 'by ear,' by an intuitive appreciation of what is actually going on. One must drop all presuppositions and dogmas and rules – for these only lead to stalemate or disaster; one must cease to regard all patients as replicas, and honour each one with individual attention, attention to how *he* is doing, to *his* individual reactions and propensities; and, in this way, with the patient as one's equal, one's co-explorer, not one's puppet, one may find therapeutic ways which are better than other ways, tactics which can be modified as occasion requires. Given a 'policy-space' no longer simple or convergent, an intuitive 'feel' is the only safe guide: and in this the patient may well surpass his physician.

I must emphasize once more – to avoid needless misunderstanding or distress – that the patients considered in this book do not constitute, nor are meant to constitute, a 'fair sample' of the Parkinsonian population-at-large; the fact that many of our patients have run into exceedingly severe, complex, and intractable problems is an index of *their* situation, which is far worse, in almost every way, than the situation of their more fortunate Parkinsonian brethren outside institutions. Their reactions to L-DOPA, in almost every way, are hyberbolic and extreme: they experience the most intense 'awakenings,' and they go on to the most intense tribulations; quantitatively, their reactions far outstrip in magnitude those likely to be seen in the vast majority of Parkinsonian patients; but the quality of their reactions is the same, and casts light on the reactivity and nature of *all* Parkinsonian patients, and of *all* human beings.

We find, in their reactions to L-DOPA, that there is another universal quality which cannot be understood in the energetic and economic terms we have hitherto used. It is necessary, but never sufficient, to speak of their reactions as 'ups,' 'downs,' 'exorbitances,' 'exhaustions,' 'recoils,' 'decompositions,' 'schisms,' etc.; for their reactions are equally imbued with a *personal* quality, which is expressed in dramatic or histrionic terms; the person shows forth in all his reactions, in a continual disclosure or epiphany of himself; he is always enacting himself in the theatre of his self. Entire memory-theatres are set in motion; long-past scenes are recalled, re-enacted, with an immediacy which effaces the passage of time; scenes past and scenes possible are called into being – presentiments and presentations of what might once have been, of what could still yet be, given an imaginable difference at any one time. L-DOPA, in this way, can serve as a sort of strange and personal time-machine, bringing to each patient time past and time possible, *his* past and *his* possible, into the palpable 'now.' Worlds past and worlds possible pass like apparitions before him, intensely real – yet not real, as ghosts tend to be. The actual, the possible, the virtual, commingle in that uncanny but beautiful coming-together, that multiplicity of being we can only call *transport* (one sees this, most clearly, in the visionary Martha N.). Rose R. awoke to *her* 1926, and not to anyone else's 1926; Frances D. was recalled to *her* long-past respiratory idiosyncrasies, which were not like anyone else's idiosyncrasies; Miriam H., in her crises, experienced a (hallucinatory) recall of an 'incident' in *her* past, not an incident in anyone else's past; Magda B. experienced hallucinations of *her* husband, his presence, his absence, his infidelities to *her,* not of anyone else's husband. How absurd to call such phenomena 'side-effects'! Or to imagine that they can be understood without reference to the experience and personality, the total make-up, of each patient.[136] We cannot understand the nature of such reactions

---

[136] The anamnestic powers of L-DOPA seem to be among its most remarkable effects, those which (in the original, Platonic sense) indicate most clearly the nature of 'awakening.' The *quality* of reminiscence induced by L-DOPA is absolutely characteristic and highly instructive. It does not consist of a vague reminiscent streaming, or the regurgitation of 'facts' deliberately learnt. It consists of the sudden, spontaneous, and 'involuntary' recall of *significant moments from the personal past,* recalled with such sharpness, concreteness, immediacy, and force as to constitute, quite literally, a re-living or re-being. The character of this living memory, in which self and world, image and affect, are totally and inseparably fused, is utterly different from that of mechanical or 'rote' memory (the literal registration of 'information' or 'data,' in the sense such terms are used with regard to computers). These sudden revocations of personal memories have nothing of the 'dead' quality of re-run documentaries, but are experienced as intensely moving re-livings of one's past, vital recollections (akin to those of the analysand or artist) by which one recollects one's 'lost' identity, one's continuity with the forgotten past. The quality of these recaptured moments shows us the quality of experience itself, and reminds us (as Proust is continually at pains to show) that our memories, our selves, our very existences, consist entirely of *a collection of moments:*

without reference to the nature of each patient; nor the nature of each patient without reference to the nature of the world: thus we are led to see (what everybody once knew) that the constitution of Nature, and all natures, is essentially dramatic ('All the World's a stage . . .') and presents itself epiphanically on all possible occasions:

> Though the World be Histrionical . . . yet be thou what thou singly art, and personate only thy self . . . Things cannot get out of their natures, or be or be not in despite of their constitutions

– as our metaphysical physician, Sir Thomas Browne, reminded us so clearly three centuries ago. One has, it is true, a number of natures, which in their totality constitute one's whole possible nature – a point raised by Leibniz in his famous example of 'alternative Adams.' This too is brought out with great clarity in responses to L-DOPA: thus Martha N., when given L-DOPA on five different occasions, showed different patterns of response on each occasion; all of these responses had dramatic unities[137] of their own – they represented a spray or bouquet of 'alternative Marthas,' although one was pre-eminent, most full and most real, and this – as she knew – was the *real* Martha-self. In the case of Maria G. – who was deeply schizophrenic – the situation on L-DOPA was more complex and tragic; for Maria G.'s *real self* only showed itself for a few days, before being decomposed or re-

---

'A great weakness, no doubt, for a person to consist entirely in a collection of moments; a great strength also; it is dependent upon memory, and our memory of a moment is not informed of everything that has happened since; this moment which it has registered endures still, lives still, and with it the person whose form is outlined in it' (Proust, *Remembrance of Things Past*).

[137] The constitution of *dramatic* (or 'organic') unities is radically different from that of *logical* (or mechanical) unities, although it at no point contravenes the latter. Thus one observes of dogs that they 'like company' or 'need company,' and one feels (if one has a dog) that this sociability is something essential and primary, which *cannot* be reduced to a question of 'reflexes,' 'drives,' 'stimuli,' 'instincts,' etc. Yet this is precisely what Descartes did – hence Sherrington's comment that Descartes writes as if he had never had, or been friendly with, a dog; and Cartesian physiology has, ever since, been a dog-less, friendless, lifeless science.

placed by swarming 'selflets' – miniature, pathological imper-
sonations of herself.[138]

Thus we are led to a deeper and fuller concept of 'awakening,'
embracing not only the first awakening on L-DOPA but all possible awakenings which thereafter ensue. The 'side-effects' of
L-DOPA must be seen as a summoning of possible natures, a
calling-forth of entire latent repertoires of being. We see an
actualization or extrusion of natures which were dormant, which
were 'sleeping' *in posse,* and which perhaps might have been best
left *in posse.* The problem of 'side-effects' is not only a physical
but a metaphysical problem: a question of how much we can
summon one world, without summoning others, and of the
strengths and resources which go with different worlds. That
infinite equation, which represents the total being of each patient
from moment to moment, cannot be reduced to a question of
systems, or to a commensuration of 'stimulus' and 'response': we
are compelled to speak of whole natures, of worlds, and (in
Leibniz's term) of the 'compossibility' between them.

Thus, we are brought back once more to our torturing 'Why?'
Why did so many of our patients, after doing so well at first, spoil,
'go bad,' move into all sorts of trouble? Clearly, they had in them
the *possibilities* of great health: the most deeply ill patients were
able to become deeply well for a time. Thereafter, apparently,
they 'lost' this possibility, and in no case were able to retrieve it
again; such, at least, is the case in all the Parkinsonian patients I
have seen. But the notion of 'losing' a possibility in such a way

---

[138] The tendency to exorbitance and the tendency to schism are clearly quite
separate (though they play on each other); they represent the two fundamental
tendencies to be seen in disease. One observes similar splits of behaviour (or,
in Pavlov's term, 'ruptures of higher nervous activity') in all organisms pushed
beyond a certain limit of stress and strain; the limit itself varies very widely and
so does the *level* at which splitting occurs. Martha N., for example, tended to a
high-level 'molar' splitting (hysterical dissociation), even before she received
L-DOPA; Maria G. tended to 'molecular' splitting (schizophrenic disintegration),
which was clearly present, though constrained, before the administration of
L-DOPA; Hester Y. had an immensely stable 'ego' or personality, but went to
pieces at a *lower* level (tics) when given L-DOPA. It seems to me unlikely that
anyone could tolerate excitement or pressures of the order of those seen in
Hester Y., and *not* show splitting at one level or another.

is difficult to comprehend, on both theoretical and practical grounds: why, for example, should a patient who retained the possibility of 'awakening,' through fifty years of the severest illness, 'lose' it, in a few days, after receiving L-DOPA? One must allow, instead, that their possibilities of continued well-being were actively precluded or prevented because they became *incompossible* with other worlds, with the totality of their relationships, without and within. In short, that their physiological or social situations were incompossible with continuing health, and therefore disallowed or displaced the first state of well-being, thrusting them into illness again.

The descent into illness, once started, may proceed by itself, moving incontinently further by innumerable vicious circles, positive feed-backs, chain-reactions – a first strain causing other strains, a first breakdown other breakdowns, perversion summoning perversion, with the dynamism and ingenuity which is the essence of disease:

> Diseases themselves hold Consultations, and conspire how they may multiply, and join with one another, and exalt one anothers force . . .

DONNE

In this spiral of deterioration, the need for illness joins hands with the liability to illness, that conjoint perversion which is pathological *propensity.* The first of these, necessarily, must be a major factor in the lives of some of our most deeply disabled and deeply regressed patients, whose illness has been the main part of their lives. In such patients, the sudden removal of illness will leave a *hole,* so to speak, a sudden existential vacuum, which needs to be filled and filled quickly with real life and activity, before pathological activity is sucked back again to fill it. The perverse need for illness – both in patients themselves, and sometimes in those who are close to them – must be a major determinant in causing relapse, the most insidious enemy of the will-to-get-better:

BURNLEY: 'How does poor Smart do, Sir; is he likely to recover?'

JOHNSON: 'It seems as if his mind has ceased to struggle with the disease; for he grows fat upon it.'

BOSWELL

Whenever . . . advantage through illness is at all pronounced, and no substitute for it can be found in reality, you need not look forward very hopefully to influencing (it) through your therapy.

FREUD

It is certain that the compensations of disease, and the destitutions of 'external' reality, can only be a *part* of the matter; but they are a part which we are well-placed to study, and sometimes to modify.

Such considerations can hardly be avoided, for instance, with regard to Lucy K., Leonard L. and Rose R. Lucy K. had spent the greater part of her life in a state of symbiotic and parasitic dependence on her mother; her mother was the most needed person in her life, and at once the most loved and most hated, and Lucy's illness and dependence, conversely, were the most important parts of her mother's life. Lucy K. had scarcely awoken on L-DOPA before she turned to me and demanded marriage, rescue, and removal from her mother; when I indicated that this was impossible, she fell back within hours into the depths of her sickness. Leonard L. had a similar if somewhat milder pathological relation with *his* mother, and she, as we have seen, herself broke down when he got better; Leonard saw, all too clearly, that his mother's well-being was incompossible with his own well-being; and shortly after this he too relapsed. Perhaps the saddest case is that of Rose R., who 'came to' joyously to the world of 1926 – and found that '1926' no longer existed; the world of 1969, into which she awoke, was incompossible with the world of 1926, and so she went back to '1926.' In these three cases, the overall situation was pathological beyond remedy: the needs of these patients were incompossible with reality. In other patients

– most clearly exemplified by Miron V. – a much happier situation eventually resulted, the 'side-effects' of L-DOPA being greatly reduced by the establishment of good feelings and relations, of central securities which had lapsed in their lives.

Thus, finally, we come to the only conclusion we can: that patients on L-DOPA will always do as well as their total circumstances will allow; that altering their chemical circumstances may be a prerequisite to any other alteration; but that it is not, in itself, enough. The limitations of L-DOPA are as clear as its benefits, and if we hope to reduce the one and increase the other we must go *beyond* L-DOPA, beyond all purely chemical considerations, and deal with the *person* and his being-in-the-world.

ACCOMMODATION

Or to take arms against a sea of troubles
And by opposing end them?

It is characteristic of many neurologists (and patients) that they mistake intransigence for strength, and plant themselves like Canutes before advancing seas of trouble, *defying* their advance by the strength of their will. Or, like Podsnaps, they *deny* the sea of troubles which is rising all round them: 'I don't want to know about it; I don't choose to discuss it; I don't admit it!' Neither defiance nor denial is of the least use here: one takes arms by learning how to negotiate or navigate a sea of troubles, by becoming a mariner in the seas of one's self. 'Tribulation' dealt with trouble and storm; 'Accommodation' is concerned with weathering the storm.

The troubles experienced are not ordinary troubles, and the weapons which are needed are not ordinary weapons:

Weapons for such combats are not to be forged at *Lipara;* Vulcan's Art does nothing in this internal militia . . .

BROWNE

The weapons of use in the tribulations of L-DOPA are those we all use in conducting our lives: deep strengths and reserves, whose very existence is unsuspected; common sense, forethought, caution, and care; special vigilance and wiles to combat special dangers; the establishment of right relations of all sorts; and, of course, the final acceptance of what must be accepted. A good part of the tribulations of patients (and their physicians) comes from unreal attempts to transcend the possible, to deny its limits, and to seek the impossible: accommodation is more laborious and less exalted, and consists, in effect, of a painstaking exploration of the full range of the real and the possible.[139]

All the operations involved in coming to terms with oneself and the world, in face of continual changes in both, are subsumed in Claude Bernard's fundamental concept of *'homeostasis.'* This is essentially a Leibnizian concept, as Bernard himself was the first to point out: homeostasis means achieving the optimum which is possible in (or compossible with) particular circumstances – in short, 'making the best of things.' We have to recognize homeostatic endeavours at all levels of being, from molecular and cellu-

---

[139] Accommodation lacks the *glamour* of Awakening. It lacks its sudden, spontaneous, 'miraculous' quality. It does not come 'of itself' – easily and effortlessly. It is *earned, worked for* – with infinite effort and courage and trouble. It does not reflect some local change in the basal ganglia, and can in no sense be regarded as localized process: it is an achievement of character, of negotiation, in its widest possible sense. What is achieved in this way, with work and difficulty, is secure and enduring – unlike the facile 'flash' of 'awakening,' which goes, as it comes, too easily, too quickly. . . . The qualities of the first DOPA-awakening are essentially those of innocence and joy – like an anomalous return to earliest childhood: the 'awakened,' in this sense, irrespective of their age, come to resemble the 'once-born' of whom William James speaks. Tribulation is an ordeal, a dark night of the soul, which challenges to the utmost those who must face it. A number are broken and fail to survive; others endure and are *forged* by their suffering. These survivors – the 'accommodated' – have (in James's words) 'drunk too deeply of the cup of bitterness ever to forget its taste, and their redemption is into a universe two storeys deep.' These, then, are the 'twice-born,' who after bitter division, physiological and social, finally achieve a real reunion, a reconciliation of the deepest and stablest kind.

lar to social and cultural, all in intimate relation to each other.

The deepest and most general forms of homeostasis proceed 'automatically,' below the level of conscious control. Such activities occur in all organisms submitted to stress, and involve depths and complexities about which we know all too little. Our deepest and most mysterious strengths are called forth from these levels.

Some of the patients described in this book – Rose R., Rolando P., Leonard L., etc. – were never able to achieve a 'satisfactory' accommodation, and were forced either to cease taking L-DOPA altogether or to accept a very miserable *modus vivendi*. Other patients described in this book – and perhaps the majority of 'ordinary' Parkinsonian patients placed on L-DOPA – did, eventually, achieve a more satisfactory coming-to-terms. Common to all such patients is a gradual diminution of the effects of L-DOPA, leading at length to a sort of plateau. The achievement of this plateau involves both a gain and a loss: a fairly stable and satisfactory level of functioning, *minus* the drama of full 'awakening' or 'side-effects.' Such patients are no longer very well or very ill; their 'awakenings' and 'tribulations' are both in the past; they have emerged into relatively even water, into a state which is nevertheless much 'better' than their pre-DOPA state. Our first history (Frances D.) exemplifies this passage.

I know of no simple way, no set of criteria, which allows one to predict whether a satisfactory coming to terms of this sort will occur. Certainly the severity of the original Parkinsonism or post-encephalitic illness is not itself a good index: thus I have seen patients with quite mild Parkinson's disease experience intractable 'side-effects' from which they never emerged, and at the other extreme one sees patients like Magda B., who do well and stay well despite the devastating severity of the original disease.

This indicated that *other* parts of the brain (or the organism) must determine or co-determine the powers and potential of deep homeostasis. It is clear, for example, that functional integrity of the cerebral cortex is such a prerequisite, for accommodation tends to be undermined if the cortex is impaired (as in Rachel I.).

But even these basic processes cannot, I think, account for the range and extent of accommodation. One must allow the possibility of an almost limitless repertoire of functional reorganizations and accommodations of all types, from cellular, chemical, and hormonal levels to the organization of the self – the 'will to get well.' One sees again and again, not merely in the context of L-DOPA and Parkinsonism, but in cancer, tuberculosis, neurosis – *all* diseases – remarkable, unexpected and 'inexplicable' resolutions, at times when it seems that everything is lost. One must allow – with surprise, with delight – that such things happen, and that they can happen to patients on L-DOPA as well. *Why* they should happen, and *what* indeed is happening, are questions which it is not yet in our power to answer; for health goes deeper than any disease.

When we rise to the level of accommodations which are accessible (in part) to consciousness, and (in part) to deliberate control, we find what we have found at every stage in our discussion: that the 'private' sphere, the sphere of individual actions and feelings, is everywhere commingled with the 'public' sphere, with the human and non-human environment. We cannot really separate individual endeavours from social endeavours, as these assist (or impede) the patient's being-in-the-world; the patient's therapeutic endeavours depend on the world's compliance, and other therapeutic endeavours depend on the patient's compliance. There must be a working together to realise the possible.

Physicians often speak of 'preventive,' 'precautionary,' or 'supportive' measures, as if these were different *in kind* from 'radical' measures. This distinction disappears the more we look into it: the therapeutic measures which we will touch on now are no less radical than taking L-DOPA, and they are an *essential* complement to taking L-DOPA. As the central concept of disease is dis-ease, the central concept of therapy is *ease:* everything which promotes the ease of the patient reduces his pathological potentials, and assists the fullest coming to terms which is possible.

All patients who continue to receive L-DOPA show a reduction of tolerance, becoming particularly in need of ease, and particularly intolerant of strain or un-ease. The need for rest becomes especially important, whether in the form of night-sleep, 'naps,' 'taking it easy,' or 'relaxation.' One invariably sees, with patients on L-DOPA, a resurgence of 'side-effects' if their rest or sleep is less than their needs. One observes this even in out-patients with Parkinson's disease, who at best show not a trace of trouble (like George W.). What is 'adequate rest' can only be found by each individual patient, and may be considerably in excess of 'normal' needs; I have under my care a number of patients who enjoy excellent health if they sleep twelve hours a day, and intractable 'side-effects' if they sleep any less.[140]

The intolerance of strain is equally marked, whether the strain is imposed by fever or by pain, disability, frustration, anxiety, or anger. One repeatedly sees, with patients who seem 'almost normal' on L-DOPA, this peculiar intolerance to all forms of stress.[141]

But life involves *action* besides 'relaxation'; one can be at ease in an easy-chair only for so long, before the impulse to move as-

---

[140] The special need for additional sleep, rest, or recuperation, in these frail, struggling, convalescing-accommodating patients must, I think, be interpreted in metaphysical as well as physical terms. One recaptures during sleep an elemental sort of strength, a reunion with the world and the grounds-of-one's being. This is poetically intimated by Sir Thomas Browne: '. . . whilst we sleep within the bosome of our causes, we enjoy a being and life in three distinct worlds . . .'; and in Lawrence's beautiful images of reunion and renewal:

> And if tonight my soul may find her peace
> in sleep, and sink in good oblivion,
> and in the morning wake like a new-opened flower
> then I have been dipped again in God, and new-created.

It is analysed by Freud, in terms of libido-theory: 'Sleep is a condition in which all investments of objects, the libidinal as well as the egoistic, are abandoned and withdrawn into the ego. Does this not shed a new light upon the recuperation afforded by sleep? . . . In the sleeper the primal state of the libido-distribution is again reproduced, that of absolute narcissism, in which libido and ego-interests dwell together still, united and indistinguishable in the self-sufficient self.' And it is experienced by us all. Physiologists have never been able to explain the need for sleep, seen in all living beings, in purely physical terms.

[141] This was strikingly exemplified on one occasion when I saw Aaron E. He had returned home at this time, and was ostensibly quite normal, but came back to see me for periodic check-ups. On one of these return-visits I was dismayed to see a rather violent chorea, grimacing, and tics, which he had never shown previously. When I inquired if there was anything making him uneasy, he replied that he had taken a taxi to hospital, and that the taxi-meter was continually ticking away: 'It keeps ticking away,' he said, 'and it keeps *me* ticcing too!' On hearing this, I immediately dismissed the taxi, and promised Mr E. we would get another one and pay all expenses. Within thirty seconds of my arranging all this, Mr E.'s chorea, grimacing, and ticcing had vanished.

sumes imperative force; and if one cannot move when one needs to, unease is extreme. Impediment to movement is a main symptom in all of these patients, and the distress thus caused is liable to call forth a variety of other symptoms. In order to break this vicious spiral of distress and disorder, various devices are needed to make movement easy. The use of such devices is an indispensable adjunct to the use of L-DOPA, and allows accommodations of critical importance.

Only a few such devices and accommodations can be mentioned. One is the use of 'auto-command' and 'pacing,' employed with such success by Frances D. and others. A variant of this is the use of external command and suggestion, where auto-command is impossible – a matter of critical importance with all Parkinsonians. The therapeutic power of music is very remarkable, and may allow an ease of movement otherwise impossible. The design of furniture, and interior design, is equally important in allowing free movement. Mechanical difficulties must be smoothed away, for they may constitute a critical danger to patients on L-DOPA.[142] In these and similar ways, the extent to which a mutual accommodation can be reached between the symptom-prone patient and his environment determines (or co-determines) the consequences of L-DOPA.

In these and a thousand and one other ways some Parkinsonian patients, and patients on L-DOPA, become astute and expert navigators, steering themselves through seas of trouble which would cause less expert patients to founder on the spot. The extent to which such ruses and wiles can be learned and employed depends, among other things, on the inventiveness and

---

[142] Thus, at the Highlands Hospital, where it is well realized that a curve rather than an angle can make all the difference to a Parkinsonian patient, the main promenade is in the form of an oval. This environmental accommodation greatly facilitates patients' walking. On the other hand, it may facilitate it so much that they *cannot stop walking.* In Mount Carmel, by contrast, where everything tends to be sharp and angled rather than curved and smoothed, Parkinsonian patients can easily walk up and down the regular stairs, but tend to get jammed in the irregular, crowded, and zig-zag corridors whenever they have to make a *shift* of direction. Thus sharpnesses and smoothnesses, steps and curves, each have their own advantages and disadvantages. A consequence of the contradictory nature of Parkinsonian symptoms is that Parkinsonian patients need a contradictory *milieu;* but this would involve them in all sorts of logical and ontological paradoxes, like those Alice encountered in the Looking-Glass World.

resourcefulness of individual patients, on their attitude and the attitude of those around them, and on the opportunities for studying one's being-in-the-world.[143] In general, post-encephalitic patients seem to be far wilier and cannier in this regard than 'ordinary' Parkinsonians; they have usually had (even before the advent of L-DOPA) decades of experience in the stormy seas of themselves; they have painfully acquired their wiles and their insight: unsung, post-encephalitic Odysseuses, dispatched (by Fate) on Odysseys of themselves.

'Deep' accommodation, rest, care, ingenuity – all of these are

---

[143] One such patient (the head-nodding patient previously referred to: n. 121, p. 245) had managed to maintain an independent life outside institutions for years, in face of almost incredible difficulties – difficulties which would instantly have broken a less determined or resourceful person. This patient – Lillian T. – had long since found that she could scarcely start, or stop, or change her direction of motion; that once she had been set in motion, she had no control. It was therefore necessary for her to plan all her motions in advance, with great precision. Thus, moving from her arm-chair to her divan-bed (a few feet to one side) could never be done *directly* – Miss T. would immediately be 'frozen' in transit, and perhaps stay frozen for half an hour or more. She therefore had to embark on one of two courses of action: in either case, she would rise to her feet, arrange her angle of direction exactly, and shout 'Now!', whereupon she would break into an incontinent run, which could be neither stopped nor changed in direction. If the double doors between her living-room and the kitchen were open, she would rush through them, across the kitchen, around the back of the stove, across the other side of the kitchen, through the double doors – in a great figure-of-eight – until she hit her destination, her bed. If, however, the double doors were closed and secured, she would calculate her angle like a billiard-player, and then launch herself with great force against the doors, rebounding at the right angle to hit her bed. Miss T.'s apartment (and, to some extent, her mind) resembled the control-room for the Apollo launchings, at Houston, Texas: all paths and trajectories pre-computed and compared, contingency plans and 'fail-safes' prepared in advance. A good deal of Miss T.'s life, in short, was dependent on conscious taking-care and elaborate calculation – but this was the only way she could maintain her existence. Needless to say, many forms of taking-care and calculation, of somewhat less elaborate kind, can become purely automatic and second nature to patients, and no longer demand any conscious attention.

This entire subject is penetratingly discussed in the last chapter of A. R. Luria's *The Nature of Human Conflicts*. Luria speaks here, and in allied contexts, of the necessity of devising 'algorithms of behaviour' – behavioural prostheses, calculated but invaluable *substitutes* for the ease, naturalness, and intuitive sureness which have been undermined by disease. Such 'algorithms' are, of course, artifices and, above all, *artificial metrics;* but they may represent almost the only way in which patients with profound disorders of force and metrication can achieve *some* control of their own incontinent tendencies.

essential for the patient on L-DOPA. But more important than all of them, and perhaps a prerequisite for all of them, is the establishment of proper relations with the world, and – in particular – with other human beings, or *one* other human being, for it is human relations which carry the possibilities of proper being-in-the-world. Feeling the fullness of the presence of the world depends on feeling the fullness of another *person,* as a person; reality is given to us by the reality of people; reality is taken from us by the unreality of un-people; our sense of reality, of trust, of security, is critically dependent on a human relation. A *single* good relation is a life-line in trouble, a pole-star and compass in the ocean of trouble: and we see, again and again, in the histories of these patients, how a single relation can extricate them from trouble. Kinship is healing; we are physicians to each other – 'A faithful friend is the physic of life' (Browne). The world is the hospital where healing takes place.

The essential thing is feeling *at home* in the world, knowing in the depths of one's being that one has a real place in the home of the world. The essential function of such hospitals as Mount Carmel – which house several millions of the world's population – is that they should provide *hospitality,* the feeling of home, for patients who have lost their original homes. To the extent that Mount Carmel acts as a *home,* it is deeply therapeutic to all of its patients; but to the extent that it acts as an *institution,* it deprives them of their sense of reality and home, and forces them into the false homes and compensations of regression and sickness. And this is equally true of L-DOPA, with the unreal 'miraculous' expectations which attend it, with its false promise of a false home in the bosom of a drug. Tribulations of every kind were at a maximum for our patients in the autumn of 1969 – a time when the hospital changed its character, when human relations of all sorts became strained or undermined (including my own relation with our patients), and when neurotic hopes and fears reached exorbitant heights. At this period, patients who had attained accommodations previously, who *had* felt reasonably at home with themselves and the world, were deprived of their accommodations, and profoundly unsettled: unsettled socially, physiologically, at all possible levels.

Many of these patients have now *re-*settled, *re-*accommodated, *re-*attained good relations, and with this are doing much better on L-DOPA. One sees this, with great clarity, in the case of Miron V., as he was restored to his work, his place in the world; and one sees it, most movingly, with regard to Magda B., Hester Y., and Ida T., who were restored to their children, and the love of their families. One sees it in *all* patients, insofar as they are able to love themselves and the world.

One sees that beautiful and ultimate metaphysical truth, which has been stated by poets and physicians and metaphysicians in all ages – by Leibniz and Donne and Dante and Freud: that Eros is the oldest and strongest of the gods; that love is the *alpha* and *omega* of being; and that the work of healing, of rendering whole, is, first and last, the business of love.

And so we come to the end of our tale. I have been with these patients for almost seven years, a considerable part of their lives and mine. These seven years have seemed like a single long day: a long night of illness, a morning awakening, a high noon of trouble, and now a long evening of repose. They have also composed a strange sort of odyssey, through the deepest and darkest oceans of being; and if our patients have not reached an ultimate haven, some of them have fought through to a staunch, rock-girt Ithaca, an island or home against the perils around them.

It is given to these patients, through no wish or fault of their own, to explore the depths, the ultimate possibilities of human being and suffering. Their unsought crucifixions are not without consequence, if they afford help or illumination to others, if they lead us to a deeper understanding of the nature of affliction and care and cure. This sense of genuine and generous, if involuntary, martyrdom is not unknown to the patients themselves – thus Leonard L., speaking for them all, wrote at the end of his autobiography: 'I am a living candle. I am consumed that you may learn. New things will be seen in the light of my suffering.'

What we *do* see, first and last, is the utter inadequacy of mechanical medicine, the utter inadequacy of a mechanical worldview. These patients are living disproofs of mechanical thinking, as they are living exemplars of biological thinking. Expressed in their sickness, their health, their reactions, is the living imagination of Nature itself, the imagination we must match in our picturing of Nature. They show us that Nature is everywhere real and alive and that our thinking about Nature must be real and alive. They remind us that we are over-developed in mechanical competence, but lacking in biological intelligence, intuition, awareness; and that it is this, above all, that we need to regain, not only in medicine, but in *all* science.[144]

In the years I have known them – and, most of all, in their years on L-DOPA – those patients have been through a range and depth of experience that is not granted to, or desired by, the majority of people. Many of them, by superficial criteria, appear now to have come full circle, and to be back where they were, in their starting position; but this, in actuality, is by no means the case.

They may still (or again) be deeply Parkinsonian, in some instances, but they are no longer the people they were. They have acquired a depth, a fullness, a richness, an awareness of themselves and of the nature of things, of a sort which is rare, and only to be achieved through experience and suffering. I have tried, insofar as it is possible for another person, a physician, to enter into or share their experiences and feelings, and, alongside with them, to be deepened by these; and if they are no longer the people they were, I am no longer the person I was. We are older and more battered, but calmer and deeper.

---

[144] James Joseph Sylvester, poet and mathematician, student of Leibniz and Goethe, speaking of an analogous awakening in mathematics ('. . . if the day only responds to the promise of its dawn . . .'), depicts in unforgettable terms the real, spacious, and *alive* quality of mathematical thinking:

'Mathematics is not a book confined within a cover and bound between brazen clasps, whose contents it needs only patience to ransack; it is not a mine, whose treasures may take long to reduce into possession, but which fill only a limited number of veins and lodes; it is not a soil, whose fertility can be exhausted by the yield of successive harvests; it is not a continent or an ocean, whose area can be mapped out and its contour defined: it is limitless as that space which it finds too narrow for its aspirations; its possibilities are as infinite as the worlds which are forever crowding in and multiplying upon the astronomer's gaze: it is as incapable of being restricted within assigned boundaries or being reduced to definitions of permanent validity, as the consciousness, the life, which seems to slumber in each monad, in every atom of matter, in each leaf and bud and cell, and is forever ready to burst forth into new forms of vegetable and animal existence' (*Address on Commemoration Day at Johns Hopkins, 1877*).

The flash-like drug-awakening of summer 1969 came and went; its like was not to be seen again. But something else has followed in the wake of that flash – a slower, deeper, imaginative awakening, which has gradually developed and lapped them around in a feeling, a light, a sense, a strength, which is not *pharmacological,* chimerical, false, or fantastic: they have – to paraphrase Browne – come to rest once again in the bosom of their causes. They have come to re-feel the grounds of their being, to re-root themselves in the ground of reality, to return to the first-ground, the earth-ground, the home-ground, from which, in their sickness, they had so long departed. In them, and with them, this is the home-coming I have felt. Their experiences have guided me, and will guide some of my readers, on that endless journey which leads to home:

> He found, on his arrival at Waldzell, a pleasure at homecoming such as he had never experienced before. He felt . . . that during his absence it had become even more lovely and interesting – or perhaps he was now seeing it in a new perspective, having returned with the heightened powers of perception . . . 'It seems to me,' he confided to his friend Tegularius . . . 'that I have spent all my years here asleep . . . It is now as though I have awakened, and can see everything sharply and clearly, bearing the stamp of reality.'
>
> HERMANN HESSE, *Magister Ludi*

> And the end of all our exploring
> Will be to arrive where we started
> And know the place for the first time . . .
>
> ELIOT

EPILOGUE (1982)

❧ Ten years have passed, now, since I completed the stories in *Awakenings,* ten years in which I have continued to work with our still-surviving but dwindling population of patients, and to observe their continuing reactions to L-DOPA. I am continually approached by people with questions of all sorts; but the central questions, which everyone asks, are: 'Those extraordinary patients of yours – are they still alive? What do you think of L-DOPA after all these years? Do you still "see" things as you did when you first published *Awakenings?*'

At the time when *Awakenings* was originally published, seven of the twenty patients whose stories I related had already died. Of the remaining thirteen patients – whose continuing stories I will now relate – ten more have died (one, Martha N., in October 1981, after I had actually written her 'story': so with her, as with Rolando P. in the original edition, I have had to add a rather melancholy ending). Thus now (February 1982), of the original twenty patients, there are left only three – Hester Y., Miriam H., Gertie C. – although these are very vigorously and *enjoyably* alive.

The twenty patients whose stories I told in detail in *Awakenings* were only a sample of a much larger number: some of these were briefly introduced, in passing footnotes or illustrations – Seymour L., Frances M., Lillian T., Lillian W., Maurice P., Edith T., Rosalie B., Ed M., Sam G., etc. – but there were a much greater number of whom I said nothing. Besides the three 'survivors' of the original twenty in *Awakenings,* there are still at Mount Carmel thirty more of the original post-encephalitic population, many of whom were admitted in the 1920s and 1930s. In addition to these, in the past fifteen years – and especially since the original publication of *Awakenings* – I have brought into Mount Carmel a further twenty patients with post-encephalitic disease. Thus, even now, sixty-five years after the start of the epidemic, we still have more than fifty survivors at Mount Carmel, most of whom require, and are maintained on, L-DOPA.[145]

In addition to this central 'colony' at Mount Carmel, I have under my care yet another thirty post-encephalitic patients, some in other homes and institutions, and others (like Cecil M.) still living outside. I know of no other physician, so many years after the sleepy-sickness, who has more than eighty post-encephalitic patients under continuing care and observation, nor one who has observed the effects of L-DOPA for so long. I am the last witness, as they are the last witnesses, to a unique situation – five decades of 'sleep,' followed by more than twelve years of 'awakening.'

In general – despite the inevitable sad toll of age, chronic illness, and death – I have become much more optimistic than I was when I first wrote *Awakenings,* for there has been a significant number of patients who, following the vicissitudes of their first years on L-DOPA, came to do – and still do – extremely well. Such patients have undergone an *enduring* awakening, and enjoy possibilities of life which had been impossible, unthinkable, before the coming of L-DOPA. A few such patients (Hester Y., Miriam H., Gertie L.) are among those whose stories I now tell; but there are known to me, in addition, dozens of such patients, who have now enjoyed more than a decade of good awakened life, and may hope to do so for the rest of their lives. I wish I could tell all these other, and often very happy, stories – but I can only make this passing general reference to them, and sometimes allude to them, briefly, in a footnote (as, for example, to Ed M., n. 97, p. 211).

Indeed, I would say, in general terms, that post-encephalitic patients with even the severest disease may ultimately do better when maintained on L-DOPA than patients with 'ordinary' Parkinson's disease (see n. 51, p. 71). There are many reasons for

---

[145] Several of these patients were transferred from state institutions and psychiatric hospitals where they had spent years or decades misdiagnosed as 'schizophrenic.' There is no doubt that this happened all over the world, to thousands of post-encephalitic patients with catatonia, thought-block, crises, etc. – patients perhaps 'schizophreniform,' but not schizophrenic (see n. 20, p. 16).

this: our post-encephalitic patients, when started on L-DOPA in 1969, were younger, by and large, than 'ordinary' Parkinsonians. Further – a paradoxical consideration! – having been ill for so long, they had become very experienced, very wise, in the ways of disease, and in all sorts of ways for combating the disease, so they were better fighters, wilier, than 'ordinary' Parkinsonians. Finally, and fundamentally, where ordinary Parkinson's disease is always progressive, post-encephalitic syndromes are often essentially static, and thus if such a patient can adjust to L-DOPA, he may then maintain an even level for the rest of his life. These general considerations are illustrated in the histories that follow.

Passing from these specific considerations to the far wider and deeper ones discussed in 'Perspectives,' I would say, by and large, that while I hold to everything I wrote at the time, while my 'feeling' or orientation remains much the same, I have struggled to reach, and have sometimes reached, rather profounder formulations – deeper, and yet simpler, than anything I could say ten years ago. Such formulations, however theoretical they may seem, have stemmed at all times from experience, and have been continually tried and tested in experience – for experience is the only touchstone of reality. The daily practice of clinical medicine, or so it seems to me, demands theoretical and even 'philosophical' viewpoints, and precisely guides one to the viewpoints one needs. That medicine provides a philosophical education – and a better and truer one than any philosopher provides! – is a delightful discovery; it seems to me strange that this is not more generally realized. Nietzsche, almost alone of philosophers, sees philosophy as grounded in our understanding (or misunderstanding) of the body, and so looks to the ideal of the Philosophic Physician. (See especially the 1886 Preface to his *Fröhliche Wissenschaft,* or *Gay Science.*)

So long as medicine consists merely of the giving of medicines, there is little call for intelligence or thought; the physician need be little more than a dispenser of physic. If L-DOPA was, or remained, the adequate or perfect remedy, if any medication or medicine, any 'purely medical' approach, could solve for ever the problems of these patients, there would no longer be 'a situation,'

or anything to consider. It is precisely to the extent that L-DOPA
is limited – that all conceivable chemical approaches, all medici-
nal medicines, are limited in power – that the singular problems
of being post-encephalitic recur, together with the scarcely less
singular problems induced by medication. With all this, then, the
need arises for other forms of understanding and therapy, which
must go beyond the medicational, and beyond what is usually or
conventionally called 'medicine.'

We need, in addition to conventional medicine, a medicine of
a far profounder sort, based on the profoundest understanding
of the organism and of life. This need is particularly clear and
pressing when we deal with neurological (and neuro-psychologi-
cal) problems and patients. The profoundest innovator in this
field, this radically new medicine, was the great A. R. Luria. But
the extraordinary patients with whom we are concerned in *Awakenings* raise problems which even Luria never considered. Such
problems were confronted, both theoretically and practically, by
an exceedingly modest and important man, James Purdon Martin, who wrote a very important and beautiful book based on his
years of minute observation and study with the post-encephalitic
patients at Highlands (Martin, 1967). He understood such patients as nobody else – and his understanding was based on a
faithful, minute, and infinitely patient observation, a pure and
disinterested love of phenomena, coupled with profound physiological knowledge and insight. His insights are, at once, of fundamental theoretical interest and of literally lifesaving importance.
He describes how patients otherwise unable to move are enabled
to do so by a variety of methods – sometimes being gently
rocked; sometimes given an object to hold; and, most fascinat-
ingly, given a sort of external regulator or command, as by regular transverse lines painted on the ground.

Such a medicine is radical because it is physiological, and deals
delicately and directly with *function*. It is radical because it is
active, rather than passive – one no longer has a patient passively
receiving, but an agent effecting his own cure. It is radical, and
rational, because it is concerned with universal procedures,
which every patient can learn and use to advantage. It is an active and collaborative physiological medicine, which joins the

patient and his physician together in learning, teaching, communicating, and understanding. Thus, with these patients, the use of L-DOPA, or any conventional and purely empirical medicine, must be supplemented by a universal and rational medicine, the medicine of Luria and Purdon Martin.

Purdon Martin, like Luria, is concerned to find *algorithms,* or universal procedures, for the neurologically disabled. Such algorithms are essential – and yet they are insufficient. I do not mean that one needs some sort of super-super-algorithm, of more and more power. What one needs, what patients need, is much simpler than any algorithm, and can allow them to move and function in a way which no algorithm can. What is this mystery which passes any method or procedure, and is essentially different from algorithm or strategy? It is art.

There is an aphorism of Novalis which I particularly like: 'Every disease is a musical problem. Every cure is a musical solution.' One finds this is literally and even sensationally so, with Parkinsonian and post-encephalitic patients: one finds patients unable to take a single step, who can dance with consummate ease and grace; patients unable to phonate, or utter a single word, who can sing without any difficulty, bringing to the music all the volume, all the richness and delicacy of intonation, all the feeling, that it demands. One sees patients with cramped or stuttering or jerky micrographia, until – all of a sudden – they 'get into' what they are doing, and then write with all their usual smoothness and style, totally regaining what Luria calls the 'kinetic melody' of writing. One sees – and I never cease to delight in it, nor do the patients themselves – how patients unable to initiate a single movement can catch and return a ball without the least trouble, with perfect accuracy, and wholly in their own style.

It is in this realm, too, that the commonest and most important phenomenon of all is seen – the importance of other people to Parkinsonians. Many a Parkinsonian cannot walk by himself, will either freeze, or stutter and festinate uncontrollably; yet he may walk perfectly if there is someone with him – not necessarily touching him, for *visual* touch is enough. Much has been written about 'contactual reflexes,' but it is certain that these are not enough, are not in the *realm* where explanation resides.

One patient, who was so eloquent on the subject of music (see n. 45, p. 61), had great difficulty in walking alone, but was always able to walk perfectly if someone walked with her. Her own comments on this are of very great interest: 'When you walk with me,' she said, 'I feel in myself your own power of walking. I *partake* of the power and freedom you have. I *share* your walking powers, your perceptions, your feelings, your existence. Without even knowing it, you make me a great gift.' This patient felt this experience as very similar to, if not identical with, her experiences with music: 'I partake of other people, as I partake of the music. Whether it is others, in their own natural movement, or the movement of music itself, the feeling of movement, of living movement, is communicated to me. And not just movement, but existence itself.' This patient is surely describing something transcendent, which goes far beyond any 'contactual reflexes.' We see that the contactual is essentially musical – as the musical is essentially contactual. One must be 'touched' before one can move. This patient, whether speaking of others or music, is speaking of just this, the mysterious 'touch,' the contact, of two existences. She is describing, in a word, the sense of communion.

Perhaps all this sounds unduly poetic, but the fact of such awakening is easily confirmed, not only clinically, but physiologically too. I have made some combined EEGs-and-videotapes which give a marvellous demonstration of the awakening and modulating powers of art. I have a fascinating such record on one patient (Ed M.) who is akinetic on one side, and frenetic on the other (whatever medication helps one side aggravates the other), and with an EEG correspondingly asymmetrical. This man is a fine pianist and organist, and the moment he starts playing, his left side loses its akinesia, his right side loses its tics and chorea, and both come together in perfect union: simultaneously, the gross asymmetry, the pathological EEG patterns, disappear, and we see in their place only symmetry and normality. The instant he stops playing, or his inner music stops, both his clinical state and his EEG abruptly decompose (see p. 330 in the Appendix: The Electrical Basis of Awakenings).

I hasten to add that with this patient, as with all patients, this strange and mysterious magic may not work. This, if nothing else, makes it quite different from a general algorithm or formal procedure, or from the action of a drug, which *does* always work, for it works in a mechanical way. Why does art, or personal interaction, sometimes 'work,' and sometimes not? There are some profound words of E. M. Forster in this matter: 'The Arts are not drugs. They are not guaranteed to act when taken. Something as mysterious and capricious as the creative impulse has to be released before they can act.'

There is no doubt of the reality of these phenomena – but what *sort* of reality is involved? Does it lie within the domain of natural science? Can science, indeed, apprehend these phenomena, which are at once so real and so difficult to conceptualize? We tend to speak of the 'eye' of science – there is something visual and structural about any scientific edifice of concepts; whereas here we are dealing with the ear, in a way – with something essentially musical and tonal, something essentially action, not structure. Can the eye of science feel the true character of music, and its unique power to animate the person? Even Kant felt this (reluctantly, perhaps!), and spoke of music as 'the Quickening Art.' If science, if thought, considers music, what will it say? It will say precisely what Leibniz said: 'Music is nothing but unconscious arithmetic . . . Music is pleasure the human soul experiences from counting without becoming aware that it is counting.' And this is fine – but tells us nothing of the sense of music, its essential inner movement – and its capacity to move: precisely what makes it both quickening and quick. It tells us nothing of the life within music.

There is a profound truth in Leibniz' dictum: music *does* contain unconscious counting. We may all feel this, vividly, if we set out on a swim or a run; we start, conscientiously, and consciously, counting every step or stroke; and then – often rather suddenly, and without our being aware of it – we have 'the feel' of it, and are running or swimming in perfect tempo, or musical inner time, without any conscious counting at all. We have leapt, unwittingly, from the metronomic to the music.

Leibniz, however, would appear to be saying that music is nothing *but* – an unconscious counting or counter, an inner pacing or metronome. Such internal pacemakers and metronomes do indeed exist; and they are indeed severely impaired in Parkinsonism – this is partly what our patient meant when she said she was 'unmusicked.'

The Parkinsonian has indeed lost, and quite fundamentally, his inner sense of scale and pace – hence the incontinent accelerations and retardations, the magnifications and minifications, to which he is prone.[146] The Parkinsonian is lost in space and time – bereft of any inner scale, or metric, at all; or with his scales, his inner metrics, fantastically capricious, warped, and unstable: earlier I called this 'a relativistic delirium.' Certainly, in the most fundamental sense, the Parkinsonian needs scale. And it is precisely in the provision of scale that algorithm and art, instruction, and action, can finally meet. But what do we mean when we speak of 'scale,' and more particularly a sense of scale? For it is sense of scale the Parkinsonian lacks, and a sense of scale he needs to regain. A scale, in the physical sense, is a constant, a convention – like a ruler or a clock. And we may say of the Parkinsonian that his inner rulers and clocks are all awry – as in the famous painting by Salvador Dali, which shows a multitude of clocks all going at different rates and registering different times – a metaphor, perhaps, for Parkinsonism (the Parkinsonism which Dali himself was beginning to feel). Purdon Martin, in effect, provides rules and clocks, to make up for the shattered, delirious, metrical chaos – the chaos of broken clocks and rulers – which is the Parkinsonian mind.

But no scale, no measure, no rule can work, unless it works, personally, livingly, for one. Posture, we may say, is a reflection of gravity, and of other physical and physiological forces acting upon one; it is the resultant and expression of such forces; but it is *one's* representation and expression, an active and absolutely personal expression, and not merely a mechanical or mathematical one. Every posture is unique and personal, as well as being mechanical and rational: every posture is an 'I' no less than an 'It.' Every posture, every action, is suffused with feeling, with grace ('Grace is the peculiar relation of actor to action,' writes Winkelman). And it is precisely this which is missing in Parkinsonism –

---

[146] See Appendix: Parkinsonian Space and Time, p. 339.

there is a loss of naturalness in posture and action, a loss of natural feeling and grace; a loss of the living 'I' – this is our other way of seeing the inert, impersonal Parkinsonian state. And this is the rationale of an 'existence' therapy: not to instruct but to inspire – to inspire with art to combat the inert (which means, quite literally, 'in-art'), to inspire with the personal and living, and, in the directest sense possible to awaken and quicken.

It is the function of medication, or surgery, or appropriate physiological procedures, to rectify mechanism – the mechanism, the mechanisms, which are so deranged in these patients. It is the function of scientific medicine to rectify the 'It.' It is the function of art, of living contact, of existential medicine, to call upon the latent will, the agent, the 'I,' to call out its commanding and coordinating powers, so that it may regain its hegemony and rule once again – for the final rule, the ruler, is not a measuring rod or clock, but the rule and measure of the personal 'I.' These two forms of medicine must be joined, must co-inhere, as body and soul. 'Where It was,' writes Freud, 'there I should be.'

What is so fundamental here is difficult to say. We can say, in a manner of speaking, that one cannot have a Parkinsonian *person;* the person, the 'I,' can never be 'Parkinsonized.' The only thing that can be 'Parkinsonized' is his subcortical 'go!', what Pavlov called 'the blind force of the subcortex.' This is not an 'I' but an 'It,' and yet the 'I' may be subjugated and enslaved by this 'It.' This is part of the peculiar mortification of the state, which the Parkinsonian may both know and detest, yet be unable, directly, to contest. This is precisely what Gaubius expressed, writing of festination *('scelotyrbe festinans')* almost a century before Parkinson: 'Cases occur in which the muscles, duly excited by the impulses of the will, do then, with an unbidden agility, and with an impetus not to be repressed, run before the unwilling mind.' It is clear that Gaubius, here, is using 'will' in two opposed senses: the will of the 'It' – that is, automatism; and the will of the 'I' – which is freedom or autonomy.

By scientific approaches, one can modulate automatism – but only by an 'existential' approach can one liberate the 'I' – the never-extinguished but dormant free will or autonomy, which has been lying passive, enslaved, in the thrall of the 'It.' We have spoken of the Parkinsonian as 'lost in space and time,' and as harbouring a 'chaos of broken clocks and rulers.' One might say that these are Kantian formulations of his state, for they correspond with the central Kantian notion that space and time are the essential forms of experience, that space and time (or, rather, the sense of space and time) are 'constructs' of the organism or mind. Thus, where we spoke previously of a relativistic or Einsteinian delirium, we might now, even more fundamentally, speak of a 'Kantian' delirium – and ultimate akinesia as being 'aKantia.'

If Kant, in his first *Critique,* dealt with space and time as the essential ('*a priori* synthetic') forms of the experience (and thus of perception and motion), he deals in his other *Critiques* with agency, the will, 'I' (and as 'I' being defined by its will – 'Volo ergo sum'). Thus the considerations we have been impelled to require *all* of Kant's thought.

Are such considerations outside the proper domain of 'science'? They are outside the domain of a purely empirical science, a Humean science, for this not only denies the ideal forms of experience, but disallows any 'personal identity.' But they point, or so I believe, to a greater and more generous conception of 'science,' which can embrace all the phenomena we have discussed. Such a 'Kantian' science, I think, is the science of the future.

Thus, in what might appear an extraordinarily small field – the study and treatment of post-encephalitic patients – we find unexpectedly vast vistas emerging. We see before us, in exemplary form, the thrilling shapes of the medicine of the future, a perfectly rational yet practical scientific medicine, and an utterly beautiful and elemental 'existential' medicine. The two are for ever separate and inseparable; not contradictory, but complementary, and calling to be conjoined – as was realized by Leibniz three centuries ago:

> I find indeed that many of the effects of nature can be accounted for in a two-fold way, that is to say by a consideration of efficient causes and again independently by a consideration of final causes . . . Both explanations are good . . . for the discovery of useful facts in Physics and Medicine. And writers who take these diverse

routes should not speak ill of each other . . . The best plan would be to join the two ways of thinking.

On one occasion I asked Luria what he considered the most interesting thing in the world. He replied, 'I cannot express it in one word, I have to use two. I would have to speak of "romantic science." It has been my life's hope to found or refound a romantic science.' I think my own answer would be exactly the same, and the peculiar joy I have known, working with my post-encephalitics for the past fifteen years, has been the fusion of scientific and 'romantic' penetrations, finding my mind and my heart equally exercised and involved, and knowing that anything different would be a dereliction of both.

When I was young, I was torn between two passionate, conflicting interests and ambitions – the pursuit of science and the pursuit of art. I found no reconciliation until I became a physician. I think all physicians enjoy a singular good fortune, in that we can give full expression to both sides of our natures, and never have to suppress one in favour of the other.

There is a passage of great pathos in Darwin's *Autobiography:*

> In one respect my mind has changed during the last twenty or thirty years . . . formerly pictures gave me considerable, and music very intense delight. But now . . . I have almost lost my taste for pictures or music . . . My mind seems to have become a sort of machine for grinding general laws out of large collections of fact . . . The loss of these tastes, this curious and lamentable loss of the higher aesthetic tastes, is a loss of happiness, and may possibly be injurious to the intellect, and more probably to the moral character, by enfeebling the emotional part of our nature.

What Darwin describes lies in wait for a science, or a scientific medicine, which is too exclusive, and does not properly include 'the emotional part of our nature.' As physicians, we may be safe from this danger if, and only if, we have feeling for our patients. Such feeling does not stand in the way of scientific precision – each, I think, is the guarantor of the other. One cannot make a minute study for many years of any group of patients without coming to love the patients one studies; and this is especially true of post-encephalitics, who while exercising an endless scientific fascination, become dearer and dearer to one as persons through the years. This sense of affection is neither sentimental nor extraneous. In studying these patients one comes to love them; and in loving them, one comes to understand them: the study, the love, the understanding, are all one. Neurologists are often seen as cold-blooded creatures, working out syndromes like crossword puzzles. Neurologists scarcely dare admit to emotion – and yet emotion, warmth of feeling, shines through all genuine work. The studies of post-encephalitics made by Purdon Martin are not coldly precise, but warmly and compassionately precise. The emotion, which is kept implicit in the text, becomes explicit in the dedication to his book: 'To the postencephalitic patients in the Highlands Hospital who have helped eagerly, in the hope that from their broken lives others might benefit.'

After spending fifteen years of my life working closely with these patients, I think them the most afflicted and yet noblest persons I have ever known. Whatever 'awakenings' have been able to hold out for them, their lives have still been shattered and irreparably broken. But I have found singularly little bitterness in all the years I have known them; instead, somehow, beyond explanation, an immense affirmation. There is an ultimate courage, approaching the heroic, in these patients, for they have been tried beyond belief, and yet they have survived. Nor have they survived as cripples, with the mentality of cripples, but as figures made great by their endurance through affliction, by being uncomplaining, and undaunted, and finally laughing; not succumbing to nihilism or despair, but maintaining an inexplicable affirmation of life. I have learned from them that the body can be tortured far more than I thought possible – that there are some Hells known only to neurological patients, in the almost inconceivable depths of certain neurological disorders. I used to think of Hell as a place from which no one returned. My patients have taught me otherwise. Those who return are forever marked by the experience; they have known, they cannot forget, the ultimate depths. Yet the effect of the experience is to make them not only deep but, finally, childlike, innocent, and gay. This is incomprehensible unless one has oneself descended, if not into post-encephalitic depths, into some depths of one's own. Nietzsche writes:

> Only great pain, the long, slow pain that takes its time . . . compels us to descend to our ultimate depths . . . I doubt that such pain makes us 'better'; but I know it makes us more *profound* . . . In the end, lest what is most important remain unsaid: from such abysses, from such severe sickness, one returns *newborn,* having shed one's skin . . . with merrier senses, with a second dangerous innocence in joy, more childlike and yet a hundred times subtler than one has ever been before.

In these words is contained the whole lesson of *Awakenings.*

FRANCES D.

Of Frances D., I wrote: 'Miss D. continues on a modest, intermittent dosage of L-DOPA and amantadine . . . She is not one of our star patients . . . but she has survived the pressures of an almost lifelong, character-deforming disease; of a strong cerebral stimulant; and of confinement in a chronic hospital' – a Total Institution – 'and remained what she always was – a totally human, a prime human being.'

This remained the case until 1976. She continued to show both a need and an intolerance for L-DOPA, neither, mercifully, as extreme as those of many other patients. She would thus do well each time she was medicated, but then require a 'drug holiday' every few months. Her responses continued to be moderate and modest – she never again showed the extravagances, the violent drama, of 1969. Over and above her physiological and pharmacological responses – though doubtless modulating these, and modulated by them – she continued to show, very beautifully, an extraordinary 'accommodation,' a transcendent valour, humour, and detachment of spirit. One felt her more and more as a person, and tended to forget that she was a patient, with pathology.

Though wretchedly handicapped in many ways, and perhaps

more so as the years passed, because she lost weight and strength, she radiated an inexplicable serenity, even happiness. In 1976, following the severe influenza – the 'swine flu' so similar to the 'Spanish flu' of 1919 – Miss D. went on to pneumonia and died. She had been ill, but triumphant, for fifty-seven years.

ROSE R.

Of all the patients I have ever known, the story of Rose R. is perhaps the strangest, the most uncanny. I felt this *before* she was started on L-DOPA: '. . . fervently as I desire her cure, I ask myself *what then will happen* when and if she finally withdraws her regard from the lightning-lit reverie of her clairvoyance, and turns it upon that battered cabman's face, the world . . .'

I felt this when she was *on* L-DOPA *('Is 1926 "now"?');* and again, overwhelmingly, when I concluded my story: '. . . she is a Sleeping Beauty whose "awakening" was unbearable to her, and who will never be awoken again.'

The years that followed 1972 were as long and empty as the years that preceded it – there had been a single wild flash in the summer of 1969, and then she fell back, for ever, into her own secret realm: whether it was darkness, lightning-lit, nothingness, or dream – *what* it was I never really penetrated or understood.[147] She was helped somewhat by L-DOPA, and continued to need it, with periodic 'drug holidays'; it remained of undoubted but very limited use – we never saw anything like the events of 1969 again. She continued to have quite terrible oculogyric crises, in many of which there was a severe *angor animi,* and she would mutter, 'I'm going to die, I know it, I know it, I know it,' or 'It'll kill me, it'll kill me, it'll kill me . . .' Horribly, uncannily, her premonition came true, and quite suddenly, in June 1979, she had a violent oculogyric and opisthotonic crisis, at dinner, aspirated a chicken-bone, and choked to death on the spot. She had been inconceivably, inaccessibly, and incommunicably ill since the nightmare-night she became ill, in 1926.

---

[147] It was, for Pinter, *A Kind of Alaska.*

HESTER Y.

Of all our 'yo-yos' (as I first described them in the *New York Times,* 26 August 1969), all our patients with 'bipolar disease,' all-or-none reactions to L-DOPA, Hester has always been the most severe and spectacular. This was evident from the start, in May 1969, when her L-DOPA had reached critical or 'threshold' level; she 'exploded,' one morning, as the nursing staff put it, and she has been exploding and imploding, countless times daily, ever since. Unlike many other patients (for example, Frances D.), who initially showed extremely violent reactions to L-DOPA, but subsequently more moderate and modulable reactions, Hester's reactions have remained unmodulably violent, like nuclear or possibly stellar explosions, fluctuating between 'black hole' and 'super-nova,' with scarcely anything in between. We have never been able to stop, or significantly reduce, her L-DOPA – attempts to do so have thrown her into respiratory depression, or coma. Almost more unaccountable than this physiological violence has been the extraordinary lack of violence, the balance, in her essential personality. In 1972 I wrote: 'She experiences violent drives, but she herself is "above" them'; 'the most extravagant in her physiological activity and reactions to L-DOPA, yet the "coolest" and sanest in her emotional attitudes and accommodations to these . . .'

This, in 1981, is still the case. She continues, and has to continue, on L-DOPA; she continues, and has to continue, her violently violent reactions; yet, indomitably, she continues all her personal activities; playing bingo (she is a whiz, second only to Miriam H.), gardening, going to poetry-readings, and excursions – having as full a life as one can have at Mount Carmel. *Her basic disease is pretty much at a standstill* – I see now that this is the case with most of our post-encephalitic patients, and it distinguishes them absolutely from patients with ordinary Parkinson's disease, who have to face a steadily downhill, if slow and progressive, course. But her severe truncal dystonia and kyphosis have got worse, which throws her off balance, and has come to make independent walking too difficult and dangerous. Fortunately she has forged a close friendship with a fellow patient, who wheels her everywhere, attends to her needs, and can understand her 'crushed' voice when nobody else can: Hester, diamond-sharp, is 'the brains' in this combine, and her companion, a little brain-damaged but mobile and very sweet, serves as 'the motor' or brawn. 'Symbiotic,' though accurate, is too crude a word for such relations; for though they are based on, and serve, the needs of both, yet there is also something 'above' this – a disinterested, a lofty kindness and goodness, which blesses both partners, and all who see them. There are a number of these friendships at Mount Carmel, which shine with a singular moral radiance in the tragic, and sometimes hellish, darkness of the place.

The matter, clearly, is extraordinarily complex – Hester has a great deal going against her, and a great deal for her. But none of this would matter, or even be known, if it were not for L-DOPA. *This, and this alone, has made possible what life she has – and in the absence of* L-DOPA *she would be effectively 'dead.'* The decisive date in Hester's life is 17 May 1969, the day she 'exploded' – 'awakened' – on L-DOPA. Before this, she was almost existence-less, 'asleep'; following this, whatever her tribulations and complications, she has been firmly awake, and most passionately and gratefully back in the world. Hester has remained alive and awakened for twelve and a half years, with no falling-off or impossibility of response; she has celebrated thirteen birthdays, with great delight, since her 'preternatural birth' in May 1969. I see no reason why she should not continue to do so for the rest of her life.

MIRIAM H.

I wrote of Miriam H. in the summer of 1972: 'all in all, she has done amazingly well . . . She draws on a strength unfathomable to me, a health which is deeper than the depth of her illness.' Very happily this remains true in 1981 – indeed, of all our post-encephalitic patients at Mount Carmel whose stories I related in *Awakenings,* Miss H. finally has done the best, has achieved and held the fullest life, and (since 1972) suffered least from complications. She remains on a very substantial dose of

L-DOPA (825 mg four times a day), which she needs and is crucially helped by, and has no complications severe enough to warrant any reduction, let alone the beastliness of 'drug holidays' or withdrawals. She has occasional attacks of mild ticcing, sometimes cursing; occasional temper-tantrums; occasional attacks of strange obsessing; and 'brilliant' attacks of calculating and figuring, which go with surges of cerebral excitement, and are accompanied by striking convulsive changes on EEG (see n. 77, p. 131). Her old enemy – oculogyric crises – which she had had weekly for more than forty years before the administration of L-DOPA, re-emerged in 1979, after a ten-year remission, but have been quite mild, quite tolerable, and only occasional.

It is clear, from both clinical observation and EEG, that Miss H. is not only 'awakened,' but somewhat 'turned on', by L-DOPA, and that even between her overt crises and tantrums and 'attacks,' she has an unusually high level of cerebral tonus and activity, which lies on the verge of the explosive and convulsive. Going with this is her great 'brightness' and acceleration of mind. She not only shows episodic 'Tourettism' (ticcing, cursing, obsessing, arithmomania, etc.), but the odd wittiness and quickness which are so characteristic of Tourette's (see Sacks, 1981 and Sacks, 1982a). It has also become clear, from many conversations with her, and the unusually detailed notes which were kept in her early days at Mount Carmel, that some (and perhaps most) of this turning-on or arousal with L-DOPA is a release of traits and propensities which preceded L-DOPA, but which had been constrained or shut up as her Parkinsonism developed – a release (and perhaps a potentiation) of an *original* encephalitic impulsiveness and ticciness, which had become hidden (and forgotten) as her Parkinsonism developed.

I had observed, in Frances D., the emergence 'of strange and primitive impulsions and compulsions, when she was acutely excited by L-DOPA,' and my feeling (and hers) that some of these were 'releases' of pre-existent and perhaps dormant post-encephalitic propensities, which had remained hidden or dormant until she (and they) were 'awakened' by L-DOPA. It has seemed to me, in regard to Miriam H. and several other patients, that I have especially seen this with continuing, and very long-term, administration of L-DOPA; and presenting not so much as a sudden uprush of overpowering feelings and urges, as a slow revelation of an entire pre-existent, psychophysiological 'repertoire' or 'character'; or, to some extent, a potential 'character' consisting of a multitude or complex of propensities partly manifest, partly latent, many years before, and becoming manifest again, and indeed 'awakened,' with the continuing stimulation of L-DOPA.

Of the twenty patients whose stories I told in *Awakenings,* the one I did least justice to was Miriam H. Perhaps it has been only since 1972 that I have penetrated past a certain shyness and reserve, and come to realize the massive personality and intelligence within, how spacious she is as a person. Perhaps, previously, there was not only shyness, but a contraction of self due to Parkinsonism and depression. If before she had to survive in face of contraction, now she must hold together in face of expansion – the centrifugal power of Tourettish excitation – convulsive and compulsive motions and notions. If she were less massive, less spacious, in her essential self, she would be carried away, or distracted, or fragmented, or contorted, by the 'false self,' the strange 'enkieness' (see n. 28, p. 26), which has developed on L-DOPA. However, she shows not the least sign of being fundamentally discomposed by this – she *is* discomposed, briefly, in her tantrums and crises, but as soon as these are over she regains her strong self: one almost feels (to use one of her own favourite words) that her attacks are a 'conduit' to deal with excitement, to discharge it harmlessly, leaving her inner economy, her basic self, undisturbed. She readily accommodates Tourettish excitement, finding room for it in the outskirts of a commodious personality, and even gaining a certain advantage and pleasure from the extraordinary swiftness of thought and invention which goes with it. She lets it be, she allows it a place, but there is never any doubt as to who controls what: there may, indeed, be a 'Tourettoma,' a false self, an 'It'; but the real self, the 'I,' is firmly in command. I find this incredible, when I think what she has been through.

Miss H. has now spent fifty years at Mount Carmel – thirty-seven years gradually sinking into a regressed, hopeless state, which could only have ended in some 'back-ward' melancholia and death; and nearly thirteen excellent years, 'awakened' on L-DOPA. Miss H., at sixty-five, looks much younger than her age, has a first-class brain, and is full of energy and good life – so full of life she almost bursts the confines of Mount Carmel. She regrets, as so many patients do, that she could not have had L-DOPA many years before; but she is not resentful, she looks to the future, and looks forward to many more good years on L-DOPA.

MARGARET A.

'Margaret A.' ends on a grim note: 'the last three years have seen her decline and fall . . . The original Miss A. – so engaging and bright – has been *dispossessed* by a host of crude, degenerate sub-selves.' I did, however, speak of the things which could bring her together: music, nature, affection, freedom, and 'life.' ('She goes mad in your madhouse because she is shut off from life.')

I could do no more than intimate, in the original edition of *Awakenings,* that there were institutional changes of a grim nature in September 1969, which had equally grim repercussions on the lives of all patients (see, for example, n. 39, p. 53 and below). Mercifully, with the coming of 1973, with the advent of a new and gentler administration, a great deal of this institutional harshness fell away; there was something of a return to the friendly, easy-going atmosphere of earlier years. This was instantly reflected, not only in the mood and morale of the patients, but in their physiological states and reactions to L-DOPA. In particular, some of the patients who had seemed hopelessly unstable in their reactions to L-DOPA now achieved a relative stability, and, with this, the potential for 'accommodation': Margaret A. – a sweet person, but emotionally frail and painfully vulnerable – was among the patients who dramatically improved in this way.

By October of 1973, when the documentary film of *Awakenings* was made, Margaret had shown a striking restabilization on L-DOPA, though remaining extremely sensitive to it, and in crucial need of it. No longer physiologically hurled to and fro, Margaret was now able to achieve what had never been possible before, what had been prevented before, first by the severity of her post-encephalitic syndrome, then by the instability of her reactions to L-DOPA: she started to achieve a remarkable serenity and depth, a personal (and artistic) unity and beauty. This was very evident in the documentary film of *Awakenings,* when she spoke with great poignancy, and sang with great beauty, astonishing the makers of the film, who were expecting a grossly pathological, hopeless, broken wreck, as she is partly depicted in the closing pages of 'Margaret A.'

In the years that remained to her, Margaret held this remarkable serenity and unity, achieved, one felt, through the long years of affliction, the cruel decades of post-encephalitic disability, and the still crueller tribulations of the first three years of L-DOPA. The last four years were the best years of her life – at least, the best she had known for more than forty years. In the last years – how sad it was not sooner! – she was released from her motor and emotional ups and downs, she made friends, she gardened, she went out on excursions. Above all, transcendently, she sang – she sang for all her afflicted fellow patients; out of the endured and survived suffering of her heart, she invented and sang the Post-Encephalitic Blues. Like so many of our patients, she was *wounded* into art.

In 1976 she fell and broke a hip, had severe post-operative complications, and died, finally, after many months of illness and pain, borne with a beautiful and serene resignation. She showed no resentment, she became spiritualized with suffering; and just as Robert O., the day before he died, asked the rabbi to read him a psalm, so Margaret, in her last days, asked for the Mozart *Requiem.* We all loved her and we wept when she died.

MIRON V.

Miron V., who had the severest 'bipolar' disease, at first seesawing constantly between pathological extremes, did very well between 1970 and 1972, and showed dramatically the healing powers of work and love. Tragically, and in a way beyond his control, he was to lose work and love, and, with this, the beneficent stability of these years.

Though Mount Carmel became gentler after 1973, in a way

which healed the gentle soul of Margaret A., it became tragically impoverished, and was to lose many of its staff and resources. We were forced to close part of our industrial workshop, and with this the cobbler's last-and-bench, which had been so crucial to the rehabilitation of this isolated, bitter man.

What happened was terrible – and terribly prompt. Mr V. fell back into melancholia and regression, and, simultaneously, into the severest Parkinsonism and catatonia. Suddenly, it seemed, the L-DOPA lost effect, and lost *all* effect, whatever dosage we used. We increased the dose to 6 gm. a day, but it could have been chalk for all the effect that it had. This sudden and terrible termination of effect, this sudden and terrible return to an infinite and imperative abyss, was almost identical with what we had seen with poor Lucy K.

Perhaps, *perhaps,* some coming-to-terms might have been reached, had one calamity not prompted another. At this terrible time, when as never before, Mr V. needed the greatest love and support, he was in effect deserted by his wife and son: their own frailty and neurosis was such that when he was most cut off, they cut him off more, recapitulating the terrible and tragic vicious circle which had obtained between 1955 and 1969.

I felt, as I had felt in the case of Lucy K., that this was the end, and that death would soon follow – but, in this, I was profoundly mistaken. Mr V. did not die; I half-wish he had. He continued to live, if it was life, for another eight years. We stopped and restarted his L-DOPA; we tried Sinemet, Symmetrel, bromocriptine, apomorphine; nothing we could do would alter his state. What he needed was life, a reason to live, and this could not be provided from a bottle. He remained virtually motionless and speechless, and he became intensely, impossibly rigid, as violently stiff as poor Lucy K., with an inseparable mixture of Parkinsonism, catatonia, and paratonia. With this continuing violent stiffness, which disallowed even passive movement of his limbs, irreversible joint-damage and ankylosis set in, compounded by emaciation, and finally skin-breakdown and decubiti. Gaunt, cadaveric, he looked like a corpse, with a sort of rigidity half-resembling *rigor mortis,* although it was partly a *moral* rigor mortis – hating himself and his poor body to death. Only his eyes were alive, burning and fixed – but looking into them was like looking into an abyss, into Hell. How he survived so long is itself unaccountable, unless he willed himself to live, to live a living death.

He had pneumonia many times, meticulously and successfully treated by penicillin. Finally, in 1980, we checked our medical reflexes and promptness, and in his last attack of pneumonia let nature take its course.

GERTIE C.

The most surprising follow-up, the only one, perhaps, which was completely unforeseeable, relates to Gertie C., who was put on L-DOPA again in 1974, after being off it for four years, and – apparently – quite unable to take it. She had a brief halcyon period when first given it, in June 1969, but thereafter had absolutely monstrous reactions, with violent delirium, thrashing movements, and multiple tics. It seemed clear, by the end of 1970, that she could tolerate neither L-DOPA nor amantadine, and was best left alone, with no strong medication. She had, however, a most peaceful spirit, and did not seem to need any awakening or stirring-up; she accepted her lot with humour and grace.

With the final wearing-off of her very persistent drug-effects, her voice reverted to an almost inaudible whisper, and she returned almost wholly to her pre-DOPA state – other than receiving kindly visits from a faithful apparition each evening. This, it seemed, was the end of her story.

When she was tried on L-DOPA again, after four years without medication, she immediately showed an excellent but intermittent reaction (a so-called 'on/off reaction'); in particular, she regained the most perfect speech, but only for a few hours a day. She can either speak perfectly – or not at all. She has no warning of the change – it may come in mid-word. When she can speak, she can move, she has freedom of action (though this is limited by long-standing dystonia and contractures); but this free movement may be stopped in a trice, and replaced by aphonia, akinesia, severe trembling, and rigidity; the reverse change also occurs in a trice (and its instantaneity may be confirmed by EEG:

see Appendix: The Electrical Basis of Awakenings, p. 327).

This situation has been maintained now for more than seven years, with no fading of effect, nor any 'side-effects' (such as the ticcing, the thrashing, she showed in 1969). The 'penalty' for this good activation is precisely its intermittency, and nothing more: Gertie enjoys five or six hours of almost normal function daily, and is totally disabled for the remaining eighteen or nineteen hours. We have tried different doses and timings of L-DOPA – it makes no difference whatever. She needs and can take 4 gm. a day, and with this can 'purchase' six good hours a day. If she has less than 4 gm., she has correspondingly less benefit – perhaps only two or three hours daily; if she has more than 4 gm., there is no increased benefit.

One cannot help thinking in economic terms, and this is precisely what Gertie herself does. She says, 'There is only so much function my brain can *afford* – it is a part-time brain, and it cannot do more. It shuts itself off when it has used up its quota – it has very good sense, it does the right thing.'

Knowing she may only expect so much 'awakening,' Gertie tries to plan her days accordingly, although there are difficulties because the 'on/off' is incalculable. All her plans are therefore contingency plans. She likes and needs conversation, occupation, recreation – but there are only certain, unpredictable times when this is possible. She has many good friends and neighbours in Mount Carmel, as well as devoted family who frequently visit, so she can usually find company whenever she 'wakes' and desires it. She does, however, have a 'contingency-recorder,' so that she can tape letters, greetings, messages, or whatever, if she finds herself alone with a limited 'quota' of movement and speech.

Now life is possible, and varied activities and friends keep her company, if only for a limited time each day, Mrs C.'s need for visitations and hallucinations has gone. 'I have real visitors now,' she says, 'real love and attention. I haven't seen my phantom-swain for more than seven years.'

MARTHA N.

Or, perhaps, every story is surprising, for no two are the same, and none is a mere continuation of what went before: for we are not speaking of cases, and uniform process, but physiology as it is embedded in people, and people as they are embedded and living in history. One may have intended the replicabilities and uniformities of science, but one encountered the vicissitudes of history or romance. This was particularly clear in regard to Martha N., and led Luria, when he first wrote to me about *Awakenings,* to single her out for particular question: 'Why,' he wrote, 'did the L-DOPA act differently each time?' I could give him no answer in 1973.

I described five (or, including amantadine, six) drug-trials with Martha, and found remarkably different reactions on all six occasions, though each reaction, once started, stayed in character: she showed strikingly little physiological constancy, but a striking dramatic unity once they were started. Her story, like Gertie's, appeared to have ended in 1970, with the decision to stop any more drug-trials, and a return to her 'pleasant, easy-going, good-humoured and sane' self. This too was her impression: 'I have had enough visions and what-not to last me a lifetime.' Perhaps this should have been the end of the story – but Martha, like Gertie, was restarted on medication in 1974. I was away myself, for much of this year, on an unusual, nearly fatal, but edifying sabbatical, which, instead of being spent in the safe lowlands of science, took me to a mountain, a fall, and six months as a patient; and while *I* was a patient, my own patients were at large, and submitted to a certain recrudescence of drug-enthusiasm. It was during this time that Gertie and Martha and many other patients (including Leonard), who seemed to have reached some accommodation, good or bad, in the absence of drugs, were restarted by an enthusiast not too swayed by experience. Re-starting Gertie turned out unforeseeably well; re-starting Martha turned out, perhaps foreseeably, badly.

Martha is still alive and well – but this would probably have been the case without drugs. She has spent the last seven years on amantadine, on and off, and has spent the last seven years in hallucinosis. Physically, she is in fair shape, with an audible voice, good swallowing, good arm movement, etc., and a great reduction in rigidity, akinesia, salivation, and oculogyria, though handicapped, physically, by severely dystonic and effectively functionless legs, and a severe and fixed torticollis. So the benefit of medication is perfectly clear: what is unclear is the cost this entails, whether, finally, she can afford its effects. 'Affording,' for Gertic C., means limits to drug-action, having six good hours rather than sixteen, and this she can very well and happily afford, the more so as she would have *no* active hours without medication. 'Affording,' for Martha N., is altogether more questionable, for it entails a chronic low-grade hallucinosis or delirium, her 'transport' out of this world, this Vale of Tears, to endlessly proliferating, preposterous false-worlds of fancy, full of romantic, whimsical, but sometimes terrifying, illusions.

She is married, she is pregnant, she has given birth to a robot. She is queen of a kingdom of rabbits and white mice. She is in Hollywood; in fairyland; with her brother in Miami. She is awaiting discharge, neurosurgery, and reincarnation. She is the Mother of God, rejected by God, and possessed by twelve devils.

Possessed and preoccupied by these fancies and phantoms, she no longer leaves the floor – she has 'other things to do.' She has virtually no converse or intercourse with others – she who was 'conspicuously sociable and affable.' We had hoped that she might do some crocheting or sewing; she was rightfully proud of her beautiful needle-work at one time. She answers, 'But I *am* sewing, don't you see,' and one sees, with a shiver, that her hands are indeed in constant complex motion, going through all the delicate motions of sewing, with a hallucinatory needle and thread. 'See what a lovely coverlet I have stitched for you today!' she said on one occasion. 'See the pretty dragons, the Unicorn in his paddock' – tracing their invisible outlines in the air. 'Here, take it!' And she placed the ghostly thing in my hands. I did not know whether to join in this courteous and graceful pantomine, or to say, 'It's not so, Martha – you know there's nothing there.'

For she knows, and she doesn't know – she keeps double books. She always knows me, knows the date, is lucid and oriented – which one would scarcely expect in an organic delirium;

and she retains clear memories of her ever-changing fancies. In this she is quite unlike Gertie C., for example, who retained no memory whatever of her acute delirium in 1970. Perhaps it is not delirium; perhaps she has gone mad.

Always and always, these dilemmas arise, in regard to the 'good' no less than the 'bad' states of these patients. Thus Hester Y., in her notebook, speaking for them all: 'Is it the medicine I am taking, or just my new state of mind?' Martha, in particular, is an adept, an old hand, at dissociation. She had had her 'Easter psychosis,' annually, for thirty years before L-DOPA; and she displayed great histrionic talent, and a complex sort of complicity and control, in the period of visitations brought on by L-DOPA in March 1970, which became so uncanny, so libidinized, for her. What goes on now? Can we call it 'drug-induced' – or is it rather that she has finally capitulated to an almost lifelong eroticized, demonized, religiose madness?

We have one clue, at least, of great importance. With the death of her parents, in 1951, Miss N.'s illness became abruptly worse – a 'precipitous deterioration' which led to her institutionalization in 1954. But I omitted to mention that there was a brother as well, something of a drunk and a scamp, but very dear to Martha's heart; with the death of her parents, and her entry to Mount Carmel, her brother remained the only deep and genuine relation, and perhaps her only mooring to emotional reality. In his absence, I think, she found herself desolatingly alone, though this was never acknowledged, but covered up by her 'affable' façade.

During 1974, her first year back on amantadine, her brother visited her frequently; but clearly, disturbingly, he was getting on in years, he was ailing, and after much indecision, which he shared with his sister, he decided to retire to Florida. Martha was herself severely torn by all this – she wanted what was best for him, but could not bear to see him go. He went down to Florida – and promptly died.

When she was given the news, Martha showed no response; she appeared not to hear, and made an irrelevent answer; she could not acknowledge the fact of his death. From this moment on, it seems to me in retrospect, she was, in some sense, hopelessly mad. The importance of this bereavement, and its total denial, was shown, hieroglyphically, in the fantasies she had: she would come down to the lobby in her chair, with a small suitcase of clothes, and say, 'Goodbye, everybody, I'm going to Florida! I'll be living with my brother. I'll write to you all!' Later, she refused to stir from the floor, and when pressed to do so, would say sharply, 'I'm leaving, don't you see . . . I'm expecting a phone call any minute long-distance from Florida.' Her life became waiting – waiting for Florida, waiting to be rejoined with her brother. With this gross denial of reality – so, at least, in retrospect it seems – she lost her anchorage in reality-at-large, had no more use for this world, the sublunary sphere, the desolate here-and-now, and started her lunatic wanderings in the whimsical other worlds of fancy.

I have never really known, none of us has known, what to say or do: should we stop the amantadine, and render her functionless? We have tried this, for six months at a time, but though she reverts to disabling Parkinsonism, she does *not* give up her strange ideas. Should we force her off the ward, to attend 'socials' and workshop, slap her hard with 'that battered cabman's face, the world'? Or should we accept the present situation, and leave her rapt, lightning-lit, in the wish-worlds of reverie? Perhaps it is not our business to choose; perhaps there is no longer any choice. As with Rose R., all ends in enigma.

In September 1981, after writing the above, I returned to New York and stopped Martha's medication. With this her psychosis instantly stopped – indeed her *imagination* instantly stopped. She became not only Parkinsonian, but profoundly forlorn, and to the Parkinsonian mask was added the mask of despair. She could hardly speak now, but what she said made me shudder: 'You've taken away my fantasies,' she said: 'I've got nothing left.' I was strongly reminded of Rolando P., and how it was when *he* lost the will to live. Every day Martha looked emptier, more ghost-like; she gazed at us with unseeing, blank eyes; and on 12 October she died. I wonder if I killed her by stopping the medication, by taking away the fantasies, which, perhaps, were all that life had left her now.

IDA T.

Ida T., while remaining decisively 'awakened,' gradually lost ground despite the continuing use of L-DOPA, despite alterations of dosage, drug holidays, etc. The beautiful freedom and fluency of movement and speech which appeared when L-DOPA was first given in 1969 never returned, and there was a gradual regression to rigidity and blockage. There was no regression in any other sense – Ida was full of life and good feeling in the last years of her life, very much a 'character,' and much liked at Mount Carmel.

In 1977 she developed a fulminating malignancy, and lost 200 pounds in a matter of months. She looked like a great dying whale – she realized she was dying, and was cheerful and resigned. I talked with her a couple of days before her death; she said, 'Thank God for the Dopey – the last years was the best.'

AARON E.

I ended my story of Aaron E. with a hope: 'He seems to have achieved a real and useful equilibrium over the last ten months, and perhaps he will continue to hold this indefinitely in the future.' These hopes proved false – and I now realize, which I did not at the time, that this is due to the fundamental difference between post-encephalitic disorders and ordinary Parkinson's disease. The former are essentially (or, at least, very frequently) *static,* so that if some sort of equilibrium *can* be achieved, this may indeed be held indefinitely in the future. This has been the case with many patients at Mount Carmel – Miriam H. provides a clear example. Parkinson's disease, by contrast, is essentially *progressive,* and this is what Aaron E. had: an advancing disease already far advanced at his admission.

Right at the start, in 1969, besides the majority of our post-encephalitic patients, I put thirty patients with advanced Parkinson's disease on L-DOPA. Now, twelve years later, all of these are dead, whereas a good number of our post-encephalitics are still alive and well.

Aaron E. lost ground from 1972 on – as, in terms of underlying disease, he had been losing ground from the start, in 1962. His reactions to L-DOPA – he was helpless without this – became feebler and briefer each time, and every few months he had to be taken off for a drug holiday. His mood and morale remained very good – there was no return to his pre-DOPA regression and depression – and he remained as active as he could and, even towards the end, was wonderfully revived by his weekends at home (fortunately he had sturdy sons and grandsons, who could lift him into the car when he could no longer walk).

By 1976, he was greatly disabled, having lost a good deal of weight and strength, as well as by the remorseless increase of Parkinsonian problems. But, finally, it was not Parkinsonism which caused his death – Parkinsonism never directly causes death – but the development of a very malignant cancer of the prostate. Surgery was performed, but the cancer had spread, and a rapidly progressive uremia set in. He died, tranquilly, in early 1977.

GEORGE W.

George, unlike most of the other patients in *Awakenings,* was not a patient in hospital, and had an unusually benign and slowly progressive form of Parkinson's disease. He went down to Florida in 1972, and was still quite active, and taking L-DOPA, in 1979. He sent me periodic letters telling me of his progress, and, on occasion, looked in at Mount Carmel to see me. In the past two years, we have fallen out of touch – so I cannot give a fully up-to-date 'follow-up' on him.

If I were to make an informed guess, based on my experience with other such patients, I would guess that he is still active, and able to get around, and still deriving clear profit from L-DOPA, even though (like Aaron) he has had Parkinson's disease since 1962. His disease was much slower and more benign than Aaron's (we are rather ignorant of the causes of such variations); second, and importantly, he was not in hospital. For reasons which are not entirely clear (though many of them, of course, are perfectly obvious), patients with Parkinson's disease tend to do rather poorly in hospital, whereas post-encephalitics, in contrast, may do rather well. We have seen this at Mount Carmel, and it is seen at Highlands too, so Dr Sharkey tells me. It seems to be a universal experience.

CECIL M.

Cecil M. does have a post-encephalitic disorder, but, like George, is an outpatient, not an inmate. (I put him into *Awakenings* out of affection, for he is not one of my own patients, but one of my father's patients, in London.) I felt I should tell his story, briefly, in *Awakenings* precisely because he was neither disabled nor an inmate, but characteristic of the thousands of post-encephalitic patients who are still able to lead very full, very active, and almost normal lives, despite clear-cut post-encephalitic disorders. This is finally made possible because their disorders are static; so if they managed to get along in 1930 or 1940, they can still manage to get along now. This, happily, is the situation with Cecil M.

Cecil M. remains vigorous and independent in 1981, able to look after himself, active, and still driving his car. He has found himself a little slowed and arthritic, with age, but shows little, if any, advance in his Parkinsonism. He has changed his mind about taking L-DOPA. He had said in 1970: 'Its effect was very pleasant at first, but then it turned out more trouble than it was worth. I can get along perfectly well without it.'

This is true; but he gets along even better if he takes it, provided he takes only the most modest doses. In particular he takes Sinemet, half a small tablet twice a day. Other Parkinsonian patients may take ten times this dose – but Cecil M. finds this small dose suits him exactly. If he takes more, he has an immediate recrudescence of his lockjaw or trismus; if he takes less, he is notably more Parkinsonian. Very fortunately for him he *can* be 'balanced,' he *can* 'titrate' himself, and not run into trouble. He is not seeking, nor in need of, a dramatic 'awakening,' but is content with the modest effects of a modest dose.

He is doing extraordinarily well, and I see no reason why he should not hold this happy stability for the rest of his life.

LEONARD L.

And, now, finally, our last patient, Leonard L. Following his eleventh and 'final' trial of amantadine in March 1972 Leonard said: 'This is the end of the line. I have *had* it with drugs. There is no more you can do with me.' And a little later, just before I wrote his story in *Awakenings:* 'Now I accept the whole situation. I've learned a great deal in the last three years. And now, I'll stay myself, and you can keep your L-DOPA.'

He accepted, we accepted, that it was 'the end of the line,' and refrained from medication for more than two years, during which time he reverted wholly to his pre-DOPA status, and seemed to have achieved an 'elegiac' detachment of mind. 'It happened,' he would tap (for he could no longer speak). 'That's all there is to it. It is over. I don't regret it. It's just simply fate.' But side by side with this feeling, he did not accept it, he could not accept it; he raged at, and pleaded with 'fate.' He thought 'fate' might relent – just a little – for him. He prayed (in the words of the Yom Kippur service) that the harsh decree might be averted, or softened for him. He thought deeply on the nature of 'mercy,' wondering whether it could transcend, without transgressing, the fixed laws of fate. He pondered on the nature of law and fate: 'Is fate law *of,* or law *for?'* he once tapped. When he saw fate as 'law of', i.e. purely natural, he found it easy to accept it, to profess *amor fati.* When he saw fate as 'law for,' i.e. purely moral, he found it infinitely harder to bear, and had to struggle to believe that it was the will of a wise God, and not the wanton cruelty of a criminal childish god. He thought a good deal about 'tempting fate': 'Is it tempting fate,' he tapped, 'to try DOPA again?' He ruminated this round and round, without resolution.

But following the remarkable and unexpected response of Gertie C., when she was put back on L-DOPA after a gap of four years, Leonard L. finally decided that if Gertie's 'fate' had changed, perhaps this had changed too. Alas! where the wonderful, the unaccountable, happened with Gertie, there was no such reaction with Leonard L. The situation had not changed, for him, in five years: in September 1974, as in September 1969, he showed the most intense and inordinate sensitivity to L-DOPA, and his response, once again, was entirely pathological – intolerable tics, and tension, and blocking of thought. 'Hopeless,' he tapped. 'Utterly hopeless. Is this really the end of the line?' He consulted with his mother – most decisions were made together – and now asked that amantadine be tried: 'It can hardly be worse,' he tapped; 'it had *some* use before.'

The years from 1974 to 1980 were essentially similar to the years between 1969 and 1972. There were endlessly repeated trials of amantadine – at first rather favourable, then less and less so. An 'average' cycle lasted six weeks: first there would be accession of alertness – a definite 'awakening' – and a reduction of Parkinsonism, though even at best, he could only whisper, and was profoundly disabled. After two to four weeks of this, he started to have sudden convulsive tics and jerks, sudden confusions and blockings of thought, and frightened darting eyes, their pupils dilated. When this happened, he had to be taken off, and with this would sink into a tremendous depth – an abyss – of Parkinsonism and near-stupor.

There was only, one felt, the merest *line* of 'health' (or 'potential normality') left, the finest, most precarious tightrope, with great abysses of pathology to either side, the abysses of stupor and frenzy. I had had this feeling with almost all of our patients who had, after a good auspicious response, lost most of the 'middle ground,' the *potential* for normality, and found themselves thrown from one pole of being (or unbeing) to another. It was only in 1977 – and first and foremost with Leonard L. – that I was able to find objective confirmation of this thought. This became possible through the use of EEGs, examining the brain-waves, the electrical activity of the brain, in a variety of different states and stages. In every such patient I found a sort of triad or tryptich: profoundly slow activity in the absence of medication, very excited and often convulsive activity with overarousal on medication, and between these, so to speak, a very attenuated, narrow band, showing relatively normal activities between the abnormals. This was strikingly seen with Leonard L. in his responses to amantadine; a fuller description and illustration appears in an Appendix (The Electrical Basis of Awakenings, p. 327).

This narrow band became narrower and narrower until it almost disappeared. We saw this clinically, we saw this electrically, we saw this horribly, again and again, with Leonard L. It placed him, it placed us, in a terrible double bind, because even his 'baseline' state became worse and worse, so that he was intolerably disabled *without* medication, but then, after perhaps a few days of improvement, would become intolerably disabled *with* medication: 'Do you suppose,' he whispered, 'that my receptors are dying off? I don't know whether medication cures them or kills them.'

Those who saw the documentary film of *Awakenings* will recollect Leonard L. as masked, motionless, and scarcely able to speak, but with a round fresh face, an excellent colour, glowing with health, and looking much younger than his fifty-two years. He retained this general health, and healthy round appearance, until about 1977. Thereafter, with intolerable medicational effects, on the one hand, and tragic reductions in nursing and other staff responsible for the basic care of our patients on the other, Leonard lost weight, became weak, choked on his food, had repeated pneumonias, urinary infections and, worst of all, breakdown of his skin. By 1978 he was an emaciated, ill man, dying by inches, and knowing this well. He was moved to the 'heavy-duty' nursing floor in Mount Carmel, in a last attempt to save his health and his life. But his bedsores got deeper and deeper, causing ceaseless pain, fever, and sepsis, and draining him of vitally needed protein.

Until this time, if Leonard 'raged,' he raged to live: it was life itself raging, raging to live. From 1978 onwards, as he grew iller and feebler, this vital rage, his will to live, was sapped, and grew feebler. And to the sapping of will, his judgement gave assent: 'What sense does it make?' he tapped in 1980. 'It's pain and pus, pus and pain. Not worth living. Not a life.'

By the end of 1980, amantadine had wholly ceased to 'work' – or, rather, produced only pathological effects. Early in 1981, therefore, after searching discussion, feeling that life was at stake, and it had to be used, we tried him once again on L-DOPA.

Now, by an extraordinary and paradoxical quirk of fate, L-DOPA 'worked,' for the first time in twelve years. Leonard suddenly became stronger, and got back a loud voice; he got back his 'rage.' But it was the rage of despair. I was in the clinic when the ward phoned to say that Leonard had 'come to.' Astounded, and fearful, I rushed to his bed. He had an enormous voice now, and he yelled his soul out: 'Hell and damnation! Fucking DOPA, fucking miracle. Look at me now – I'm falling apart. I'm dying, almost dead, and *now* you resurrect me with L-DOPA! This is a *stinking* miracle – obscene – a lot worse than Lazarus . . . For Christ's sake stop it, and let me die in peace.'

I stopped it, of course, and let him be. He reverted again to motionless silence, giving no external sign of life. I had no idea what went on inside him – but I felt he was conscious, though turned to Last Things. He seemed immensely composed and prepared – I was reminded of how Donne composed himself for death. I often sat by his bed and watched his peaceful face. Death, when it came, was gentle and insensible – he gave up the ghost, willingly, gladly, leaving the poor body which had been his long purgatory.

Dear Mrs L.:   June 24, 81
I have been trying to get you by phone since hearing of Leonard's death, but never succeed. I hope this letter will reach you.

I was deeply saddened – and, although he had been so ill for so long, deeply shocked – to hear of Leonard's death; and my first thought was for you, who had nourished him, and given him life, in every way, all these years. It seems so inadequate to say that I feel the deepest sympathy for you – but, finally, this is all one human being can say to another. I only met Leonard's brother a couple of times, but I hope you will convey my condolences to him too.

Only the passage of years can give one perspective – and it comes to me that I have known Leonard – and you – for fifteen years; which is quite a long time in anyone's life. What I felt in 1966 I felt more strongly every year – what a remarkable man Leonard was, what courage and humour he showed, in the face of an almost life-long heart-breaking disease. I tried to give form to this feeling when I wrote of him in *Awakenings* . . . but was conscious of how inadequate and partial this was: perhaps even more so to you, for you were such a *life-giver* to him . . . Perhaps this only became clear to me in the years afterwards . . .

I have never had a patient who *taught* me so much – not simply about Parkinsonism, etc., but about what it means to be a human being, who survives, and fully, in the face of such affliction and such terrible odds. There is something inspiring about such survival, and I will never forget (nor let others forget) the lesson Leonard taught me; and, equally, there has been something very remarkable about *you,* and the way in which you dedicated so much of your strength and life to him . . . he could never have survived – especially these last years – without your giving your own life-blood to him . . . You too are one of the most gallant people I know.

Now Leonard has gone, there will be a great void and a great grief – there has to be where there has been a great love. But I hope and pray that there will be good years, and real life, ahead for you yet . . . you have a great vitality, and you should live to a hundred! I hope that God will be good to you, and bless you, at this time, give you comfort in your bereavement, and a kind and mellow evening in the years that lie ahead.

With my deepest sympathy and heartfelt best wishes,
    Oliver Sacks

Dear Dr Sacks,

My son and I wish to thank you for the most expressive condolence letter you have sent me.

Yes, Leonard was very courageous and even more so. His passing left a great void in my life, and I don't know how to live without him. I haven't stopped crying since he's gone. I love him so, and don't know how to form a life for myself after being so close to Leonard in so many years.

I never made close friends with anyone and I wouldn't know how or care to now at my age (83), so you see, dear friend, I'm lost and am a nothing now that I'm not needed any more.

I love my other son and his family but Leonard was always special in my heart. Again I thank you for that heart-warming letter and hope you will have a chance to call me.
    Tina L.

POSTSCRIPT (1990)

℺ In the past nine years I have continued to see a diminishing number of post-encephalitic patients at Mount Carmel, and at other places where I work in New York, and to keep in frequent touch with the post-encephalitics at the Highlands Hospital and elsewhere.

Hester Y., Miriam H., and Gertie C. remained in good health and spirits until 1984, when – with several other post-encephalitic patients (and dozens of other, non-post-encephalitic patients) they died in a tragic and protracted hospital strike (or in consequence of this). Such patients are very frail, and need the most assiduous nursing care. Breakdown of this for a single day can pave the way to a breakdown of skin, and contractures, the formation of bedsores and decubiti – and it was precisely such hazards which led to the deaths of our patients. A few post-encephalitic patients survived 1984, continued to receive L-DOPA, and continued to lead as full a life as possible; the last of these (Mary S.) died in the summer of 1989.

One former Mount Carmel patient – the head-nodding, trajectory-computing, and altogether astonishing Lillian T. (see n. 143, p. 271), who was the most articulate spokesman for our post-encephalitic patients in the 1973 documentary of *Awakenings,* is still very much alive, although she has developed hyperbolic reactions to L-DOPA – changing within seconds, unpredictably, several times a day – from motionless akinesia to reasonable function (sufficient for speech, for slow walking, for reading and writing) . She is kept on a very modest dose of L-DOPA (only 250 mg. four times a day); if she is on a larger dose (which she prefers), she has 'wild' periods, with extreme pressure of thought, speech, and movement, multiple tics, hooting, touching, and tossing objects all around her – a sort of 'Tourettism' which she enjoys, but the institution finds hard to handle.

I have half a dozen post-encephalitic patients at the Little Sisters of the Poor where I work, all maintained on L-DOPA, and all in excellent shape. One of them, Mary T., has severe Parkinsonism on one side, but a tendency to tics on the other – and has to receive a carefully-calibrated 'compromise' dose of L-DOPA (for whatever helps the Parkinsonism exacerbates the tics). I have often wished there were some way of delivering dopamine independently to the two sides of her brain.

I have continued to see the post-encephalitic patients at the Highlands Hospital: there were ninety of these when I first visited them in 1969; now, sadly, there are only nine left. Several of them are maintained on small doses of L-DOPA – but several prefer to go without it (or its 'side-effects'). These patients are on the whole younger and more active than those at Mount Carmel.

Cecil M., also living in London, continued active, through his seventies, on a small dose of L-DOPA, able to take care of himself, to drive his own car, to be quite independent. He died, of a massive heart attack, in April of last year. He felt the last, excellent twenty years of his life were a 'gift' of L-DOPA.

Although these patients are the last of the last, the last survivors of the great epidemic, there have appeared, over the years, reports of occasional 'sporadic' cases of *encephalitis lethargica* and post-encephalitic syndromes (see Appendix: A History of the Sleeping-Sickness, p. 319). Very recently (February 1990), through the courtesy of my colleague Dr Margery Mark, I have been enabled to see such a patient for myself – a woman in her early fifties who, after a severe febrile illness with somnolence (called 'flu') on Thanksgiving 1986, developed a rapidly advancing syndrome of akinetic Parkinsonism, rigidity, loss of postural reflexes, catatonia, and (most recently) a state of intense neck-retraction with a suggestion of oculogyria. This patient has shown a singular (and pathological) sensitivity to L-DOPA, developing tics, grimacing, and hooting in response to a very modest dose.

Writing the Epilogue in 1981, I spoke of post-encephalitic syndromes as being static, or at most very slowly progressive, in distinction to the invariably and relentlessly advancing course of 'ordinary' Parkinson's disease. But this is not always the case now, with the further ageing of the few post-encephalitic patients remaining. Thus, Lillian T., who appeared as an extremely youthful 48-year-old, with good motor abilities and extremely clear speech, in the 1973 documentary film of *Awakenings,* is far more disabled now – and shows not only exacerbated Parkinsonism, with extreme sensitivity to L-DOPA, but striking palilalia (a typical post-encephalitic symptom, of which there was no trace fifteen years ago). This highly specific impairment of her speech and motor function is in great contrast to her perfect preservation of intellectual function and personality: she shows all the wit, the vividness, the pungency, the humour, she used to show (which were so remarkable in the documentary film, and which were to be so moving and amazing to everyone in the feature film of *Awakenings* seventeen years later) – the deterioration has been solely in certain aspects of motor regulation. There has been a similar, highly specific deterioration in about three-quarters of the post-encephalitic patients whom I have followed through the 1980s.[148]

A few of the post-encephalitic patients under my care have not shown *any* deterioration – one such patient, Joseph F., whom I have followed since 1975, and who was followed by Dr. Duvoisin for ten years prior to this, still walks around and talks just as he did in the late 1950s. Others have shown only minimal changes.

Such is the continuing pathology and physiology of these last-

---

[148] My observations here are in accordance with those of Calne and Lees (1988), who recorded similar, highly specific losses of motor function (without any comparable loss in intellectual function) in ten out of eleven post-encephalitic patients at the Highlands Hospital who had been closely followed since Purdon Martin's studies in the mid-sixties.

They discuss various possible reasons for the late, age-related motor deterioration which seems to affect a majority of post-encephalitic patients as they get into their seventies: a selective dying-back of collateral nerve terminals formed in the acute stages of the disease; a decreased 'life-expectancy' of the affected neurons; or the effects of an age-related decay of dopaminergic neurons superimposed on the specific damage caused by the encephalitis.

It has been postulated that such age-related changes, as well as the progressive neuronal decay seen in ordinary Parkinson's disease (and perhaps other degenerative diseases), may be due to the accumulation of free radicals such as superoxide, and that the use of anti-oxidants, perhaps, may retard or prevent this (see Appendix: Beyond L-DOPA, p. 333).

remaining survivors of the great epidemic. If their lives were nothing but pathology, these last few years would have been miserable for them – and *Awakenings* itself no more than a chronicle of misery. But what has been so striking throughout is still striking now – the humour, the affirmation, the transcendence these patients show. A similar 'inexplicable' gaiety and good humour, and a continuing interest in life, characterise the remaining patients at Highlands. When I visited them in August 1989, I was once again astounded that these patients, who had been admitted as adolescents in the early 1930s, and had spent nearly 60 years there, were so lacking in bitterness and so richly appreciative of life.

Appendices

A HISTORY OF THE
SLEEPING-SICKNESS

I am often asked whether the great pandemic of 1916–27 was unique – whether there had ever been cases of epidemics of sleeping-sickness prior to this time, and whether there have been cases of undoubted or probable *encephalitis lethargica* since 1927. Above all, whether there is any possibility of a new epidemic . . . Such questions occurred to me, of course, as soon as I started working with our post-encephalitic patients at Mount Carmel, and in 1971 I wrote a letter to the *British Medical Journal* detailing the 2,000-year history of some past cases and episodes. The following extract is taken from this.

The older literature is full of vivid accounts of feverish somnolent illnesses followed, within months or years, by the development of characteristic slowness, poverty, and difficulty of movement, masking, rigidity, tremors, and, on occasion, torticollis, dystonias, oculogyria, strabismus, blepharoclonus, myoclonus, catatonus, somnolence, etc., etc. The unique symptomology of such cases, so circumstantially described in the older literature, is scarcely compatible with any other illness *but encephalitis lethargica* with Parkinsonian and other typical sequelae. Many such accounts are collected and scrutinized in the encyclopaedic works of von Economo and Jelliffe. Von Economo, while allowing that such retrospective diagnosis can only be tentative, concludes: 'We may assume with some degree of certainty that *encephalitis lethargica* had already appeared *repeatedly* before the Great War, both sporadically in the shape of isolated cases and in epidemics which again and again attracted notice for a short period on account of the . . . singular combinations of symptoms displayed . . .'
A few of these former cases and epidemics may be recalled. In

1580, Europe was swept by a serious febrile and lethargic illness ('Morbus epidemicus per totam fere Europam *Schlafkrankheit* dictus . . .'), which led to Parkinsonian and other neurological sequelae. A similar serious epidemic occurred in London between 1673 and 1675, and is described by Sydenham as 'febris comatosa'; hiccough was a prominent symptom in this epidemic (as in the Vienna encephalitis of 1919). Albrecht of Hildesheim, in 1695, provided an elaborate account of oculogyric crises, Parkinsonian symptoms, diplopia, strabismus, etc. following an attack of somnolent brain-fever in a 20-year-old girl ('De febre lethargica in strabismo utriusque oculi desinente'). A severe epidemic of *Schlafkrankheit* occurred in Tübingen in 1712 and 1713, and was followed in many cases by persistent slowness of movement and lack of initiative ('aboulia'). Minor epidemics of 'coma somnolentum' with Parkinsonian features occurred in France and Germany during the latter half of the eighteenth century, alternating with hyperkinetic epidemics of hiccough, myoclonus, chorea, and tics. Many isolated cases of *juvenile* Parkinsonism, variously associated with diplopia, oculogyria, tachypnoea, retropulsion, tics, and obsessional disorders were described by Charcot, and were almost certainly post-encephalitic in origin. In Italy, following the great influenza epidemic of 1889–90, the notorious *'nona'* appeared – a devastatingly severe somnolent illness which was followed by the development of Parkinsonian and other sequelae in almost all of the few survivors.

A knowledge of such historical accounts, and of the peculiar comings and goings of *encephalitis lethargica* in previous centuries, is of more than academic importnce. A graphic description of the *'nona,'* given by his mother to the young von Economo, enabled him to recognize and characterise this illness when it re-appeared in its catastrophic form in 1917; this is movingly described in the preface of his book. Jelliffe, in his many writings at the time of the great encephalitis epidemic, asks again and again how it could happen that a disease which had obviously existed since the days of Hippocrates could be 'discovered' only *now,* and how it was possible for an illness which had been described unmistakably innumerable times to be 'forgotten' anew by each generation. Such forgettings are as dangerous as they are mysterious, for they give us an unwarranted sense of security. In 1927, with the virtual cessation of new cases of *encephalitis lethargica,* the medical profession heaved a huge sigh of relief, and did its best to forget the horrors of the previous decade. Von Economo warned against this, saying that the causative virus was not extinct, but only in a dormant or non-virulent phase, from which it would inevitably re-emerge as it had done innumerable times since the dawn of recorded history.

There has been nothing like a widespread epidemic of *encephalitis lethargica* since 1927, although there was probably a small epidemic in the concentration camp at Theresienstadt during World War II (the documentation here is clinical only). There have, however, been repeated reports of *sporadic* cases – many of them very well authenticated – appearing at different places around the world: among recent reports one may cite the careful account of four cases seen at the National Hospital in London between 1980 and 1985 (Howard and Lees, 1987); the intriguing report of two cases near Manchester, both presenting as catatonic stupor (Johnson and Lucey, 1988); the eight cases reported by Rail et al. (1981); a report of a striking case with oculogyric crises, seen at Mount Sinai Hospital in New York (Clough et al., 1983); and a very detailed account from Japan of *encephalitis lethargica* coexisting with general paresis (Mitsuyama et al., 1983). A detailed clinical description of an *encephalitis lethargica*-like picture in a child has been reported by a former student of mine (Richard Shaw, personal communication); and I have very recently (February 1990), with my colleague Dr Margery Mark, been able to examine a young post-encephalitic patient whom Dr Mark has been following and videotaping for three years.

It is clear that *encephalitis lethargica* is still around, and that it may indeed be undiagnosed or greatly underdiagnosed at the present time (this is strongly suggested by Greenough and Davis, 1983). And if this is the case, there must certainly be the potential of a major recurrence, in the form of either a confined or widespread epidemic. The former probably occurred in the terrible conditions of the concentration camp at Theresienstadt. The latter was feared in 1976 with the anticipation of an epidemic of swine flu and possible encephalitic sequelae (200,000,000 doses of vaccine were prepared in the United States alone, but the epidemic never materialised). Pandemics of viral diseases, as Lederberg points out, are a natural and almost predictable phenomenon (Culliton, 1990), and there is certainly no reason to think that *encephalitis lethargica* is extinct. Our best protection, as von Economo stressed, is a continuing vigilance, so that we are never again, as in 1918, taken unawares.

'MIRACLE' DRUGS:
FREUD, WILLIAM JAMES,
AND HAVELOCK ELLIS

The notion of a drug which will banish sadness and fatigue, increase energy, expand consciousness, imbue or reimbue the world with wonder, has always excited desire and imagination. As I worked with our patients, and heard and saw their reactions – especially Leonard L.'s identification of L-DOPA as 'resurrecta-mine' and 'power' – I could not help being reminded of certain historical parallels, parallels equally of enchantment and disillusion. Freud, William James, and Havelock Ellis come to mind.

Freud and Cocaine

The astonishing story of Freud's dalliance with cocaine is brilliantly related in Ernest Jones's biography (see volume 1, pp. 86–108: 'The Cocaine Episode'). The following quotations and paraphrases are taken from this.

Freud, in the mid-1880s, in the midst of arduous labours of every kind, poor, scarcely known, and hungry for fame, 'was constantly occupied with the endeavour to make a name for himself by discovering something important in either clinical or pathological medicine.' One of the endeavours which beguiled him was the notion of giving the world a wonderful drug. The 'side interest' which so enthralled him sprang from the notion that depression, lassitude, and neurotic suffering were due to a deficiency in the brain – a 'neurasthenia,' and that this deficiency could be made good by the administration of cocaine. Cocaine, indeed, could scarcely be thought of as a drug at all – it merely restored one to normality: thus Freud wrote of the 'exhilaration and lasting euphoria, which in no way differs from the normal euphoria of the healthy person . . . In other words, you are simply normal, and it is soon hard to believe that you are under the influence of any drug.' Not the least desirable of its effects was to restore the sense of energy and virility: thus, in a letter to his fiancée, Freud wrote: 'Woe to you, my Princess, when I come . . . you shall see who is the stronger, a gentle little girl who doesn't eat enough or a big wild man who has cocaine in his body. In my last severe depression I took coca again and a small dose lifted me to the heights in a wonderful fashion. I am just now busy collecting the literature for a song of praise to this magical substance.'

This 'song of praise' aroused enormous interest, and was couched in a style which never recurred in his writings: in Jones's words, '. . . with a personal warmth as if he were in love with the content itself. He used expressions uncommon in a scientific paper, such as "the most gorgeous excitement" . . . he heatedly rebuffed the "slander" that had been published about this precious drug.'

Freud's active interest in cocaine lasted from 1884 to 1887 and passed through three phases: extravagant enthusiasm; anxiety and doubt, concealed by his dogmatic rebuffs of all 'slanders'; and, finally, a relinquishing and repudiation of his notions followed by a long-lasting sense of reproach.

William James and Nitrous Oxide

William James was deeply interested throughout his life in the 'mystagogic' powers of alcohol and drugs. The following personal account is taken from *The Varieties of Religious Experience*, pp. 304–8.

'The next step into mystical states carries us into a realm that public opinion and ethical philosophy have long since branded as pathological, though private practice and certain lyric strains of poetry seem still to bear witness to its ideality. I refer to the consciousness produced by intoxicants, especially by alcohol. The sway of alcohol over mankind is unquestionably due to its power to stimulate the mystical faculties of human nature, usually crushed to earth by the cold facts and dry criticisms of the sober hour. Sobriety diminishes, discriminates, and says no; drunkenness expands, unites, and says yes. It is in fact the great votary of the *Yes* function in man. It brings its votary from the chill periphery of things to the radiant core. It makes him for the moment one with truth. Not through mere perversity do men run after it. To the poor and the unlettered it stands in the place of symphony concerts and of literature; and it is part of the deeper mystery of life that whiffs and gleams of something that we immediately recognize as excellent should be vouchsafed to so many of us only in the fleeting earlier phases of what is in its totality so degrading a poisoning . . .

'Nitrous oxide and ether, especially nitrous oxide, when sufficiently diluted with air, stimulate the mystical consciousness to an extraordinary degree. Depth beyond depth of truth seems revealed to the inhaler. The truth fades out, however, or escapes, at the moment of coming to . . . Some years ago I myself made some observations on this aspect of nitrous oxide intoxication. One conclusion was forced upon my mind at that time, and my impression of its truth has ever since remained unshaken. It is that our normal waking consciousness, rational consciousness, as we call it, is but one special type of consciousness, whilst all about it, parted from it by the filmiest of screens, there lie potential forms of consciousness entirely different . . . No account of the universe in its totality can be final which leaves these other forms of consciousness quite disregarded . . . they forbid a premature closing of our accounts with reality. Looking back on my own experiences, they all converge towards a kind of insight to which I cannot help ascribing some metaphysical significance. The keynote of it is invariably a reconciliation. It is as if the opposites of the world, whose contradictoriness and conflict make all our difficulties and troubles, were melted into unity . . . To me (this sense) . . . only comes in the artificial mystic state of mind.'

Havelock Ellis and Mescal

The following is taken from 'Mescal: a Study of a Divine Plant,'
a paper written by Havelock Ellis for *Popular Science Monthly,* May
1902, pp. 52–77.

'Under mescal, as far as I have been able to observe, [the exuberant motor manifestations of hashish] seldom appear. Mescal may
at one stage produce a sense of well-being, vigour and intellectual
lucidity, but there is no actual motor exhilaration, or loss of self-
control . . . Every sense is affected . . . Mescal seems to introduce
us into the world in which Wordsworth lived or sought to live.
The "trailing clouds of glory," the tendency to invest the very
simplest things with an atmosphere of beauty, a "light that never
was on sea or land," the new vision of even "the simplest flower
that blows," all the special traits of Wordsworth's peculiar poetic
vision correspond as exactly as possible to the actual and effortless
experiences of the subject of mescal.'

Havelock Ellis notes that no sooner were the effects of the
'divine plant' described, than attempts were made to use mescal
therapeutically, especially (as with cocaine) in the treatment of
neurasthenia. The shortcomings of such therapeutic endeavours
Havelock Ellis ascribes to energetic and economic considerations, above all others: 'Mescal,' he writes, '. . . rapidly overstimulates and exhausts the nervous and cerebral apparatus, more
especially on the sensory side . . . The day has gone by when it
could be supposed that a stimulant put anything into a system. It
acts not by putting energy into the system but by taking it out
. . . So that by the use of [mescal and] other stimulants . . . we
not only draw on our capital, we actually dissipate and waste it.'

THE ELECTRICAL BASIS OF
AWAKENINGS

Since 1977, with my colleague P. C. Carolan, I have been able to study in great detail the electrical activity of the brain in those *Awakenings* patients who still survive (see Epilogue), and in several other post-encephalitic patients, on and off L-DOPA, and in a variety of circumstances and conditions (Sacks and Carolan, 1979).

Electro-encephalography (EEG) allows, so to speak, a direct access to the electrical activity of the brain – it allows (as its name implies) the brain to write its own electrical signature. With the development of highly portable equipment it is now possible to do EEGs under the most varied conditions – even with patients playing the piano! In so doing we can *directly* observe 'the expressions on the face of the nervous system' (Jonathan Miller). Such EEGs show us, as nothing else can, what 'goes on' inside the heads of our post-encephalitic patients.

Rose R., after her fabulous 'awakening' in 1969, returned again to a trance-like state which could no longer be altered by giving her L-DOPA – returned, in effect, to her pre-DOPA state. She would stay like this all day, utterly motionless with her head forced back, unless something or someone called her to life. The moment one spoke to her, or called her name, she would emerge from this strange and empty state, show a charming smile, warmth and intelligence, and a tantalizing glimpse of her old animation and personality, before falling back again into the abyss of trance.

Her EEG while in her 'trance' (figure 1) shows exceedingly slow and irregular, almost formless, brain activity, similar to that seen during stupor. The instant she is called – which brings her to life – this stupor-like activity is replaced by a lively, well-organized, very

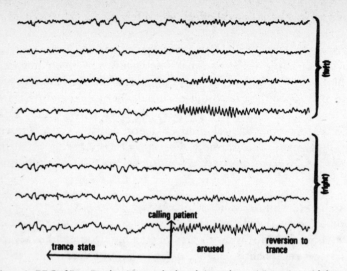

Figure 1. EEG of Rose R., showing grossly slowed, irregular activity, going with her state of 'trance.' The instant she is called, a lively normal alpha-rhythm appears. But within a second or two this disappears, and she falls back into 'trance.'

regular 'alpha rhythm' – such as one sees in a normal, alert, and awake brain. But then the moment passes, and with the passing of her momentary awakening and animation, her alpha rhythm disappears, and she reverts to the grossly pathological electrical picture of 'trance.' This EEG, then, shows a precise consonance with her clinical states – shows how the pressure of sickness keeps her entranced, and yet, tantalizingly, how human contact, or anything of interest, can 'awaken' and 'animate' her – but only for a moment. This was essentially the situation for all of these patients before the coming of L-DOPA – it had been their situation for decades before 1969.

L-DOPA (or similar drugs) is uniquely effective in evoking a sustained 'awakening'; but, as we have seen in every case, this initial effect is always complicated, after a while, by 'tribulations.' This was especially clear with Leonard L. who, after the extraordinary summer of 1969, could never tolerate L-DOPA or similar drugs for very long – showing not only a grossly exaggerated sensitivity to them, but a grossly pathological effect after a few weeks (as described on p. 218). Leonard L.'s EEG, in the absence of any drug activation, is profoundly slow – even slower than that of Rose R. – of a slowness never seen in the deepest normal sleep (figure 2a) – even though he is himself, at these times, not asleep, though bereft of motion, feeling, and will. When he is put on amantadine (figure 2b) he does quite well at first, and his EEG becomes much faster, better organised, and more rhythmical – indeed almost normal. However, with the continuing use (and now, *stimulation*) of the drug – and this occurs in three to four weeks – he develops sudden, convulsive-compulsive motions and notions, and his EEG becomes grossly excited and convulsive, with repeated bursts of high-voltage paroxysmal activity (figure 2c). Finally, he becomes so violent and explosive that the amantadine must be stopped – but with this he returns within hours to his motionless, apathetic, almost-stuporous state (figure 2a).

The essential problem is to find a stable 'middle' position in a patient whose behaviour and cerebral states always tend to extremes

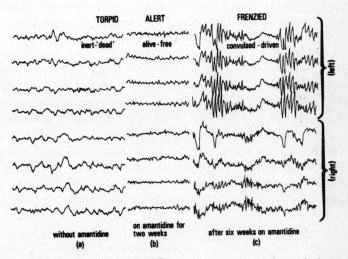

Figure 2. EEG of Leonard L. in three different states. In (a) we see the grossly slow and irregular electrical activity, in the absence of any medication; in (b), much faster, livelier, normal cerebral rhythms, with the initial 'awakening' effects of amantadine; in (c), very excited activity, with convulsive bursts, especially on one side, with the continuing and now pathogenic effects of medication.

– who has, in effect, a 'bipolar' disorder. Leonard L.'s EEG – like a dozen others we have – gives exact objective confirmation of this clinical dilemma; it shows how the continuing use of any awakening or stimulant drug in such patients comes to exert an increasing pressure, which is finally too great to be borne – so that they can no longer stand what they so greatly need. We see, not just clinically, but in their EEGs as well, that such patients have only the narrowest *base;* that they walk, as it were, a tightrope of health, with abysses of sickness to either side – the abyss of stupor and the abyss of frenzy. What might seem to be a mere (or extravagant) figure of speech is seen, in their EEGs, to be a terrible physiological reality. For such patients there is only a physiological Ixion's Wheel, which whirls them round and round from one extreme to another – the extremes, so to speak, of a physiological hell.

Mercifully, what medication cannot achieve, music, action, or art can do – at least for the time that it lasts ('you are the music/While the music lasts'). We have observed this, too, in many EEGs – most strikingly in two patients (Rosalie B. and Ed M.), who are highly musical, and performed in the documentary film of *Awakenings.* Both of these patients have grossly abnormal EEGs, with both stuporous and convulsive features. (Ed's is very slow on one side, and convulsive on the other; as he himself is catatonic on one side, and wildly ticcy and Touretty on the other.) But, in a way which is wonderful to see, their EEGs – like their clinical states – become entirely normal when they are playing or listening to music; only to fall back into the grossest pathology when the music stops. This normalisation of the EEG occurs even if the music is only played *mentally:* thus with Rosalie B., who knew all Chopin by heart, and had eidetically vivid musical imagery, one had only to say (for example), 'Opus 49,' and her EEG would instantly change, as the F-minor Fantasie started to play itself silently inside her; the moment this inner performance was over, her EEG would instantly become abnormal again.

These studies show us how the physiological and the existential go together. The end of physiological processes, as Claude Bernard taught, is the provision of a constant *milieu intérieur* – this being, in his words, 'la condition de la vie libre.' At the highest level there must be constancy of cerebral rhythms – perhaps this constitutes a final condition for the free life. Experience with these patients, and their EEGs, shows the profound truth of this: that the physiology of one's cerebral rhythms and 'tone' must at least be reasonably constant and correct in order to provide a base for action and freedom; that one is in bondage, held captive, passive, unfree, if one's cerebral physiology is *too* abnormal; and that both L-DOPA and music, by calling forth a steadier and more rhythmic activity of the brain, give to the patient the possibilities of freedom.

At the time I started EEG studies of our patients, I was not aware of any other such studies on a comparable group of institutionalized post-encephalitic patients. To be more accurate, I had forgotten about Onuaguluchi's fascinating work with the post-encephalitics in Glasgow, which I had not read since its publication many years ago (Onuaguluchi, 1964). It is evident at a glance that some of Onuaguluchi's patients have extraordinarily slow EEGs, but that this is far from common: he notes slowish (theta) activity, on occasion,

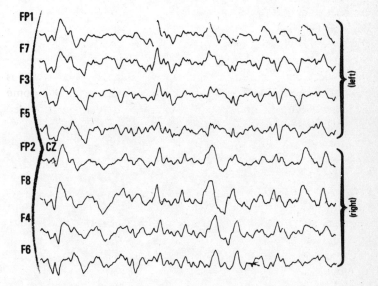

Figure 3. Sample of EEG on a post-encephalitic patient (Leonora di P.), who was admitted to Mount Carmel in 1980 without ever having received L-DOPA. The entire record shows the most profound (delta) slowing, as is usually only seen in the deepest sleep or coma, even though the patient was perfectly conscious and alert throughout the EEG recording.

in 60% of his patients; whereas profoundly slow (delta) activity was found scarcely at all.

By contrast, in our population, more than half of the patients show profound and persistent delta activity (see figure 3) – the sort of picture more usually seen in deep sleep or stupor. This discrepancy, like the clinical discrepancies between the Highlands patients and our own, confirms the much higher incidence of profound arousal-disorders ('sleep') in our own patients – and, with this, the necessity, and the possibility, of a much more drastic 'awakening.'

BEYOND L-DOPA

The late 1960s and early 1970s saw tremendous enthusiasm for the use of L-DOPA, and a sense that its 'side effects' could be easily conquered. But then – as it became evident that there was no simple solution to these 'side effects' or the sudden on/off reactions which, sooner or later, almost all patients maintained on it showed – a mood of disappointment and disillusion set in. New dopamine agonists were discovered or devised, some facilitating the production of dopamine (at presynaptic terminals), others blocking its release (at postsynaptic ones). Different receptors (D_1 and D_2 terminals) were delineated. But still the situation remained essentially the same – so that in the third (1982–3) edition of *Awakenings,* I could report little positive other than a greater realism about L-DOPA's powers and limitations.

The last eight years have seen some wholly unexpected and exciting new developments, which, though they have emerged from a highly specific (and even bizarre) situation, may promise to shed the most general light on the genesis and treatment of all sorts of Parkinsonism, and perhaps of neurodegenerative disease in general.

In the summer of 1982 there appeared in California a number of young people (including some teenagers) who had become virtually 'frozen' overnight. Some were misdiagnosed as having 'catatonic schizophrenia' or 'hysteria' (as had happened sixty years earlier with some of the first victims of the sleeping-sickness), but were then realised to be suffering from an unprecedented, acute, and overwhelming form of Parkinsonism. Physicians had occasionally seen cases of severe juvenile Parkinsonism (these were commoner in the last century), but never the development of profound Parkinsonism literally overnight.

This remained a medical mystery, until brilliant detective work by William Langston and his colleagues showed that all of those affected had taken a synthetic opiate, a so-called 'designer drug' supposed to have effects similar to heroin.[149] In each case of sudden-onset Parkinsonism the offending agent was identified as 1-methyl-4-phenyl-1,2,3,6-tetrahydropyridine, or MPTP.

Those affected by this new form of Parkinsonism showed all the classical signs – tremor, rigidity, bradykinesia, salivation, micrographia, etc. – but to a quite overwhelming degree. They had Parkinsonism of a severity almost never seen in ordinary Parkinson's disease – and hitherto seen, indeed, only in post-encephalitic Parkinsonism. The damage to the substantia nigra which had caused this Parkinsonism was permanent and irreversible. But once they were diagnosed, fortunately, these young patients proved to be extraordinarily sensitive to L-DOPA, showing spectacular, sudden responses after quite modest doses. But then, very rapidly, instabilities set in: innumerable 'side effects' of all sorts rapidly proliferated, and the patients moved into sudden, unpredictable, on/off oscillations. Such patients, in the words of the documentary, 'live on a narrow ledge between being completely frozen and having terrible side effects.'

Interestingly, when Langston described this extraordinary sensitivity to L-DOPA, followed by the extremely rapid development of oscillations and side effects, his observations were strongly criticized and doubted – precisely as happened in 1970 when I first wrote about the equally dramatic and hyperbolic reactions of post-encephalitic patients to L-DOPA.[150] The reason for the similarities of Langston's findings and my own, is extremely simple, but its discovery had to await the development of PET scanning, which can directly visualize living brain tissue.[151] An 'ordinary,' moderately Parkin-

---

[149] A powerful documentary of this, 'The Frozen Addicts,' presented by Langston, was produced by the PBS series 'Nova' in 1986.

[150] I had described very prompt and often sudden 'awakenings' in my patients, followed, sometimes within days, by the appearance of intractable 'side effects' and on/off reactions – all in response to exceptionally small doses of L-DOPA (Sacks et al., 1970c). These observations aroused incredulity among my colleagues (see letters in response to my paper, *JAMA*, December 1970). It was only later that I realised that our experiences had been quite different – that they had never seen such responses themselves, and so could neither imagine nor believe that they might actually occur.

[151] The similarity between Langston's patients and my own was dramatically shown in 1986 when his tapes, and the documentary film of *Awakenings*, were shown together at a meeting of the American Academy of Neurology in San Francisco.

sonian patient, it has been established, may still have 5% of the normal dopamine levels in the substantia nigra, while a post-encephalitic or MPTP patient might, startlingly, have less than 0.1%. This degree of degeneration is simply never seen in the usual form of the disease.

Langston established that MPTP has an absolutely specific effect on the neurons of the substantia nigra (and not only in man, but in many animals, thus for the first time making an animal model of Parkinsonism available for researchers). He further determined that it was not MPTP as such which was toxic, but a derivative (MPP+) into which MPTP was transformed within the nigral neurons – and importantly, that this lethal transformation could be prevented by a mono-amine oxidase (MAO) inhibitor. Such inhibitors (there are two forms of MAO, A and B, and it is only the MAO-B inhibitors which are effective) had a dramatic effect, safeguarding exposed animals from the toxic effects of MPTP, so that they neither developed Parkinsonism nor showed any depletion of dopamine or cell death in the substantia nigra. It was further established that such agents not only protect animals exposed to MPTP, but they can, seemingly, slow the advance of the disease process in 'ordinary' Parkinson's disease.[152]

Several different ideas have emerged from this. One is that ordinary ('idiopathic') Parkinson's disease may itself be the result of a toxin, if not of MPTP then of other, allied compounds which could be converted to MPP+ or other lethal agents in the brain. (Parkinson's essay was written in 1817, and it seems that Parkinson's disease may have become more common with the industrial revolution.)

Another is that an insult to the nigral cells early in life (whether from MPTP, or a hypothetical industrial toxin, or *encephalitis lethargica*) might fail to produce any clinical effects at the time–for Parkinsonism only becomes clinically manifest when destruction of cells in the substantia nigra reaches about 80% – but later lead to Parkinsonism with the further loss of nigral dopamine and cells which occur with normal ageing. This might explain what has always been a mystery (see n. 81, p. 161): why post-encephalitic syndromes may develop so many years after the original encephalitic insult, and why,

---

[152] After discussing this with Langston, I looked back on the records of our own post-encephalitic patients, several of whom had been given MAO inhibitors as anti-depressants in the 1950s, and felt that there was a suggestion that these might have retarded the disease process in these patients as well.

once the syndromes have developed, they often progress. There is a vital therapeutic corollary to this – namely, that one might intervene, with the use of an MAO-B inhibitor like selegiline (Deprenyl or Eldepryl), very early in the disease, and prevent it from getting worse.

With PET scanning, it has been shown that some patients who took only a single small dose of MPTP, and did not become clinically Parkinsonian, nonetheless showed marked reductions of nigrostriatal dopamine. This, while producing no Parkinsonism at the time, could still be considered a dangerous situation, in that further doses of MPTP, or just the decline of striatal dopamine which occurs with age, might bring on manifest Parkinsonism. There was a strong demand, by 1986, for prospective trials of an inhibitor like Deprenyl – and now, in 1990, the first results are in, and it appears that Deprenyl may indeed have a real and substantial effect in delaying the advance of Parkinsonism.

The substantia nigra, prior to 1980, was an inaccessible nucleus of cells buried in the midbrain. We can now visualise these cells and their dopamine, in life; we can destroy them, selectively; and we can protect them against such destruction, and perhaps too against the slow degenerative destruction which may be common to both idiopathic and post-encephalitic Parkinsonism. These are all achievements of great moment, which were not even on the horizon ten years ago.

But there is another, quite different but equally fascinating advance, or at least work in progress – namely the idea of *transplanting* dopamine-rich cells into the brain as a 'cure' for Parkinsonism. Various techniques have been employed, from transplanting adult cells from the adrenal medulla to transplanting dopaminergic cells from foetal brain tissue. Such cells, it is hoped, might not only serve as a source of dopamine, as a sort of dopamine pump, in the brain, but might actually form a morphologically organised organ or structure, a neuronal as well as chemical replacement for the nigrostriatal system which has been damaged. It remains to be seen whether it is possible or practicable to have such a *structural* replacement in the brain.

Thus as we enter the 1990s there is great excitement and great hope in the field of Parkinsonism, a sense that we have now entered a new era. If the 1960s were the great era of replacement therapy

– and it was such a therapy which made my patients' 'awakenings' possible – we may now be fairly launched on an era where Parkinsonism, and other degenerative diseases, can be suspected or diagnosed *before* they become manifest, and treated so that they never become so.

PARKINSONIAN SPACE AND TIME

Frances D. (like half a dozen other highly articulate post-encephalitic patients under my care) has often depicted for me the strange and deeply paradoxical world in which she lives. These patients describe a fantastical-mathematical world remarkably similar to that which faced 'Alice.' Miss D. lays stress on the fundamental distortions of Parkinsonian *space*, on her peculiar difficulties with angles, circles, sets, and limits. She once said of her 'freezing': 'It's not as simple as it looks. I don't just come to a halt, I am still going, but I *have run out of space to move in* . . . You see, *my* space, *our* space, is nothing like *your* space: our space gets bigger and smaller, it bounces back on itself, and it loops itself round till it runs into itself.'

We may first take a brief historical look at notions of 'space.' An essential difference (one might almost say, *the* essential difference) between the philosophies of Newton and of Leibniz hinges on their differing notions and uses of the word 'space' – the Newtonian concept of 'motion' versus the Leibnizian one of 'action.' For Newton space and time were absolutes – absolute media in which motion occurred; they were not hypotheses *('Hypotheses non fingo'),* or, as we would say now, frames-of-reference. For Leibniz, in contrast, 'space' and 'time,' and all such notions of continuity and extension, were simply ways of speaking, ways of picturing and measuring *the size of actions:* they were concrete and actual, not absolute and abstract, i.e. they were convenient (or conventional) constructions or 'models,' figurative language (albeit of a very special sort). (These essentially relativistic concepts of Leibniz are fully spelled out in his correspondence with Clark – a correspondence interrupted only by Leibniz's death, and not published until many years later.) The notion of 'space' as a way of speaking and looking at the world, rather than as a Euclidean or Newtonian absolute, was revived by Gauss in his famous papers on the possible curvatures of possible spaces, and then by the great Russian geometers in their 'alternative geometries.' These, then, combined with Maxwellian dynamics, were the intellectual antecedents of Einstein's thought, his notions of coordinate-systems in motion relative to each other, of the possibility of countless, individual, variable space-times . . .

Let us now come to practical examples, familiar and unfamiliar, of 'personal space' and 'personal time,' which indicate how our judgements and our actions may be at variance with the abstract measure of clocks and rulers, or the judgements and actions of other human beings. First, a familiar and universal example, which all of us have experienced when impatient, hurried, or 'pressed for time': 'a watched pot never boils,' as the old saying has it – if we are impatiently awaiting its boiling, it seems to take 'unduly long,' and we may feel that the very watches we wear have become unreliable; again, if we are hurrying to catch a bus or train, the distance we must traverse seems 'unduly long,' and the time we have 'unduly short.'

Thus we may experience illusions (or misleading conjectures) about space-time when we are hurried or festinant; and equally we may have illusions when dawdling or procrastinant. Now let us examine Parkinsonian behaviour in this light, concerning ourselves especially with *illusions of scale.* I have had letters from Frances D., and other Parkinsonian patients, which showed singular (and often comic) disparities of scale: I remember one such letter from Frances D., of which the first page was in a perfectly formed but microscopic hand (so small I needed a magnifying-glass to decipher it), while at the start of the second page (which was in normally sized script) she had written: 'I see that what I wrote yesterday was far too small, although I didn't see this at the time. Today I have borrowed a ruler and ruled lines on this page, and I will use the lines to guide my writing, so that I don't inadvertently make it tiny again.' Other letters from Frances D., and certain other patients, were sometimes marked by enormous (though perfectly shaped and formed) writing, and this too would be done in seeming ignorance of its abnormal magnitude.[153] Similar disturbances were common in speech: most

[153] If one observes Parkinsonians with sufficient minuteness – for example in the act of writing – one may say that there are indeed changes of scale, but that these

Parkinsonian patients tend to speak softly, and often to do so without knowing they are doing so; but if asked to 'speak up,' they may find no difficulty in raising their voices; on the other hand Cecil M., who had 'megaphonia,' habitually spoke in a Brobdingnagian voice, and felt everyone around him was speaking too softly (I should add that his hearing was perfectly normal – it was his *judgement* of sounds which showed aberrations).

Again, in walking, one may see 'microambulation' *('marche à petits pas')* in Parkinsonian patients; if such patients measure themselves against regular marks or clocks, or the framework of dimensions around them, or against the movements of other persons whom they take to be 'normal,' they may perceive (and perhaps correct) their own tiny steps; but this may not happen, or may be prevented from happening – the patient may be engrossed in his own scale of walking, and fail to realize that either the walking or the scale is 'wrong.' Parkinsonian patients often make 'macro-' or 'micro-gestures' – gestures of the right *sort,* but on the wrong *scale* (too large, too small, too fast, too slow . . .); these they may perform completely unwittingly, unaware that the gesture is inappropriate in scale. I am often able to show a beautiful example of such 'kinetic illusions' when I demonstrate Aaron E. (a deeply Parkinsonian, but not post-encephalitic, patient) to my students: 'Mr E.,' I say, 'would you be kind enough to clap your hands steadily and regularly – *thus?*' 'Sure, doc,' he replies, and after a few steady claps is apt to proceed into an incontinent festination of clapping, culminating in an apparent 'freezing' of motion. 'There, doc!' he says, turning to me with a pleased smile. 'Didn't I do it nice and regular, just like you asked me?' 'Gentlemen!' I say to the students. 'You be the judges. Did Mr E. clap his hands steadily and regularly, as he says?' 'Why, of course not!' exclaims one of the students. 'His movements kept getting faster and faster, and smaller and smaller – like *this!*' At this point Mr E. leaps to his feet in indignation: 'What do you mean?' he cries to the student. 'What do you mean by saying my movements got faster and smaller – in that crazy way you did it yourself? *My* move-

---

consist of *sudden, incalculable jumps:* within a couple of seconds, for example, there may be a dozen such 'jumps' – so what we observe is not, in fact, a continuously *warped* metric, but an infinitely stranger *twitching* metric; not a smooth geometrical or topological transform, but a sudden algebraic or statistical one.

Festinant clock, warped by Parkinsonian pressure; lilliputian handwriting, unwarped but minute. Both were felt as 'normal' by the patient, though only truly normalised by L-DOPA.

ments were perfectly regular and stable – like *this!*' And, concentrating fiercely, totally absorbed in his own activity, he falls once again into the grossest festination. This demonstration (when it works! and this depends on how much Mr E. is enclosed in his own frame-of-reference, versus how much he can stand outside it and make comparisons and corrections) is – in the charming idiom of my New York students – 'mind blowing,' 'mind boggling,' 'wild!', 'out of sight!' It is, indeed, literally *shocking,* because of the clarity with which it shows that what Aaron E. clearly perceives in others, he cannot perceive in himself; that he may use a frame-of-reference (or coordinate-system, or way of judging space-time) which departs from 'the normal' in an ever-increasing and accelerating way; and that he may be so enclosed within his own (contracting) frame-of-reference, that he is unable to perceive the contracting scale in his own movements. Thus, the curious 'dialogue' between Mr E. and the students comes to resemble an imaginary Einsteinian dialogue between people in lifts (or frames-of-reference) which are moving or accelerating relative to each other; and the entire demonstration provides the clearest manifestation of relativity in action, the clearest vindication of Frances D.'s insights when she speaks of different 'spaces,' and says: '... *my* space, *our* space, is nothing like *your* space.'

Such a demonstration certainly establishes that individuals may have varying experiences of space and time – and (a point continually stressed by Richard Gregory) that their experiences are themselves hypotheses or conjectures. It does not, by itself, show that the false conjectures of Aaron E. are of a relativistic kind, rather than of a simpler kind, involving simple visual or kinaesthetic or motor illusions. We are all subject to the latter – as shown by the 'queer feeling' (or continually violated delusion of motion) we may experience if we walk on an escalator which has stopped. Patients with cortical apraxias and agnosias are especially liable to misperceptions (misconjectures) of this sort, and so too, for a while, are patients who have sustained peripheral injuries (e.g. an injury which has de-activated, hence de-realised, a leg or a foot): such patients may make *individual* misjudgements, or a series of these, with regard to the size of individual objects, especially meaningless, geometrical objects like *steps,* because of an uncertainty or deficiency in their own inner scales, secondary to a mutilation or distortion in part of their body image, of their own biological measuring-apparatus . . . But such errors, which all of us are prone to when faced with new motor tasks (skiing, pole-vaulting, riding bicycles, etc.) are different in kind from Parkinsonian misjudgement.

I vividly remember, from my first month with these patients, the following event in 1966. As I was writing notes at my desk, I perceived through the open door Seymour L. *careering* down the corridor; he had been walking pretty normally, and then, suddenly, was accelerated, festinant, precipitated. I thought he was going to fall flat on his face. He recovered himself, however, and was able to proceed without further incident to the nursing station near my desk. He was obviously in a rage, and a panic, and bewildered: 'Why the hell do they leave the passage like that?' he spluttered.

'What do you mean, Mr L.?' the nurse rejoined. 'What's wrong with the passage? It's no different from usual.'

'No different from usual!' Seymour shouted, going red in the face. 'It's got a bloody great hole in it – they been excavating or something? I'm walking along, minding my business, and the ground suddenly falls away from my feet at this crazy angle, without reason. I was thrown into a run, lucky I wasn't thrown flat on my face. And you say there is nothing wrong with the passage?'

'Mr L.,' the nurse replied. 'You're not making sense. I assure you the passage is perfectly normal.'

At this point I got up, agog at the whole thing, and suggested to Mr L. and the nurse that we walk back together, to find out about the 'excavation.' Seymour walked between us, unconsciously attuning his pace to ours, and we walked the length of the passage together without any incident – and without any hint of festination or precipitation.

This absence of incident left Seymour confounded. 'I'll be damned,' he said. 'You're perfectly right. The passage is quite level. But' – he turned to me, and spoke with an emphasis and a conviction I have never forgotten – 'I could have *sworn* it suddenly dipped, just as I said. It was *because* it dipped that I was forced into a run. You'd do the same if you felt the ground falling away, in a steep slope, from under your feet! I ran as *anyone* would run, with such a feeling. What you call "festination" is no more than a normal reaction to an abnormal perception. We Parkinsonians suffer from illusions!'[154]

The Parkinsonian – unlike the cortical apraxic-agnosic – *understands* perfectly well what is meant by a 'foot'; he has in no sense lost his *ideas* of dimension. What we observe, however, is that all his space-time judgements are *pushed out of shape,* that his entire coordinate-system is subject to expansions, contractions, torsions, and warps; and that such generalized distortions of his metrical field are produced by pulling, pushing, and twisting forces – by the tractions, pulsions, and torsions of being which constitute the very essence of his illness. The apraxic-agnosic patient may make errors of action or cognition, but he is not *driven* into misperformance or miscognition

---

[154] Such illusions of space are common in Parkinsonism – this was well understood a century ago. Thus Michael Foster, in the 1883 edition of his *Textbook of Physiology* (London: Macmillan), writes:

Persons who have experienced similar forced movements as a result of [basal gangliar] disease report that they are frequently accompanied, and seem to be caused by disturbed visual or other sensations; thus when they suddenly fall forward they say they do so because the ground in front of them appears to sink away beneath their feet.

through being the subject of violent deforming forces; he may, so to speak, have forgotten his tape-measure or pocket-watch, but he has not had all his measuring devices, his metrical judgements, warped by forces which he may be unable to recognize, because the judgement by which he might judge his judgements is itself warped, and so on . . . The Parkinsonian engrossed in his Parkinsonism can no more judge the 'abnormality' of his own state than could a self-conscious rod, accelerated towards the velocity of light, which had itself undergone a Lorentz contraction. It is for reasons of this sort that it is insufficient to speak of Parkinsonism as a simple *'dyskinesia'* (motor disorder). One must speak of it as a systematic disorder of space-time parameters, a systematic warping of coordinate-systems; indeed one must go further, and say that this misjudgement or warping is secondary to a systematic disorder of 'will' or *force,* which has the effect of warping Parkinsonian 'space' and making it a dynamic, field, or relativistic disorder.

Frances D.'s ability to climb stairs in a regular and controlled fashion, which stood in the most dramatic contrast with her irregular and uncontrollable tendencies to hurry or freeze in her walking, is an example of the use, and indeed the necessity, of *external means* to activate Parkinsonian patients, and to regulate or control their activity. Such direct methods of activation and regulation – direct in that they concern themselves directly with the actual behavioural and experiential disorders of Parkinsonism, and not with its chemical or anatomical substrate – are of fundamental importance, both theoretically and practically, in helping us to understand, and through understanding to help, Parkinsonian patients. Such direct methods are discovered, or can be learned (and should be learned!) by all Parkinsonian patients, by their friends and relatives, by their physicians and nurses, by all who come into close contact with them; they are easy, and often delightful, to learn; they can make a literally vital difference to the lives of Parkinsonian patients; and they form an essential complement to the use of L-DOPA.[155]

The central problem in all Parkinsonian disorders is *passivity* – passivity *and* pulsivity, i.e. inertia – as the central cure for them all is *activity* (of the right kind). The essence of this passivity lies in

---

[155] See also n. 45, p. 60 and n. 47, p. 63.

peculiar difficulties of self-stimulation, and initiation, not in the capacity to respond to stimulation. This means, in the severest cases, that the patient is totally unable to help himself, although he can very easily be helped by other people, or other means, outside himself; in less severe cases (as Luria has never ceased to stress) the Parkinsonian patient *can* help himself in a limited fashion, by using his normal and active powers to regulate his pathological or 'de-activated' ones. Thus a Parkinsonian patient may be totally mute unless spoken to, when he may be able to reply with perfect facility; he may be motionless unless motioned to, when he immediately makes a motor reply (waving, gesticulating, rising to meet one); he may be mute and motionless in a silent environment, but sing and dance perfectly if music is provided; he may (like Frances D.) remain frozen in one spot, or helplessly festinant, unless steps are provided, or regular marks, in which case he may use them with perfect facility.

The problem, then, is to provide a continual stimulus of the appropriate kind – and if we can achieve this we can recall Parkinsonians from inactivity (or abnormal activity) into normal activity, and from the abyss of unbeing into normal being. *'Quis non agit non existit'* (writes Leibniz); when the Parkinsonian is not active he does not exist – when we recall him to activity we recall him to life.

We may use alternative terms, and say that the problem of activation is one of *order* or *organisation,* of finding forms of order or organisation which will combat the specific *disorders* and *disorganisations* which constitute Parkinsonism. We observe of Parkinsonians that either they fail to move at all, or they move wrongly, and that the wrongness of their movements is a wrongness of *scale* – their movements are too large or too small, too fast or too slow. Thus what the Parkinsonian needs, and what we must give him, is *measure* (or metric), so that he can overcome his peculiar deficiencies or distortions of measuring (his *'ametria'* and *'dysmetria'*).

What is a measure – and how do we measure? We create and use two sorts of measure: measures that are abstract, absolute, and formal (measuring-sticks and pendulums, rulers and clocks, the C.G.S. measures of engineering and physics); or measures that are concrete, actual, and active – measures that relate to our environment and ourselves. ('Man is the measure of all things,' said da Vinci.) Both come together, for example, in the concept of 'a foot,' which was at first a living, practical measure, based on the size of a human foot, and then a precise and abstract measure, the distance between two marks on a rigid, lifeless rod.

So, in the most general terms, we find that ametric-dysmetric Parkinsonian patients can be activated and regulated, ordered and organised, by either sort of measure: by regular marks in a conventional, formal (and linear) space-time, e.g. stairs, steps painted on the ground, clocks, metronomes, and devices that count in a simple, regular, and orderly manner; or by co-action and co-ordination with a concrete, living activity or agent. Thus, in the case of Miss D., the chalking of regular lines on the ground enabled her to walk stably, but like a puppet or robot; but taking her arm, and strolling with her, enabled her to stroll like a normal human being. The first form of treatment is *kinetic,* the second *mimetic.* The first is directed to *the scale of motion,* the second to *the shape of action.* Parkinsonism, at its severest, presents itself as an akinetic amimia (as opposed to certain cortical disorders which are amimic akinesias). Since right mimesis entails right kinesis, whereas kinesia *per se* entails only itself, the best form of therapy is mimetic, kinetic therapy constituting a second best – a prosthetic or algorithmic substitute (like a wooden leg, or an artificial pace-maker).

Thus Hester would rush and dart when alone in a room, but move at a more 'normal' pace if she were moderated by other things or other people; similarly Miriam would only speed up in her speech when she 'forgot' the presence of others, when she was, as it were, enveloped in monology. At such times, they *felt* they were moving and talking 'normally,' i.e. they suffered a sort of tachyscopic illusion which blinded them to their own tachykinesia and tachyphemia. Could not such a tendency and such an illusion be countered by the introduction of a commensurate resistance or retardation in the medium of their movements, or a commensurate illusion of 'bradyscopy'? Such measures do work, in a limited way: thus Hester's tendency to walk too fast was moderated if she had to walk uphill (as it was aggravated if she had to walk downhill); it was also moderated if she *thought* she was walking uphill (when, in reality, she was walking on the level). Indeed she once asked me if it might not be possible to make a special pair of glasses for her which would distort appearances so that all the level corridors would seem to her to be going uphill. (I was unsure whether this would be ontologically possible, let alone optically possible.)

We have repeatedly referred to the usefulness of steps, lines, ticks, clocks, routines, pacings, etc. – scales, measures, series, patterns, disposed in a fixed and regular and conventional space-time. All of these can provide (in Luria's terminology) 'syntagms' or 'algorithms' for the structuring and coordination of experience and behaviour; they provide (again in Luria's terms) 'logico-grammatical' or 'quasi-spatial' paradigms or schemes.

All of us (by 'us' I mean *human* animals, as opposed to non-human animals, who are so admirably guided by their own, biological, 'clocks' and 'scales') require and use artificial, abstract, conventional measures – *standards* – of this sort, standards for consensus and communication. The Parkinsonian, who is 'far out,' whose behaviour has become so different from, so incommensurable with, ordinary conduct, stands in special need of such formalities and conventions; but he also stands in special peril from them. A subtle and sensible balance is needed, a propriety of relation, so that the Parkinsonian patient can have the mechanical and the systematic *at his service, without himself becoming enslaved to them.*

Complementary to the artifices and algorithms which can so help Parkinsonian patients is the real world, infinite in variety, aspect, and depth, infinitely concrete, infinitely metaphorical, infinitely formal yet infinitely expressive, infinitely ordered yet infinitely free. The real world, whether in Nature or Art or social relationship, is – finally – the only thing which can give the Parkinsonian (which can give any of us) that fullness, ease, and spontaneity of action which constitutes happiness, health, freedom, and life.

The true ideal would be the restoration of a 'natural' rhythm and movement, the 'kinetic melody' (in Luria's term) natural and normal to each particular patient: something which would not be a mere scheme or diagram or algorithm of behaviour, but a restoration of genuine spaciousness and freedom. We have seen, again and again, that patients' own kinetic melodies *can* be given back to them, albeit briefly, by the use of an appropriate flow of *music:* one is reminded here of Novalis's aphorism: 'Every sickness is a musical problem, and every cure a musical solution.' Other 'natural' motions of Nature and Art are equally potent if experienced visually or tactually. Thus, I have known patients almost totally immobilised by Parkinsonism, dystonias, contortions, etc., capable of riding a horse with ease – with ease and grace and intuitive control, forming with the horse a mutually influencing and natural unity; indeed, the mere *sight* of riding, running, walking, swimming, of any natural movement whatever – as a purely visual experience on a television screen – can call forth by sympathy, or suggestion, an equal naturalness of movement in Parkinsonian patients. The art of 'handling' Parkinsonian patients, learned by sensitive nurses and friends – assisting them by the merest intimation or touch, or by a wordless, touchless moving-together, in an intuitive kinetic sympathy of attunement – this is a genuine art, which can be exercised by a man or a horse or a dog, but which can *never* be simulated by any mechanical feedback; for it is only an ever-changing, melodic, and *living* play of forces which can recall living beings into their own living being. Such a subtle, ever-changing play of forces may also be achieved through the use of certain 'natural' devices, which *intermediate,* so to speak, between afflicted patients and the forces of Nature. Thus while severely affected Parkinsonians are particularly dangerous at the controls of motorcars and motorboats (which tend to amplify all their pathological tendencies), they may be able to handle a sailing boat with ease and skill, with an intuitive accuracy and 'feel.' Here, in effect, man-boat-wind-wave come together in a natural, dynamic union or unison; the man feels at one, at home, with the forces of Nature; his own natural melody is evoked by, attuned to, the harmony of Nature; he ceases to be a *patient* – passive and pulsive – and is transformed to an *agent* – active and free.

CHAOS AND
AWAKENINGS[156]

The pathological physiology of Parkinsonism is the study of an organised chaos.

–MCKENZIE (1927)

The early days of L-DOPA were a delight to us all – our patients got wonderfully better, and we, their physicians, got a heady sense of power: it was in our power seemingly to 'fix' Parkinsonism, to banish its symptoms, to offer our patients an apparently unlimited cure (or at least an unlimited remission from their symptoms). And when, to our surprise, unexpected complications occurred, we were quick to call these 'side-effects,' to see them as insignificant, or easily controlled. If 'akinetic episodes' occurred (advised Cotzias), one could just drop the dose of L-DOPA by ten percent: the myth of control, of titratability, of predictability, still held. These were nothing but 'side-effects,' surely we could fix them.

I certainly shared this wish myself – how could I not? But soon after the 'honeymoon' period (which, with my post-encephalitic patients, sometimes lasted only a few weeks, sometimes only days), complications set in: new phenomena – chorea, tics; over-excitement – mania, akathisia, drivenness; fluctuations, rapidly deepening to sudden and catastrophic oscillations, as, for example, in Hester Y.:

---

[156] The work described here was undertaken in collaboration with Dr. Ralph Siegel (of the Thomas J. Watson Research Center, IBM, and Rutgers University). A fuller version of it will be published by us later.

Her reactions to it have become . . . entirely all-or-none in character – she either reacts totally or not at all . . . She leaps from one physiological extreme to another in the twinkling of an eye, in a flash, in a fraction of a second. . . . Such transitions . . . are no longer 'correlated' in any predictable way with the timing of her L-DOPA doses – indeed, she is apt to make somewhere between 30 and 200 abrupt physiological reversals a day . . . The abruptness and totality of these reversals scarcely give one an impression of a gradual, graduated process, but of sudden reorganisations or transformations of *phase*. (p. 107)

Already, by August of 1969, I had to speak of such 'yo-yo' reactions as occurring in a majority of my patients; and, along with this, there increasingly occurred an extreme and ever-increasing sensitivity to L-DOPA; and extraordinary (and unpredictable) sensitivity to all sorts of conditions and circumstances which would normally have little or no disturbing effects. The broad base, the resilience, of health was lost; the patients all became, sooner or later, 'unstable,' 'brittle,' impossible to titrate, liable to gross destabilisation at the drop of a hat. 'At best,' George W. wrote, 'I feel completely normal . . . but I've become very over-sensitive, and the moment I over-exert myself or over-excite myself, or if I am worried, or get tired, all the side-effects immediately come back . . . I'm *perfect* when everything is going smoothly, but I feel like I'm on a tightrope, or like a pin trying to balance on its point' (see pp. 200–201).

Things would go smoothly, during the administration of L-DOPA, *up to a certain point,* a certain critical point; but then instabilities would set in, instabilities which tended to amplify from then on, and then to split, to become more numerous and bizarre:

. . . total recoils or rebounds or reversals of response, which fling patients, in an almost incontrollable trajectory, from pole to pole of their being or 'space' . . . [these] extremities tending to *increase,* in a frightening paradigm of positive feedback or 'anti-control' . . . [then] with the continuation of such states . . . further splits or decompositions . . . behaviour refracted into innumerable facets (pp. 256–257).

Reducing or even stopping L-DOPA was often of no use in these circumstances. One might indeed, by greatly reducing or stopping the dose, bring this apparent turbulence, bring *everything*, to a stop, but then, more often than not, an unstable and turbulent re-action would re-occur as soon as one reinstituted L-DOPA. Thus even the most radical treatment – so-called 'drug holidays' – would often fail to restore the original, stable state and responses. Something had happened to 'the system,' it was clear: one could no longer predict, even after a drug holiday, exactly what would happen. And what might happen, with a second use of L-DOPA, might be qualitatively (as well as quantitatively) different from what happened the first time, as in the case of Martha N., who responded to medication, on six occasions, in six different ways (p. 175).

The sense of anxiety and helplessness produced by this was ex-treme; I kept wondering if I was doing something wrong (as sev-eral of my colleagues suggested, when I first published my gen-eral results and thoughts in 1970), but try as I might, I could not alter the situation. What I was seeing could not be dismissed as anomalies, 'side-effects,' or errors. They had an obstinate, irre-movable reality of their own. Some of this anxiety was (with me, as with my colleagues), epistemological too; for science, as I had learnt it, was based on the predictable, on everything being, in principle, predictable and reversible. 'In some sense,' writes the chemist Prigogine, 'this unlimited predictability is an essential part of the scientific picture of the physical world. We may perhaps even call it the founding myth of classical science.' And this was being deeply shaken. My perspective, not merely with regard to the effects of L-DOPA, but with regard to the world in general, had been the classical or Laplacian one of perfect predictability. But something wholly unclassical, unLaplacian, was happening in front of me, and happening, terrifyingly, with all of my patients. I was seeing the invasion, or even replacement, of predictability, of law and order, by an apparent indeterminacy, anarchy, disorder.

I was thrown into a crisis. The effects of L-DOPA should have been straightforward – but weren't. They were straightforward at first, but then something happened . . . My feelings, I later realised, were not unlike Prigogine's, when he started to encounter unpredictability and non-reversibility – the non-classical – in the hitherto classical realm of physical chemistry. 'Is this a defeat for the human mind?' he started wondering. 'Is this the end of classical thought?' I found myself wondering this too – but my vision was more of complexity than anarchy.

For there is a world of difference between complexity and anarchy. The weather is complex, it is not anarchic. I found myself frequently comparing the L-DOPA situation to the weather (see p. 258).[157] Turbulence, another concept I was constantly drawn to, is complex, but it has obvious structure. I sometimes thought of the L-DOPA response as a calm stream, at first, with smooth, laminar flow; then breaking up, as it increased in force and accelerated, to a torrent with innumerable whirlpools and eddies – but a torrent which surged in a non-linear space (n. 133, p. 256).

I felt intuitively that there had to be some way of understanding and describing these enormously complex situations or systems which had been set into motion by L-DOPA. They could not, it was clear, be understood (much less controlled) as long as one thought in reductive, linear terms; one needed different terms, terms suitable for describing complex, dynamical systems. I used the term 'non-linear' several times in *Awakenings;* I referred to Cantor; I spoke of 'trajectories' and 'phase-space' and 'reversals' and 'splittings'; I spoke of the 'relativistic,' the 'macro-quantal,' the jumping of scales, the constant meeting of 'micro' and 'macro' – but all this was intuitive and vague; it was no more than metaphor, groping in the darkness.

I was not mathematician enough to discover the right concepts at the time – and, importantly, *no one* was thinking of the right concepts at this time. The mathematical concept of 'chaos' – not as randomness, not as disorder, but as a special sort of order, or a special sort

---

[157] Indeed, little did I know that the first formally-worked-out example of inherently unpredictable, 'chaotic' behaviour, in fact, related to the forecasting of weather – but Lorenz's pioneering work here was not even known to most mathematicians at this time (see Gleick, 1987, pp. 11–31).

of simplicity which coexisted with disorder in these complex, non-equilibrium situations – the formal concept of chaos, in this sense,[158] was not yet in the air, had not spread beyond the papers of a very few scattered mathematicians and physicists, and was certainly not known to the scientific community at large.

My own first glimpse of the new theory of chaos came only in 1980, when I read of it in a physicochemical context, in Prigogine's 1980 monograph *From Being to Becoming*.[159] His book was a jungle of differential equations, and I picked my way between these to paragraphs of text I could understand. Prigogine introduces his text by a consideration of the 'breakdown' of classical, Newtonian mechanics towards the end of the nineteenth century, with the consideration – for the first time – of more complex systems (e.g. of a dynamical system containing three moving bodies – or, mathematically, three variables). He describes how Poincaré, who was the first to do this, soon found that the equations needed to describe the behaviour of such complex systems were non-linear in type, and that such equations *could not be solved,* in the ordinary, analytic sense: they did not approximate, or converge, to a fixed solution. The dynamical behaviour of such systems could change, by degrees or suddenly, to appearing 'random,' or at least erratic, once a certain critical point was reached. Prigogine speaks here of 'dan-

---

[158] The term 'chaos' has countless colloquial meanings, but is very specific and precise in its scientific usage. It refers to the behaviour of a system – biological, physical, or mathematical – with extreme sensitivity to small (and even infinitesimal) changes in the initial condition of the system. An example of such a system is a leaf floating down a swiftly-moving stream – where the slightest displacement of the original position of the leaf (a breath of wind) will lead to dramatic changes in its final trajectory. Such systems become unpredictable very quickly, and move deeper and deeper into the unpredictability of chaos. (A clock pendulum, by contrast, is stable and non-chaotic; any small disturbance in the pendulum will be rapidly lost.) In classical mechanics, it seemed that if the state of a system at a given time were known with sufficient accuracy, one could forecast its future with perfect accuracy and certainty; but this is precisely what one cannot do if a system is chaotic.

[159] I had, however, in the 1970s, been intrigued by what I had read of 'catastrophe theory,' in semi-popular accounts such as those of Zeeman (1976) and Woodcock and Davis (1978). Interestingly, Richard Hardie, in a very recent article, comments on how many of the descriptions in *Awakenings,* published before catastrophe theory was conceived, are nonetheless suggestive of its topological formulations (Hardie, 1990, pp. 579–580).

gerous' behaviour, of 'anomalous' behaviour, and of the occurrence of non-analytical, 'pathological' functions; and he speaks of the critical point at which these occur as the 'Poincaré catastrophe.' 'In this way,' he writes, 'the problem of irreversibility now appears at the very heart of physics. It is remarkable,' he adds, 'how prevalent Poincaré's catastrophe is. It appears in most problems of dynamics starting from the celebrated three-body problem' – and indeed, as is evident from Prigogine's own work in physical chemistry, in many problems outside classical dynamics; and, perhaps most exciting of all, in all sorts of biological systems. I was intrigued as I read Prigogine's study of complexity and irreversibility in physical systems, for it seemed to me that it was just such a situation – the occurrence of a critical or 'catastrophic' point; the breakdown of titratability, reversibility, symmetry, beyond this point; the emergence of pathological, anomalous, and dangerous behaviours – that I was seeing in my patients.

A mathematical device invaluable in the solution of the behaviour of such non-linear equations involves the creation of *representations* – abstract 'maps' or 'spaces' (so-called 'phase-spaces'). One can represent *linear* equations in a phase-space – a simple point, for example, would represent the convergence of behaviour to a fixed and steady value; a circle would represent an oscillation. In *non-linear* equations the phase-space itself becomes highly complex, or split, when one tries to work out the full extensions (or 'consequences'). Such 'phase-space representations,' indeed, were quite intractable when Poincaré first perceived them, and so disquieting that he later abandoned their study, saying, 'These things are so bizarre that I cannot bear to contemplate them.' It was only with the advent of the first digital calculators, and then of high-speed computers, that it became possible to visualise the behaviour of such equations, to visualise in real (or computer) time the *evolution* of such irreversible, non-linear dynamical systems (whether these were planetary, meteorological, hydrodynamic, or whatever), and their inner structure. When this was done (by Lorenz, in the 1960s), it became evident that it was not randomness which appeared, but a strange new domain to which the formal term 'chaos' was applied. The realm which was seen, by Poincaré, as irrational and intolerably bizarre, could now be re-examined in a positive way, with the aid of computers, and (no less important) in light of crucial new concepts, in particular Lorenz's concept of 'attractors.'

In such a 'chaotic' domain, where non-linearities are fully expressed, an infinitesimal cause may result in an enormous effect (as a vanishingly-small change in the dosage of L-DOPA may have incalculably large effects); there are continual changes, fluctuations, oscillations; there tend to be repeated splittings or bifurcations of an already complex dynamic, which cause new phenomena, innovations, to appear; and one finds, characteristically, 'islands' of complete order in the middle of, enveloped by, chaos, or vice versa (as one may have brief moments or islands of 'normality' entirely surrounded by Parkinsonism or tics). This, then, is strongly reminiscent of the sort of domain which may be induced by continued administration of L-DOPA. But is this a mere metaphor, or can chaos theory provide a formal model as well? Can McKenzie's vision of Parkinsonism as 'an organised chaos' be given an unexpectedly accurate and rich interpretation in terms of the mathematical theory of chaos?

The structure of chaos is not static but dynamic; it must be understood in terms of orbits or trajectories in a phase-space, orbits whose motion is determined by what chaos theorists call 'attractors.' But to show that this is so – that there is, indeed, a hidden structure within an apparently disorderly stream of data – one needs to display the data as moving, as trajectories in an abstract, suitable phase-space representation. And when this is done, a strange new sort of picture or image emerges, which shows graphically that the data are not random, but constrained and determined by an attractor (Figure 1).

Very recently (in early 1990), with my colleague Ralph Siegel, I have tried to re-examine the sort of data one gets from Parkinsonian patients once they pass the critical point and start showing unpredictable reactions to L-DOPA. In an astonishing, rare stroke of luck, we have been assisted in this research by a mathematically-inclined patient, who has been able to note and measure his own reactions with great accuracy and provide us with suitable data for analysis.

Figure 2 shows the reactions of Ed W., who was taking 150 mg. of L-DOPA (admixed with 15 mg. of DOPA-decarboxylase) at ninety-minute intervals from 4:30 a.m. to midnight each day. His reactions, judged on a ten-point scale, are first plotted against time. Here, in this first plot, we see a suggestion of oscillations between 'high' and 'low' with a periodicity of about ten hours.[160] But if we then make a phase-plot, plotting his state against derivatives of his state, in a treatment similar to that which Lorenz did with his weather data, we get a graphic view of the 'trajectories' of the data, and we see that these seem to form a figure-of-eight, to circle or cycle indeed around an attractor. We now see, graphically, that there is in fact no simple linear process at work—but a most complex, chaotic process, one that involves *nonlinear* determinants in at least three dimensions.

To show more minutely the structure of the underlying dynamical

---

[160] These findings relate only to short-term fluctuations, but there are striking long-term fluctuations too. Though Ed W. has been on exactly the same dosage-schedule of L-DOPA (in the form of Sinemet) for more than two years, his responses to it are erratic, and fluctuate not only hourly, but daily, weekly, monthly. Sometimes he may have a week or two, even a month, with excellent general function; at other times he may have entire days, and sometimes an entire week, in which he stays at a very low and disabling level. He has kept detailed calendars throughout this time, and has tried to correlate these gross fluctuations with mood, diet, activity, stress, bowel action, depth and length of sleep, etc. Sometimes he *does* find clear correlations – especially with sleep, of which he must have enough (see pp. 268–269) – but, as frequently, he cannot make any correlations, and has to accept that some of the fluctuations come 'out of the blue,' and defy explanation in ordinary terms.

Such long-term fluctuations and periodicities are commonly seen with disorders like migraine or epilepsy, which may have peculiar and puzzling patterns of occurrence. When I see migraine patients I always encourage them to keep a calendar, and striking (and sometimes very unexpected) correlations may be found. Yet sometimes the most minute research fails to find a 'cause' for an attack, or a cluster of attacks; they have, apparently, come out of the blue. Sometimes there may be long periods of health or normality in which attacks do not occur, despite adverse life-circumstances and other 'precipitants'; and at other times attacks do occur, either 'spontaneously' or in response to what would normally be the most trifling events. Though alterations of 'threshold' are usually summoned to account for these, it is not clear that such considerations are sufficient. Periodicity over many time scales, however, is a feature of chaotic systems, and strongly suggestive that the system is chaotic.

Ed W. has observed that when in the midst of sustained 'bad' periods he may have a very brief, unexpected 'island' of normality; and in the midst of sustained 'good' periods, similarly, he may have very brief, unexpected accesses of disability – he sometimes feels there is health 'buried' in his sickness; and likewise, sickness 'buried' in his health. There may be similar islands of normality embedded in severe migrainous states – and, as recently stressed, 'islands of clarity' in the deepest psychosis (Podvoll, 1990). Such embeddings, such islands, are hardly explicable unless one thinks in terms of temporal structure, and sees all of these as dynamical disorders.

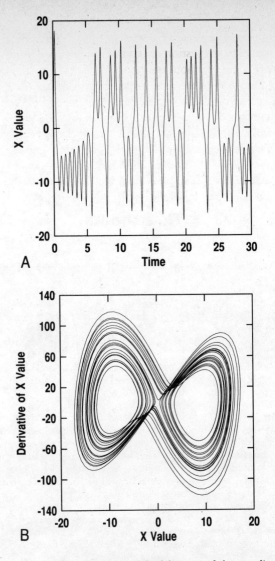

Figure 1. The Lorenz attractor is defined by a set of three nonlinear interdependent equations that were originally defined to describe the weather; the behaviour of these equations can be studied on a computer. (a) The progression of one of the three variables may be plotted as a function of time. This variable changes erratically, although there appears to be some hint of regularity–actually, there is a fair amount of order, which can be visualised using phase-space representations. (b) In such a phase-space representation, the variable is plotted against its rate of change (i.e. its derivative). The loops that emerge result from the presence of a strange attractor. It is said that the system is chaotic; there is order, although it will always be difficult to predict the next value.

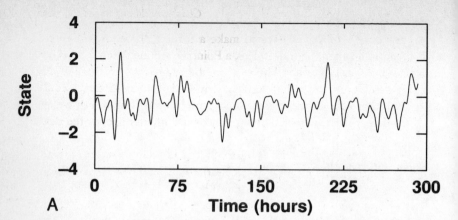

A

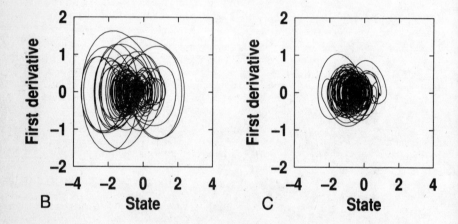

B   C

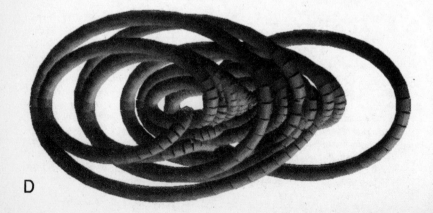

D

processes, we would have to make a further procedure—a cross-section through the trajectories, a Poincaré section. With this, as we get more data, we might hope to see the beginnings of structure, an internal structure within the apparent disorder (such a structure as Poincaré guessed at, the sort of structure Lorenz found, but which could hardly be revealed before our own computer age, or the new concepts of non-linear dynamics).

These first results are, of course, slight and preliminary; they stand in need of amplification and confirmation, and we must analyse thousands, not hundreds, of points.[161] Yet they suggest that once patients have gone past the critical point, it is not randomness, but chaos (in its formal sense) which enters and comes to dominate the situation. Such a conjecture would certainly be easy to test. What is curious is that it has never, apparently, been tested before.[162]

---

[161] Within the relatively gross periodicities measured and plotted here are countless finer periodicities which have not been 'caught.' Thus, if one stays with Ed W., it is obvious that his state changes many times in an hour – it may change profoundly as he is crossing the room; he may 'turn off' in mid-sentence, and 'come to' seconds later. One needs to obtain data at every time scale, from seconds to months (and this, indeed, we hope to do).

[162] It is quite possible that such quantitative data already exist–for the 'on/off' and 'yo-yo' responses I observed in my post-encephalitic patients in 1969 were

---

Figure 2. Opposite. Analysis of Ed W.'s state. Ed W. scored his degree of Parkinsonian motor symptoms on a scale of −5 to +5. A value of 0 was defined to represent 'normalcy'; −5 indicated complete stoppage; +5 indicated hyperkinesia. Ed W., who has had Parkinson's for more than a decade, evaluated and recorded his state roughly every ninety minutes over a period of three months. We performed a mathematical procedure (convolution of 'state' with a Gaussian function with a standard deviation of two hours) in order to interpolate a smoothly varying function of his state. (a) Ed W.'s state as a function of time. Like the Lorenz attractor (Figure 1), the progression is irregular, although there are hints of some periodicities. (b) A phase-space representation of Ed W.'s state, plotted against the numerically computed derivative of state, results in a plot with multiple loops–suggesting that there is some underlying attractive process restricting his dynamics. (c) A control for the interpolation process. The state values were randomized as a function of time and then the interpolation procedure was performed. Although loops are still present (and arise from the interpolation process), they are disorderly. (d) A three-dimensional plot of Ed W.'s state for the first month. The horizontal and vertical axes are as in Figure 2c; however, the depth is given by the second derivative of the state. Now the source of the irregularities in Ed W.'s condition over time is clear: his state depends on the movement of some process in at least three dimensions; his state variable may turn up, down, left, right, into or out of the page under the influence of the proposed attractor.

An important phenomenon, seen in several patients but most clearly in Martha N., and the phenomenon which especially fascinated Luria, is the way in which different reactions may be elicited at different times. I observed with her that 'given the *initial* form of behaviour – whether tongue-pulsing, therapeutic, catatonic, ticcy-palilalic, formicatory, or hallucinatory – the rest of the reaction would follow this form' (p. 175). Martha, clearly, had potentials or dispositions for all of these; they were all equally 'available.' What is striking is the dependence on 'chance' – i.e. on the particular, but wholly fortuitous, circumstances at the *start* of her reactions. This 'sensitive dependence on initial conditions,' as chaologists call it, is highly characteristic of non-linear dynamical systems, and has been called (in weather forecasting) 'the butterfly effect.'

But chaos theory, which is only now coming into general view (see Gleick, 1987 and Briggs and Peat, 1989), has been very little noticed by physicians, except in the special instances of cardiac and electroencephalogram rhythms, and the rhythms of nystagmus and certain tremors[163] – oscillations with a period of less than a second

being very generally observed, in *all* Parkinsonian patients, by 1974 (they simply occurred, in some post-encephalitic patients, within days rather than years). There have been many quantitative observations and accounts in the literature since this time, from the early papers of Fahn (1974) and Marsden and Parkes (1976) to Richard Hardie's work (Hardie, 1984; Hardie, Lees, and Stern, 1984; Hardie, 1990); but these have looked at the phenomena only in *physiological* terms (as reflecting altering plasma levels of L-DOPA, altering sensitivities of dopamine receptors, etc.) and not in *dynamical* terms–and hence have not submitted their observations to the sort of phase-space plotting and Poincaré sectioning which are necessary to bring out an underlying chaotic pattern.

[163] Parkinsonism – and especially the much more complex and various syndromes seen in post-encephalitic disease – has a great range of phenomena of differing periodicities: first and foremost Parkinsonian *tremor,* which has been minutely observed since Gowers first timed it (in the 4 to 7 Hz. range) more than a century ago (Fine et al., 1990). Post-encephalitic patients may show rapid ticcing at rates up to 300 per minute. On a somewhat longer time scale we see palilalic and verbigerative repetitions, and cycles of complex tics and stereotypies, with a periodicity of one to twenty seconds. One sees (as in Rolando) a variety of circadian and diurnal cycles, and, at a still longer time scale, oculogyric or other crises coming with periodicities of 3 to 50 days. All of these, in principle, could be submitted to careful quantitative investigation – and this has been done recently, with Parkinsonian tremor, by Beuter et al. (unpublished), who find that its oscillations are indeed suggestive of chaotic dynamics.

Another aspect of chaos is the appearance of fractional dimensions (or 'fractals'; see Mandelbrot, 1977 and 1982). Kraus et al. (1987) have recently found (but see Winfree, 1980, for the vast range of phenomena, with periodicities up to decades, in which oscillations and chaos may occur). Glass and Mackey proposed, as long ago as 1977, that diseases characterised by abnormal temporal organisation be called *dynamical diseases* (Glass and Mackey, 1988), but there has been almost no examination of long-term *neuro*dynamical disorders, of the sort which seems central in long-term reactions to L-DOPA.[164]

If Parkinsonian patients are so easily thrown by continued L-DOPA into these 'dynamical disturbances,' is Parkinsonism itself a dynamical disease? I had been struck from the first, before I had ever heard of L-DOPA, by certain curious instabilities in Parkinsonism itself, by the fact that it seemed to have a number of very different 'phases,' and could be thrown between these even in the absence of L-DOPA (see p. 12). Such transformations are especially seen in the remarkable phenomenon of *kinesia paradoxa,* in which a state of profound Parkinsonian akinesia is suddenly replaced either by 'normality,' or *hyper*kinesia, for a few seconds, or, on occasion, minutes. *Kinesia paradoxa* is rather rare in 'ordinary' Parkinson's disease (though Ed W. himself occasionally shows it), because, paradoxically, this is rarely severe enough. It is most apt to occur when there is intense akinesia, where there seems to be an intense constrained or curled-up pressure, which can suddenly explode into hyperkinesia – or normality. One may see similar phenomena, on occasion, in catatonia – when catatonic immobility or stupor is suddenly replaced by catatonic frenzy ('amok'). And equally with the 'phases' of tics, which can suddenly turn from tonic or cataleptic to darting and

---

that finger-tapping in Parkinsonian subjects appears to have a fractal dimension; and one has to wonder whether post-encephalitic patients, with their forced or delirious imagery of 'maps within maps' (n. 54, p. 76), ever-enlarging yet ever-reiterating patterns, and other such images of self-similarity, may not be projecting, in a quasi-hallucinatory way, fractal qualities in their own perceptual and thought processes.

[164] There have been some studies of long-term fluctuations in certain other physiological systems, in particular those of diabetes. 'In some instances,' write Glass and Mackey, 'it can be difficult to establish schedules for insulin administration ... [and] periodic insulin administration, combined with eating and exercise schedules, is ineffective in maintaining blood glucose within normal limits.' In such patients, they conclude, 'it will be necessary to develop protocols for insulin administration based on . . . an understanding of the dynamics of the glucose control system' (Glass and Mackey, 1988).

precipitate; or vice versa (p. 108). It is as if *Parkinsonism itself* can be visualised as a sort of surface, a curved surface, bipolar, like a figure-of-eight. The transformations we see with L-DOPA are *already* inherent in Parkinsonism itself, as if L-DOPA can serve to release a tendency already built into the topological shape of Parkinsonism; or, more likely, to change the shape of the (Parkinsonian) attractor, making it sharper or steeper, with higher peaks and deeper valleys.[165] The patient with Parkinsonism is, so to speak, enthralled on this surface, which is a dynamical surface, an orbiting surface in time. Every so often this orbiting will take him, tantalisingly briefly, through a few seconds of 'normality,' or into the mirror-state of hyperkinesia, only to return him to the immense 'gravitational' attraction of that powerful attractor which (in dynamical terms) is the 'cause' of Parkinsonism.[166]

When I first found that my patients' reactions to L-DOPA were becoming erratic and unpredictable – that what had been clear was clear no longer, that something strange and unintelligible was gradually taking over – I felt fear, guilt, and a sort of revulsion. This attitude changed when I first read Prigogine and gained the sense that there could be a hidden order, a new sort of order, in the midst of disorder. A most vivid sense of this new order – new, but also old, because it is the order of trees, of landscapes, of innumerable natural features – was given to me, visually, when I saw Mandelbrot's book,

---

[165] Sometimes I put this image in topological terms: 'The "shape" of behaviour . . . becomes that of an hour-glass, with a "waist" fined down to almost-zero proportions . . . a space, moreover, which allows no exit, for it runs into itself like a Möbius strip' (n. 132, p. 256), and sometimes in terms of an imaginary 'landscape': 'One feels of such patients . . . that they no longer dwell in a world of gentle slopes and gradients . . . but have been transported . . . to a sort of moonscape of fearful pinnacles and precipices' (n. 91, p. 201). I compared this 'acicular' world to Newton's image of an infinity of needles trying to stand on their points, an image which could be the quintessential image of chaos.

[166] In 1972, in 'The Great Awakening,' I wrote: 'The qualities of dynamical being (or disorder) . . . are relativistic . . . being those of a highly-structured, anisotropic continuum, in which the space-deforming curvatures are determined by Parkinsonian or other "ontological" forces which take the place of gravitational potentials.' I was groping in the dark, then, looking for some image, some metaphor, of what I intuitively felt. I think now that what I then tended to call 'relativistic' was really a sense of a *temporal* structure, an orbit or trajectory determined and constrained by the presence of an attractor – but this was not a concept which was available to me at the time.

The Fractal Geometry of Nature, although I did not then grasp the relation between these two books which so pleased me. 'There are no Grotesques in Nature,' Sir Thomas Browne says, and 'Nature Geometrizeth in all things.' One of the things which was at first so alarming about chaos, when I only apprehended it as breakdown and disorder, was the breaking of this classical world, this timeless and Platonic world; and the intrusion into it, seemingly, of the anarchic and the bizarre. But as our insight into chaos has grown, we have started to see that it is not anarchic or bizarre, but rather that it constitutes a new, beautiful, dynamical world, a geometrizing in time more wonderful than anything which Browne dreamed of. Prigogine speaks of this as 'the re-enchantment of Nature.'

I spoke earlier (in the Epilogue) of the need for a rational medicine, one based on the deepest understanding of natural law. The 'chaos' which occurs as patients continue on L-DOPA at first seems to threaten the overthrow of natural law; but then, beautifully, establishes a yet deeper law. The chaos which first seemed impervious to understanding, and to threaten complete intellectual defeat, excites us, entices us, with a new sense of challenge. Chaos, which first seemed the enemy of reason, now serves as the basis of a new rationality, a new reason.

At first, when chaos entered, we had no idea of the rational thing to do; the old rationality (of 'titration') had become inapplicable or useless. But a new rationality, and perhaps a rational treatment, is perfectly possible, *provided one understands the dynamical systems involved.* And it is this, to study the minutiae of the non-linear determinants, precisely this, which we now have to do. The idea of doing this is exciting and challenging not only theoretically, but practically as well, for it may give us new therapeutic strategies, new powers we have scarcely imagined, and may perhaps open to us new horizons of the possible.

AWAKENINGS ON
STAGE AND SCREEN

The central themes of *Awakenings* – falling asleep, being turned to stone; being awakened, decades later, to a world no longer one's own – have an immediate power to grip the imagination. This is the stuff that dreams, nightmares, and legends are made of – and yet it actually happened.

Awakenings has inspired short stories, poems, novels in the seventeen years that have passed since its publication; but it is especially the dramatic or dramaturgic imagination that it has stirred. The reality *was* a sort of drama – perhaps nearer Greek tragedy than any other, with a singular disease, finally, playing the role of Fate (certainly this is how Leonard L. saw it). It is the imagination of other people's worlds – worlds almost inconceivably strange, yet inhabited by people just like ourselves; people, indeed, who might *be* ourselves – that forms the centre of *Awakenings*. Every reader brings to *Awakenings* his own imagination and sensibilities, and so too does every writer, every actor, every director, who has been inspired by it and gone on to create a version of his own. Thus there have emerged, in the past decade, several radically different versions of *Awakenings* in dramatic form. But the best of these, while so different in style, and varied in detail, have always shared a faithfulness to the *truth* of the story, the inner truth of the patients' plights and lives. This, for me, is the ultimate touchstone of truth – a sense that the actual patients, if they could be shown these versions, would exclaim: 'Yes, that's amazing – that's just how it was!'

When *Awakenings* first came out (in England) in June 1973, it aroused much interest and curiosity and compassion – and, in particular, a desire to *see* and to *hear* the actual patients of whom I had written. I was not sure of the propriety of this, of my patients being shown, undisguised, on film; nor did I know how *they* would feel about this. What passes between physician and patient is confidential – and even to write of it, in some sense, is a breach of this confidence; but writing allows one to change names and places and certain other details. No such disguise is possible in a documentary film; faces, voices, real lives, are all exposed. And so I asked my patients how they would feel about this. They had encouraged me, earlier, about publishing the book: 'Go ahead; tell our story – or it will never be known.' And now they said: 'Go ahead; film us. Let us speak for ourselves.'

I was approached by several producers of documentary films, and was particularly impressed by one of them, Duncan Dallas of Yorkshire Television, especially by his combination of scientific strength and human feeling. Duncan came to Mount Carmel for a visit in September 1973, and met all of the patients. Many he recognised, from having read their stories in *Awakenings*. 'I know you,' he said to Sylvie, and others. 'I feel I've met you before. It's like I've known you for a long, long time.' He would have recognised them, doubtless, from photos, but not with this intense sense of *knowing* them, as familiars, with a history, as people.

Almost all of the patients warmed to Duncan, realised he would see them – and, if they permitted, film them – with objectivity and a discreet compassion, neither over-medicalising nor over-sentimentalising their lives. They felt too that he would approach them as a discoverer or explorer, and show them as human beings who had entered, been forced to dwell in, a deeply strange land. Thus, mutual understanding and respect was established, and the filming of the documentary film of *Awakenings* was done the following month.

The documentary has much of the same overall structure as the book, with a prologue (given extra power by marvellous archival footage from the days of the epidemic); portraits of patients' 'awakening' as they were given L-DOPA, and then as they suffered bizarre 'tribulations' of all types (incorporating some of the Super-8 film I myself had shot in 1969); and finally, deeply moving interviews with the patients, as they looked back on these events, and described how now, in their 'accommodations,' they were living their lives after having been 'dead' and out of the world for so many years.

Many of the same 'characters' in the book appeared in the documentary: Hester Y. (her real name is Lola), Rose R. (Sylvie), Margaret A. (Mary B.), and Leonard L. (Ed); and (somewhat more briefly) Frances, Miriam, Miron, Gertie, and Martha. Other patients are shown who are mentioned only very briefly in the book – Seymour, Sam, Rosalie, and Lillian W. – but who emerge, in the film, as full-fledged characters. One of them, indeed – Lillian T. – becomes the spokesman, in the documentary, for all of the patients.

The documentary film of *Awakenings* was first shown in England early in 1974, and has since been seen around much of the world. It is the only documentary account of these last survivors of a forgotten epidemic, and how their lives were transformed for a while by a new drug; of how intensely human they were, throughout all their vicissitudes. The documentary has a great power, not only to instruct, but also to bring home, as perhaps only actual images can, how these patients actually lived and endured. I regard it as the cinematic equivalent of the book, and wish it could be packaged together with the book, tucked into its jacket.

Early in 1982 I received a packet from London, containing a letter from Harold Pinter and the manuscript of a new play, *A Kind of Alaska*, which, he said, had been inspired by *Awakenings*. In his letter, Pinter said that he had read *Awakenings* when it had originally come out in 1973, and had been deeply moved; but that he had then 'forgotten' it, and that it had stayed 'forgotten' until it suddenly 'came back' to him eight years later. (I was reminded here of the genesis of Rilke's *Duino Elegies*, which had submerged for so long, and then re-emerged, explosively, ten years later.) Pinter had awoken, he said, one morning the previous summer, with the first image of the play – the patient awakening – and the first words of the play ('Something is happening') clear and pressing in his mind; and the play had then 'written itself' in the days and weeks that followed.

A Kind of Alaska is a one-act play, in which the entire development and action is condensed into a single afternoon. It opens with the awakening of Deborah, a patient who has been 'asleep,' or in some deeply strange, inaccessible, frozen state ('a kind of Alaska') for 29 years. She is now 45 – but feels she is 16. She has no idea of her age or what has befallen her. She thinks the grey-haired woman near her is some sort of cousin, or 'an aunt I never met' – and the revelation that this is her sister, her younger sister, shocks her into the reality of her situation.

When I showed the play to Margie Kohl, who had worked so closely with me in 1969, when our patients were 'awakening,' she made a fascinating comment: 'It's not like Pinter,' she said, 'it's just like the truth.'

But Pinter, I replied, *is* just like the truth.

Pinter had never seen my patients, nor even their images in the documentary of *Awakenings;* and yet–I was in total agreement with Margie – what he had written, uncannily, was just like the truth. My immediate thought, indeed, was of my patient Rose R., who had clearly (despite all the differences) been a model for his Deborah; I imagined Rose reading and seeing the play, and saying: 'My God! He's got me. He's got me to a T.' I felt Pinter had somehow perceived more than I had written, had penetrated, divined, inexplicably, into the heart of the matter, the inmost truth. Despite what Margie said, it was a very Pinterish play: his mind, his language, were everywhere apparent – no one but Pinter could have written the play. And then again, paradoxically, it was in another sense not really Pinterish, for the play was utterly transparent and transcendent; the author was there, invisibly, behind it, above it, but (to paraphrase Joyce) he had refined himself out of existence.[167]

These same paradoxical considerations arose for me when I saw the play's first performance, at the National Theatre, in October of 1982. It gave me, it gave everyone who saw it, an uncanny sense of being present at the awesome moment of a patient's 'awakening.' And Judy Dench, who played Deborah: her performance, a great one, was simply . . . truthful. I was amazed at this, as I had been amazed at the verisimilitude of Pinter's conception. Dench, like Pinter, had never met a post-encephalitic patient; indeed, she said, she was not sure whether she wanted to (she did see the documen-

---

[167] I could not help contrasting this with a play I had been sent four years before – on exactly the same subject, and indeed the same patient. This too was accompanied by a letter, in which the author said he had been 'obsessed' by the subject, had thought of it 'day and night for two years.' And yet this play, though literally and factually closer to what I had written, gave me a strong sense of unreality, and untruth. Moreover I found the author's 'obsessions' all too clear, intrusive on every page. It was like *him* – but it was not like the truth. And I was agonized at the thought that Rose R. might see it, and be beside herself, and say: 'No, no, it's all wrong, it's nothing like the truth.'

tary and visit Highlands, later). She felt she could imagine the patient sufficiently from Pinter's portrayal. This struck me as extraordinary, but her performance was gripping, and what she said, I had to
admit, seemed indeed to be so.

I wanted to say: But Pinter's Deborah is two removes from reality
– first there is the actual, original Sylvie; then my portrayal or conception of her as Rose R. in *Awakenings;* and now Pinter's, as Deborah, in *A Kind of Alaska.* But it was clear this was not the right way
to see things, for each had an original force of its own. My Rose, one
might say, was inspired by Sylvie, yet she is not literally, documen-
tarily, objectively Sylvie – but Sylvie seen through my eyes and
sensibility, suffused with my own emotion and subjectivity. (When
Sonia Orwell read the original edition of *Awakenings,* she was disturbed at the Polaroid photographs of Sylvie as the frontispiece – 'So
bald,' she said. '*Your* picture is much richer.')

Prior to receiving Pinter's play I had reservations about 'dramatic
representations,' or anything else 'based on,' or 'adapted from,' or
'inspired by' my own work. *Awakenings* was the real thing, I felt;
anything else would surely be 'unreal.' How could it be real if it
lacked direct contact with the patients, if there was only indirect
contact, at a remove? Yet Pinter's play showed me that there is no
necessary dilution of reality in representation; quite the opposite, if
the representation has power. Reality is conferred, re-conferred, by
every original representation. I felt Pinter had given me as much as
I gave him: I had given him a reality – and he had given me one
back.[168]

1987 saw two productions and the start of a third, all of these
dramatizations of *Awakenings.* Early in the year, John Reeves, a
producer with the Canadian Broadcasting Corporation, approached
me about adapting *Awakenings* as a drama for radio, and soon afterwards he sent me a script. This script, for a two-hour play, read by
eight or nine actors, had the same general structure as the book:
eight or nine cameos of patients, with their families, or doctors; and
a prologue and epilogue, spoken by the doctor (I myself was to read
this part). Indeed, 99 percent of the radio play used the language of
the book, with relatively slight changes, allocating words to the

---

[168] *A Kind of Alaska* has been performed in many countries and languages
(although it has not yet been performed in Sign). At its most recent (1989)
performance in London, Pinter himself played the part of the doctor.

'characters' in the book. I had never thought of a dramatic structure when I wrote; I thought in terms of case-histories . . . and meditation. Yet, to my amazement, this worked.

As I and the other actors read our parts, we became patients and doctor, under John's direction (direction which, at times, seemed to me no less musical than dramatic). I kept having the uncanny sense that my patients, my old patients, were actually coming to life – I had turned them, and their lives, into words; and now the words, miraculously, were turning back into people. I felt, and we all felt, an extraordinary poignancy, sadness, joy: I wanted to reach out and embrace them – 'Hi, Leonard! Rose!' Leonard and Rose and Lucy and Miron and Hester and Magda were all incarnated before me; illusion had become reality, they were there, they were alive, they were flesh again. It was not just the individual performances which were so moving; the actors performed as a community, as a troupe, and collectively we became the 'characters' of *Awakenings,* collectively we played it, lived it, made it alive in a new medium.

John Reeves's production, which was broadcast that March, excited a large radio audience in Canada – hundreds of phone calls and letters came in from listeners, who said they had been completely transported, that they felt they knew the patients themselves, had been present and shared their lives, and lived through their 'awakenings.' Many of these listeners had not read the book; many said, indeed, they were not 'readers'; that reality, for them, came through the ear, not the eye. This new intermediary of speech, the human voice, had given the words a physicality, a body, a presentness they lacked on the page. And even though writing is (perhaps) 'written speech,' and 'converted' in the mind of the reader to speech; yet speaking aloud has a directness which no writing has. The radio version of *Awakenings* showed the power of the word, and specifically the power of the spoken word, to represent, to convey, to evoke, a reality. Listeners said they could 'see' Leonard, Rose, and the others, even though the medium of communication was auditory, verbal. This modified my own attitude to *Awakenings:* I continued to hope that people would read it, but I started to feel that other modes were valid, and needed, too.[169]

---

[169] At this point, with Carmel Ross, an actress and producer, I selected parts of *Awakenings* and read these aloud, spoke them, performed them, for an audiotape version. I had never read aloud before, nor listened much to recorded speech – but now, suddenly, it seemed right, and indispensable.

* * *

In September of 1987, Arnold Aprill, artistic director of Chicago's City Lit Theater Company, which specialises in near-verbatim dramatisations of written works, put on a stage dramatisation of *Awakenings.* I was not quite prepared for what I saw – I had thought this would be a dramatic reading of *Awakenings,* as with the CBC radio production; I did not realise it would be an actual staging.

Listeners to the radio play often wrote that they could 'see' the patients and characters, but this meant 'imagine' or 'in the inward eye.' But here the characters were actually visible. I (perhaps alone in the audience) knew what the patients actually looked like, knew that the real Leonard, or Rose, or Lucy, looked quite different from the stage versions. This discrepancy perturbed me – for all of five minutes – and then ceased to matter, for what I was seeing had great verisimilitude, was truthful, was *also* real, despite the actual and factual differences. That this could be so quite fascinated me: the Chicago Miriam H., a wonderful actress, was a great, busty, gutsy, ebullient black woman – whereas 'my' Miriam H. was an ageing, and somewhat deformed, Ashkenazi-Jewish white woman. None of this mattered – indeed the reverse: Jackie Samuels was an absolutely perfect Miriam, a deeply creative, deeply *right* characterisation such as the original Miriam H., had she been alive, would have delighted in. And Samuels, while sticking closely to the text of *Awakenings,* made Miriam her own, charged her with her own vitality, exuberance, idiosyncrasy. She invented, or created, a Miriam all her own; and yet this Miriam was fundamentally true – it was my Miriam, and the original Miriam, too.

The stage version took liberties which the radio version had not. It invented a certain amount of dialogue (though three-quarters of the dialogue, and the general structure, were still those of the book), and it used a certain amount of invention and dramatic licence in the creation of characters and situations. It was not just a dramatic reading, it was Arnold Aprill's vision or version of the book. It was more of a departure, certainly, than the radio version had been, but a fascinating and creative one which never departed from the truth.

Just a month later, now from Los Angeles, I received the first version of a film script of *Awakenings.* Its producers, Walter Parkes and Larry Lasker, had approached me as far back as 1979; they had visited Mount Carmel the following year, and had met Leonard L. and many of the patients I had written of in *Awakenings*. There were to be many more visits, and there was much discussion over the years – but Hollywood is slow to move, and I remained unsure if anything would actually happen, until finally, in 1987, a film script came.

The script, written by Steve Zaillian, was very different in structure from the book, concentrating on a single patient (Leonard L.). The background of a whole ward of post-encephalitic patients, and the hospital they were in, was vividly sketched in; all of these patients had their own, individual 'awakenings.' The script centred on the close bond between Leonard L. and his doctor (who bore some relation, but only some relation, to myself!), a bond which gets closer as the film develops, as the doctor himself develops, from being a little academic, a little withdrawn at first, to intensely and humanly concerned for his patients. Many unexpected things occurred – some tender, some violent – and there was a fine dramatic ending which moved me as I read it, even though, factually, it was completely untrue. I was not quite sure how I felt about the script, for while in some ways it aimed at a very close reconstruction of how things had been, it also introduced a plot, several plots, which were entirely new. But I saw that this was necessary, and I liked many of the dramatic inventions (though I had reservations about the creation of a violent psychiatric ward – no such ward ever existed at Mount Carmel – and a certain tendency to portray the institution, and the other doctors, as unimaginative and repressive). What I could respond to, clearly and positively, was the emotional truth of the portrayals, the imagination and depiction of the inner lives of the characters. And what I was especially pleased with, and determined to watch closely, were the neurological portrayals demanded by the script – the portrayals of a profound illness, with innumerable strange forms; of the ways in which the patients endured and coped; and, of course, of their 'awakenings' and thereafter.

Though I was to be intimately involved with this film as a consultant, I had to renounce the notion that it was, in any way, 'my' film – it was not my script, it was not my film, it would be largely out of my hands. It was not entirely easy to say this to myself; and yet it was also a relief. I would be able to advise and consult, to ensure medical and historical accuracy; I would do my best to give the film an authentic point of departure, so that it *could* depart, so that the filmmakers and actors could realise their own creative work.

The following October I met the film's director, Penny Marshall; she too came to Mount Carmel, and we spent days walking round the Botanic Garden just by Mount Carmel, discussing the patients and the film. In June of 1989 I heard that Robert De Niro was to play the patient, and the following month I heard that Robin Williams would play . . . *me,* or at least the doctor character in the film who was, in part, to be based on me.

Bob, Robin, Penny, and Steve were all eager to see as many patients as possible, to get the feel of Mount Carmel, and to get it right. We spent many hours and days visiting various hospitals where I work, talking to patients with Parkinsonism, and to the few remaining post-encephalitics. And the documentary film of *Awakenings* was to be studied in minute detail by all the actors who would play post-encephalitics. This became the primary visual source, the source of images, for the feature film. There were, in addition, miles of Super-8 film and audiotape which I had taken myself in 1969 and 1970. And finally, there was archival film taken at the time of the great epidemic.

Robert De Niro's passion to understand what he is going to portray, to research it in the minutest, most microscopic detail, is legendary among actors; and now I was to see this for myself. I had never before witnessed, much less played any part in, an actor's investigation of his subject – the investigation which would finally culminate (as Tom Conti once said to me) in the actor's *becoming* his subject, knowing him, knowing it, in his own body, from the inside.

Learning that there were still nine post-encephalitic patients remaining at the Highlands Hospital in London – patients who had been admitted there as adolescents, and been there for almost sixty years – Bob felt it important to visit these, so in August of 1989 we went to see them together. He spent many hours talking with these patients, and taping them (he always liked to make research tapes which he could study at length). This was the first time I had actually seen him with patients, and I was impressed and moved at his powers of observation and empathy. He came to them not as a doctor concerned with their medications, not as a scientist concerned with their physiology, but as one human being approaching another. He approached them also as an artist and actor, as someone determined to make an accurate portrait, determined to *become* an accurate portrait. This was fully realised by the patients themselves, who were intrigued and moved at a sort of attention they had never had before – and one which, curiously, they felt akin only to the best sort of scientific study. 'He really observes you, looks right into you,' one of them said to me the following day. 'Nobody's really done that since old Purdon Martin. *He* tried to understand what was really going on with you – and Mr De Niro, he's a bit like him, he's trying to understand too.'

By the time we returned to New York, Robin Williams had arrived, and now I was to meet the man who was to be me. This was not entirely easy, at first, for either of us: I had seen with what precision Bob had observed and studied the Highlands patients, and now, I feared, I was to be observed and studied in equal detail. But Robin wanted chiefly to see me in action, to see me in my own role as explorer and physician – and, equally, to see the sorts of patients I had worked and lived with in *Awakenings*. So, with Penny, we went off to the Little Sisters of the Poor, where I had two post-encephalitic patients I had followed for fifteen years. Here, as with Bob, I was fascinated to see how immediately at ease Robin seemed to be in a situation which was wholly new to him; how open and easy he was with the patients; and how his spontaneity put them at ease. He is very different from Bob, clearly, as a person and an actor – gregarious and outgoing, where Bob is brooding and intense – yet they share the same intensity, yet tact, of care; the passion, the minuteness of observation.

This hit me explosively a few days afterwards, when Robin, Bob, and Penny all came along with me to Bronx State Hospital. We had spent a few minutes in a very disturbed geriatric ward, where several of the patients were shouting and talking bizarrely, at one point at least six of them together. Later, as we all drove away, Robin suddenly exploded with an incredible playback of the ward, imitating everyone's voice and style to perfection. It was incredible to hear this: I felt that he must have taken in everything which went on, all the different voices and conversations together, and held them in his mind with total recall – and now he was reproducing them, or, almost, being possessed by them. This instant power of apprehension and playback, a power for which 'mimicry' is too feeble a word (for they were funny imitations, feeling ones, and full of creativity), was developed to an enormous degree in Robin. It constituted, I came to think, the first step in his actorial investigation; the one which provided an intense and minute sensory and motor corporeal image, which he could then scan internally and analyse, and then finally imbue with himself, deepen, subjectivise.[170]

The three of them – Bob, Robin, and Penny – went to Mount Carmel several times, to get the atmosphere and mood of the place, and most especially to see patients and staff who remembered the 'awakenings' of twenty years before. One evening especially moving to me (and to many of us) personally was a gathering together of all of us – doctors, nurses, therapists, social workers – who had been at Mount Carmel in 1969, all of us who had seen, and participated, in the 'awakenings.' Some of us had long since left the hospital, and some of us had not seen each other for years; but that evening in September, we swapped memories of the patients until early the next morning, each person's memories triggering others. We realised again how overwhelming, how historic that summer had been, and equally how funny, how human its events. It was an evening of laughter and tears, nostalgia and sobriety, as we looked at each other, at our twenty-years-later faces, and realised the many years that had passed – and, most sadly of all, that almost all of the patients were now dead.

All, that is, save one – Lillian Tighe, who had left Mount Carmel in 1975 to go to another chronic care hospital nearby, and who showed such eloquence in the 1973 documentary film. Lillian was, is, the only survivor, the only "Awakenings" patient still left. In September we visited her – Bob, Robin, Penny, and I – and we all marvelled at her toughness, her humour, her lack of self-pity, her realness. She has retained, despite advancing disease, and unpredictable reactions to L-DOPA, all of her humour, her love of life, her spunkiness. Bob, Robin, and Penny, although they had lived for months now with the reality of book and script, were overwhelmed

---

[170] I was soon to find this in regard to myself. After our first meeting, Robin 'had,' or mirrored, some of my mannerisms, my postures, my gait, my speech; all sorts of things of which I had been hitherto unconscious. It was uncanny, and disconcerting, at first, to see myself in this living mirror. We would talk – and the way we stood, and our cadences, our gestures, were the same: it was like suddenly acquiring an identical twin. But then this too-explicit mimesis gave way to a much profounder, much more subjectivised, actor's portrait of me – or rather of a being half-Robin, half-me, one created by his imagination and feelings, no less than by his observation of me; and finally, to a new character, neither Robin nor me, but one with a life and personality of its own.

(as Bob had been earlier at Highlands) by the reality of flesh and blood, by the mixture of terrible disease with gay, laughing transcendence. Indeed, Lillian was to remain a powerful inspiration and presence throughout the actual shooting of the film, visiting the set several times and even playing a part in a scene with Bob.

This careful research did not stop with pre-production but continued into the months of filming in the fall and winter of 1989. Particularly important was another person with firsthand knowledge of the disease, Ed W., a brilliant man in his forties, exactly Bob's age, who has a youthful form of Parkinson's disease and spectacular reactions to L-DOPA. Ed could describe eloquently – and even more importantly, *demonstrate,* in his own person – many of the phenomena Bob, and the other actor-patients, would have to show: he could show, and describe, exactly what it is like to be frozen in one's chair, or bed, for hours, unable to leave it; how it felt to be 'high' on L-DOPA; and how it felt to have, at times, a 'chemical personality' not one's own. Bob spent a great deal of time with Ed, sometimes spending whole days with him on weekends, in his apartment, or walking outside, or travelling – continually taking in more and more of what such a disease, such a changing neurological state, such a life, is actually like.[171]

---

[171] The question of how a dramatic representation compares with reality – the clinical reality of my patients – always comes to my mind, perhaps even when it shouldn't. I once went with a cousin, Carmel Ross, to see the play *Wings* (in which one character is supposed to be aphasic). I was disappointed by the performance, and said to my cousin: 'But this is nothing like aphasia – it isn't real.' She replied: 'Stop talking about "real"! Can't you forget you're a neurologist? Can't you appreciate it as a wonderful performance – *emotionally* true?' But I remained unconvinced.

On another occasion I went with her to see Tom Conti acting the role of a quadriplegic in *Whose Life Is It, Anyway?* This struck me, besides everything else, as being full of verisimilitude, as being clinically real. I spoke to Tom Conti at length about this later: I was fascinated to learn how he had spent hundreds of hours amid quadriplegic patients, and how he himself would spend hours daily imagining himself to be quadriplegic, at least imagining how, say, he could get his hair out of his eyes, if he happened to be paralysed from the neck down. 'You're an investigator,' he said to me. 'But acting is investigation too. We investigate from the inside, we investigate by *becoming.'*

On yet another occasion I saw Peter Barnes's short play, *Drummer,* based on my case-history of a Tourettic drummer, *Witty Ticcy Ray.* I went along with a Tourettic friend. The actor playing the 'drummer' himself, I learned later, as he was waiting in the wings, was very taken aback at hearing a *real* Touretter in the audience, and thought, 'How will this appear to *him?* Will *he* think it's convinc-

There were, besides Bob, fifteen other actors playing post-encephalitic patients in the film, and I had to show them what Parkinsonism, and other symptoms, looked like and felt like. These were intriguing classes, oddly similar, in a way, to my classes for medical students – and then again, of course, completely different. For the medical students needed to gain a medical and physiological knowledge, to gain a general picture of Parkinsonism, a picture from the outside. Whereas the actors needed a concrete picture of Parkinsonism from the inside, so clear and concrete, so motorically precise, that they would be able to simulate, and in a sense *become,* Parkinsonian.

I showed them how Parkinsonian patients sat – immobile, with masked face and unblinking eyes; the head perhaps pulled backwards, or torqued to one side; the mouth tending to hang open, with spittle drooling from the lips (drooling was felt to be difficult, and perhaps too ugly, for the film, so we did not insist on this). I showed them common dystonic postures of hands and feet. I showed them tremors, and tics. (I found, interestingly, that the actors naturally divided themselves into 'shakers' and 'jerkers,' those who found it easier to tremor and shake, and those who found it easier to jerk and tic; I could not help wondering if there was some physiological disposition behind these different mimetic faculties.)

I showed the actors how Parkinsonian patients stood, or tried to stand; how they walked, often bent over, sometimes accelerating and festinating; how they might come to a halt, freeze, and be unable to go on. I showed them different sorts of Parkinsonian voices, and noises; Parkinsonian handwriting; Parkinsonian *everything.* I counselled them to imagine themselves locked in small spaces, or to imagine themselves stuck in glue ('It's like being in a vat of peanut butter,' said Ed, graphically).

We practised *kinesia paradoxa* – the sudden release of Parkinsonism into normality. We practised the release of Parkinsonism by music; and by spontaneous responses, such as catching a ball (the actors loved practising this with Robin, whom we felt might make a great ballplayer were he not committed to acting). We practised catatonia, and post-encephalitic card games: four patients completely frozen, clutching hands of cards, until someone (perhaps a nurse)

---

ing?' as well as 'Will he think this decent – or will he see it as a cruel take-off, an exploitation of his condition?' But my Tourettic friend was impressed, and delighted, with the performance and play.

made a first move, and how this precipitated a tremendous flurry of movement – the game, first paralysed, now finishing itself within seconds (I had seen and captured this on Super-8 film in 1969, and now it was to become a scene in the feature film).

Sometimes special tricks are invaluable in allowing actors to simulate Parkinsonian symptoms which, otherwise, they could not have done. I have described how Miriam H. was able to talk at 500 words a minute *without fudging or missing a single syllable* – something which no 'normal' person can ordinarily do. But Jackie Samuels, who played Miriam in the stage adaptation, found that she could do this if she thought of Miriam's words as *music,* as musical phrases, operatic arias, recitations to be conceived (though not actually sung) in musical terms, as a series of musical impulses, rather than a series of words or sentences (perhaps auctioneers use a similar trick).

These singular, almost Zen-like exercises – becoming immobile, emptying oneself, or accelerating oneself, perhaps for hours on end – were both fascinating and frightening to the actors. They started to feel in their own persons, and with frightful vividness, what it might be like to be actually stuck in this way.

The one thing I could no longer directly show the actors was the impulsive, witty, ticcy, 'hyper' states so many of the post-encephalitics had been in when young – the 'enkieness' they had shown before their Parkinsonism closed in on them, and which so many of them were to show, extravagantly, when they got over-excited by L-DOPA. To show them this I brought a number of young people with Tourette's syndrome to the set – for this was the nearest thing to the enkieness I could no longer show them. I had described enkieness and Tourettishness to the actors, but description is pallid; they needed to be *seen.* One of the Touretters, Shane F., in particular, showed the sort of 'motor genius,' zaniness, and acceleration of thought which had been so characteristic of many enkies (p. 24), as well as explosive gusts of joking, mimicry, ticcing. All of this amazed, delighted, and above all, taught the actors, as no verbal descriptions or films could possibly do.

But perhaps none of them came to know Parkinsonism in as much depth and detail as Robert De Niro did, in his intensive playing of Leonard L. Can a neurological syndrome be acted? Can an actor with, presumably, a normally-functioning nervous system and physiology 'become' someone with a profoundly abnormal nervous system, experience, and behaviour? Can he have the experience – psychological, or indeed, physiological – which would enable him to do this? There can, obviously, be a sort of imitation or mimesis – but this is not acting, this is not the level at which Bob works. He himself had said, right at the beginning, 'It's never just a method, just a technique – it's a *feeling*. You have to feel what's right, feel it out of your own experience and self-knowledge.'

Ed W. told Bob that sometimes he might be completely frozen for hours, completely unable to get out of his chair or bed. Bob told me that he would sit and think of being frozen like this, of not being able to get out of bed – he would think about this intensely, almost hypnotically, for hours; he would imagine the inner quality of frozenness, at such times. Bob also had to imagine what Ed described as 'the challenge of not being able to do anything directly, the need to break it down into a series, a task.' One of the greatest, and most paradoxical, challenges of all was imagining *nothingness,* which Leonard L. himself, and many other post-encephalitics, would often experience. Bob and I spent hours talking about nothingness, and the different sorts of nothingness patients might experience (see Rose R., n. 54, p. 75); this was a challenge Bob took very seriously – he quoted Beckett to me once: 'Nothing is more real than nothing.'

Bob's method, as far as I could see, was to take in everything he learned about Parkinsonism, absorb it silently, without any external sign; let the images he had taken in sink down into his unconscious, and there ferment, unite with his own experiences, powers, imagination, feelings – and only then would they return, become visible, so deeply infused with his own character and subjectivity as to be, now, an integral part, an expression of, himself. (So it was with Harold Pinter; the processes of creation seemed very similar, whether within the writer's or the actor's mind.) This process, it was clear, could not be hurried. Sometimes there was, it seemed to me, a tension between the brisk timetable of the shooting schedule and the slow, unhurryable pace of the creative process. And yet, through incessant inner work and rehearsal (and I had the impression that Bob was occupied with these, consciously or unconsciously, almost 24 hours a day), he would always come up with the needed image, the matured performance, on time.

One morning, when everyone was busy in another building filming a scene, I caught sight of Bob, alone in a corner of the set, with a look of rage on his face; he looked extremely formidable. A few seconds later this gave way to a look of suspicion, a look of the most terrible, deepest, almost paranoid distrust. And then, the look of rage once again. When I first saw him I thought he *was* beside himself with rage, and then with suspicion. Now, I realised, he was *playing* with expressions of rage and suspicion, rehearsing privately for a coming scene. He clearly thought himself unobserved, so I hushed my breath and tiptoed away. It was amazing to see this; it was like overhearing a man *thinking* – but thinking with his body, experimenting, thinking in action. Thinking is not normally visible, but for the actor, for Bob certainly, it may be. Jerome Bruner (1966) speaks about three sorts of representation: iconic, symbolic, and enactive. The actor represents *enactively,* though in a very special, uniquely sophisticated sense. ('I learned to make of my body,' said Gielgud, 'a vessel to receive the text.')[172]

On one occasion Bob and Robin were depicting a scene in which the doctor is testing Leonard's postural reflexes (which can be severely impaired, or absent, in Parkinsonism). I took Robin's place for a moment, to show how one tested these – one stands behind the patient and, very lightly, pushes or pulls him off balance backward (a normal person would accommodate to this, but a Parkinsonian or post-encephalitic might fall backward like a ninepin). As I demonstrated this on Bob, he fell backward, completely inert and passive, with no hint of any reflexive reaction. Startled, I pushed him gently forward to the upright position – but now he started to topple, incontinently, forwards; I could not balance him. I did not know what to do; I had a sense of bewilderment admixed with panic. In that moment I forgot he was an actor; I thought he *had* suddenly lost all his postural reflexes, that there had suddenly been a neurological catastrophe. And then I remembered, and said to myself: 'Don't be silly, he is only acting.' But even when I bore this in mind, I still found it uncanny, I still thought he had somehow managed to override all his postural reflexes. At this point I started to wonder how

---

[172] A couple of years ago, I had a visit from Dustin Hoffman, who was then researching for the film *Rain Man.* We had visited an autistic patient of mine in hospital, and were now strolling outside in the Botanic Garden. I was chatting with his director, and he was walking by himself a few yards behind. Suddenly I thought I heard my patient. I was extremely startled, and turned round – and saw it was Dustin thinking to himself, but thinking with his body, thinking enactively, thinking of the young autistic man he had just seen.

deep, with Bob, acting might go. I knew how deeply he might
identify with the characters he portrayed, but I had to wonder now
how *neurologically* deep he might go – whether he might actually, in
his acting, *become* Parkinsonian, or at least (in an astoundingly controlled fashion) somehow duplicate the neurological state of the
patient. Does acting like this, I wondered, actually alter the nervous
system?

The next day I was talking with him in his dressing room before
the day's shooting began – and, as we talked, I noticed that his right
foot was turned in, turned in with precisely the dystonic curvature
it was held in when he portrayed Leonard L. on the set. I commented
on this, and now Bob seemed rather startled. 'I didn't realise,' he
said. 'I guess it's unconscious.' I knew that Bob sometimes stayed in
character for hours or days – he might make comments at dinner
which belonged to Leonard, not himself, as if 'residues' of the 'Leonard' mind and character were still adhering to him – but I had not
realised that this might include the sustained holding, unconsciously,
of *neurological* characteristics, such as this persistent, dystonia-like,
inward turning of the foot. (I observed this sort of thing also with
some of the other actors playing 'enkies,' especially those who had
to maintain a very abnormal and fixed head or eye posture for hours;
some of them seemed to be getting a wry-neck even off the set.)

There was one grand and (neurologically) climactic week in January when Bob portrayed two sorts of post-encephalitic crisis – an
oculogyric and a respiratory crisis. He studied for these with extreme care, reading and rereading the descriptions in *Awakenings,*
going over and over bits of film and tape, and questioning me
endlessly as to what they were like. But when he actually did them,
entered them, it was with a power and a conviction that seemed to
exceed representation: he gasped, he stiffened, his eyes rolled tor-
turedly upwards, he turned such a color I feared he would pass out.
And here again – all of us watching him were appalled and spellbound – it seemed to us that he was no longer 'acting,' that he was
actually in the throes of a terrible crisis. I thought, 'He is actually
having an oculogyric crisis,' and wondered what altered state his
nervous system was now in; I wanted, half-seriously, to get an EEG,
an electroencephalogram, on him at this time, wondering whether
it might not be (as it tends to be in an actual crisis) grossly slowed,
or perhaps convulsively abnormal. And his respiratory crisis, for me,

at least, was deeply moving and nostalgic. I had not seen a respiratory crisis for twenty years, not since the stormiest days, the tribulations, of 1969. I was delighted to see one once again – I thought, 'You dear old thing'; it was like seeing an old and missed friend. And so real, so real, it made me *think* about respiratory crises, which I had not had occasion to do for twenty years (ever since I had published a short paper in the *Lancet* about them); it made me look through my tapes again, reread the classic papers of Turner and Critchley, and then write a new footnote for this edition of the book (p. 46). Here, then, the flow was reversed: it was not I teaching the actors neurology, but the actors beginning to teach me – at least making me *see* it, see the nervous system, in an unusual and fresh way.[173]

But there were many revelations for me in the film – it was not merely, for example, that I was made to think about neurology and acting in a new way; I saw whole events anew from the perspective of their portrayal in the film. One such event – a very central one – sticks in my mind. The enkies, the post-encephalitics, have all 'awakened' one night (for dramatic reasons this was condensed, although in real life some of the patients had come to at different times, over the course of several weeks), and the next day are seen, all awake, in the dayroom. It is a complex scene, for there are fifteen patients there, and each of them has awakened, indeed, *to a world of his own.* They do not, at this point, form a community, in the least – every patient is still alone, almost autistic, in his own singularity. There are fifteen Rip van Winkles, fifteen intense egos, each totally absorbed with the wonder, and the problems, of their own, individual, and totally separate 'awakenings.' All of them have their own, completely different needs and demands. The staff is rushing from one to the other, answering a score of questions at once, dealing with a dozen and more completely different lives – intensely excited, intensely individual, intensely importunate new lives.

This is an amazing scene, in every way – it is, as a start, one of enormous physical complexity, for so many people are moving and doing different things at the same time. Penny has many special gifts,

---

[173] Jonathan Miller, who is both a theatre director and a neurologically trained doctor, has often made comparisons of patients and actors, how both have an implicit, unconscious knowledge of neurology – not in the formal, medical sense of 'savoir,' but in the intimate, personal knowledge of 'connaitre.'

but her choreographic gift – her power of directing twenty people doing twenty things simultaneously, of visualising and directing all their movements like a ballet – this choreographic power reached its height in this scene; all was movement, all was confusion, and yet everywhere, at the same time, all was focus, all was sense. But what was overwhelming for me was the *truth* of this scene. Steve Zaillian had invented it, but he had invented it right. For one reason and another (some of this to do with the form of the book, my presenting individual patients one by one, rather than the evolution of a social situation, as a whole), I had never described such a scene as now unfolded before me. But Steve, with his strong dramatic sense, had seen that such a scene must have occurred, and in this he was joined by Penny's strong dramatic sense too. They created this scene, then, with nothing to go on – nothing, that is, except their sense of what was dramatically necessary and right. And they were right, they had imagined absolutely correctly – there had been such a scene, several such scenes. I recollected this, as soon as I saw *their* scene. 'Dammit!' I thought, 'They've got it – that's what happened. That's just like the truth.'

By February, we were tired – there had been four months of filming, to say nothing of the months of research that preceded this. We were all tired, dog-tired, until an event that galvanized everybody into life. I made notes in my journal:

Thursday morning: Arrival of Lillian T. – the only living survivor of *Awakenings.* She has come to the set, where she will play *(be)* herself in a scene with De Niro . . . What will *she* think of the would-be 'enkies,' the film post-encephalitics, around her? And what will they feel about her, the last survivor, the real one among them? As she enters there is a feeling of awe – everyone recognises her from the documentary – and a sudden, almost frightening sense of reality – not that anything was unreal before, but it was the reality of stage, of script and book, these *constructed* realities. But now Lillian enters, the aboriginal reality – like Caesar entering a set of *Julius Caesar,* like someone stepping out of the pages of a history book . . .

However much the actors immerse themselves, identify, they are merely playing the part of enkies; Lillian has to be one, is one, for the rest of her life. They can slip out of their roles, she cannot. How does she feel about this? (How do I feel about Robin playing me? A temporary role for him, but lifelong for me.)

As Bob is wheeled in, and takes up the frozen, dystonic posture of Leonard L., Lillian T., herself frozen, cocks an alert and critical eye. How does Bob, acting frozen, feel about Lillian, scarcely a yard away, actually so? And how does she, actually so, feel about him, acting so? She has just given me a wink, and a barely perceptible thumbs-up sign, meaning, 'He's okay – he's *got* it! He really knows what it's like.' . . .

Everyone has been in to see Lillian, or talk to her. The entire set, steeped in make-belief, is moved to the depths. She shines with reality, in this make-believe world. People come in and touch her, grounding themselves, touching the rock.

Past and present had come together, model and representation had come together, to produce an extraordinary sense of reality, of completeness. The film – or at least the filming, the moral act of filming – needed Lillian's actual presence to culminate and complete it. We all had a feeling, now, that the circle was completed.

GLOSSARY

A book such as this necessarily uses a number of unfamiliar words referring to its special subject matter. In general, I have tried to indicate the meanings of these, by context, as they occur. The following short glossary is designed as a reader's companion, to help him visualize the peculiar disorders of movement, posture, will, appetite, sleep, etc., which constitute a major part of the subject matter of this book. Such terms are analogous to the much more familiar words with which we discuss emotional and neurotic disorders. The following words merge and overlap in meaning, as do the disorders they denote.

ABOULIA.   Lack of will or initiative. Especially favoured, at one time, in descriptions of neurotic 'paralyses of the will,' true aboulia is perhaps only seen with organic disease or damage to the brain – as in *encephalitis lethargica,* following extensive leucotomy, etc. It is often, but not necessarily, associated with profound apathy. The opposite of aboulia is *hyperboulia* – excess of will, wilfulness, urgency, appetency.

AGRYPNIA.   Total inability to sleep, absolute resistance to sedation – the acme of insomnia. This disorder, fatal if it lasts much longer than a week, is also only seen in diseases and intoxications – especially *encephalitis lethargica* and ergot-poisoning.

AKATHISIA.   Inability to keep still; intense urge to move; restlessness or fidgets in their most extreme degree.

AKINESIA.   Total lack of movement, or inability to make voluntary movements, for any reason whatever – seen in its most profound degree in post-encephalitic illness. One speaks, similarly, of *aphonia* (inability to make sounds), *amimia, aphrenia* (stoppage of thought), etc.

ALGOLAGNIA.   Lust for inflicting or suffering pain.

AMETRIA, AMORPHIA. Deficiencies, respectively, in judgement of *scale* and judgement of *form* (as *dysmetrias* and *dysmorphias* are systematic misjudgements of these). The causes and varieties of such aberrant or misjudged movement are multiform.

AMIMIA. Literally a loss of *mimesis,* of mimetic, histrionic and expressive capacities. The term is often used of the fixed and rather inexpressive face *(masking),* voice, and posture of many Parkinsonian patients. It should be stressed that this 'amimia' is secondary, not primary: Parkinsonians may have a full repertoire of *internal* expressions and gestures which have been denied full external expression due to the constraint (or enfeeblement) of akinesia. Sometimes, radiantly and unexpectedly, vivid expressions *do* 'break through' (see photo insert). Parkinsonians overdriven by L-DOPA (like patients with Gilles de la Tourette syndrome) may become *hyper-mimetic* – full of histrionic excesses, grimaces, and gesticulations, very suggestible, and prone to involuntary imitations, tics, mannerisms, etc.

ANABLEPSY. Forced upward gaze – the opposite of *catablepsy:* disorders especially seen in the *oculogyric crises* of sleeping-sickness, but also in hysteria, hypnosis, ecstasy, etc.

ANACLITIC. Literally 'leaning on' – used for relation of infant to mother.

APHAGIA. Inability to swallow.

APHONIA. Inability to make sounds.

APHRENIA. Stoppage of thought.

APNOEA. An arrest of breathing.

APRAXIA, AGNOSIA. Difficulties in action or perception due to inadequate understanding. Such difficulties are often associated with damage to the cerebral cortex, and may occur with brain tumours, strokes, senility, etc. They do *not* occur in Parkinsonism, where the difficulties are in *undertaking,* not in *understanding.*

ATHETOSIS. 'Mobile spasm,' in Gowers's term; involuntary writhing movements of the face, tongue, and extremities – a form of *dystonia.*

AUTOMATISM. Forced obedience to external stimuli or commands, as opposed to *command-negativism:* seen most dramatically in catatonia, but also in Parkinsonism and obsessive or hysterical neurotic disorders (see also *echolalia, palilalia,* etc.).

BLEPHAROSPASM. Spasm of the eyelids, which may be continuous *(blepharotonus)* or fluttering *(blepharoclonus).*

BLOCK. Resistance (at any level) to thought or movement. Seen most strikingly in catatonia, often associated with command-negativism; but also in Parkinsonian 'freezing,' and in neurotic impediments of thought, feeling, speech, and action. 'Involuntary' at lower levels, but associated with a sense of 'stickiness' or reluctance at higher levels.

BRADYKINESIA. Slowness of voluntary movement, extremely characteristic of Parkinsonism; one speaks, similarly, of *brady-phemia, bradyphrenia,* etc. Similar slowings are common in depression.

BRADYPHRENIA. Slowness of thought.

BRUXISM. Grinding of the teeth, allied to *trismus* (forced clenching). Common not only in post-encephalitic illness, but in states of neurotic tension, and in response to amphetamines.

BULIMIA. Literally 'ox-hunger.' A violent and insatiable appetite. Bulimia – like all exorbitances – easily switches to its opposite – violent refusal to eat, loathing of food, *anorexia,* voracity-in-reverse (see also *orexia*).

CATALEPSY. The tireless, timeless, effortless maintenance of postures – including perceptual postures and thought-postures (fascination, enthralment, etc.). As characteristic of hysteria and hypnosis as of catatonia; but also seen, at a lower level, in Parkinsonism.

CATATONIA. So-named about a century ago, but described and depicted since the dawn of recorded history: comprising, in its most familiar forms, catalepsy and the holding of statuesque postures, command-automatism or negativism, extreme suggestibility (either positive or negative), etc. Less familiar is *catatonic frenzy* ('amok'), to which catatonic immobility may suddenly turn. Although common in schizophrenia (especially schizophrenic panic), catatonia is also common in non-schizophrenic post-encephalitic patients, and may also be induced by hypnosis or drugs. Accompanied by an arrest, a deepening, and an intensification of attention, catatonia is perhaps more familiar as ecstasy, trance, rapture, and extreme 'concentration.' Catatonia may be regarded as 'intermediate' in level between Parkinsonism and neurotic disorder.

CHEMOPALLIDECTOMY. An operation to destroy part of the *globus pallidus,* formerly much used in the treatment of Parkinsonism.

CHOREA. An involuntary, desultory, flickering movement (or motor scintillation), which tends to dance from one muscle-group to another: a movement more primitive than tics, but more highly organised than jactitations and myoclonic jerks.

CLONUS.   A vibrato-like reaction to forced muscle stretching.

COGWHEELING.   See *hypertonia.*

COMA.   A state of deep unconsciousness, with loss of awareness and all higher activities: a state only seen with severe brain-damage or intoxication. It is opposed to *stupor* (in which there is preservation of crude protective responses, and sometimes mental activity of a disorganised, delirious type); and to states of abnormal lethargy *(torpor),* from which patients can be fully, if briefly, aroused.

CONTRACTURES.   Permanent contraction at joints (knees, hips, etc.), due to immobility and lack of (passive or active) exercise.

COPROLALIA.   Exclamatory swearing and use of hostile and obscene epithets, in a compulsive and convulsive manner, interlarded with *sotto voce* muttering and cursing. Especially associated with ticcing, and other over-active and impulsive states.

CUNCTATION.   Dawdling, delaying, resisting, hindering – the opposite of *festination* (haste).

Cunctation-festination form the corresponding opposites of Parkinsonian behaviour, as procrastination-precipitation form the opposite poles of neurotic behaviour.

It is in similar terms ('obstructive'-'explosive') that William James analyses 'the pathological will.'

DYSTONIA, DYSKINESIA.   Generic terms for abnormalities of muscle-tone and movement, and thus including such disorders as Parkinsonism, *athetosis, torticollis,* etc.

ECHOLALIA.   The forced repetition of someone's words again and again; *palilalia,* similarly, is the repetition of one's own words, phrases or sentences; *echopraxia* and *palipraxia* are forced repetitions of movements or actions. Such symptoms are common in catatonia and are analogous to *catalepsy* (which is a forced repetition or echoing of postures).

EMPROSTHOTONOS.   Forced flexion of the head on the chest, as opposed to forced throwing-back of the head *(opisthotonos).*

ERETHISM.   Pathological excitement of an itching, goading, urging type – especially used of onanistic and venereal excitements.

EXOTROPIA.   Divergent squint (or *strabismus*) of the eyes.

FESTINATION.   Forced hurrying of walking, talking, speech, or thought – perhaps the most characteristic feature of Parkinsonism.

Festinating steps tend to become smaller and smaller, until finally the patient is 'frozen' – stepping internally, but with no space to step in:

> '. . . movement which moves not
> and going which goes not . . .'

LAWRENCE

GEGENHALTEN. Sometimes called *paratonia.* A forced resistance or reluctance to passive movement, akin to, yet distinct from Parkinsonian, negativistic, and neurotic resistances. Its antonym (I suppose) would be 'mithalten' (going-with, compliance), though I am not sure that I have ever heard the term used.

GLABELLAR TAP. Tapping on the glabellum, just above the nose, which can elicit uninhibitable blinking in Parkinsonism.

HYPERKINESIA. Increased force, impetus, speed, violence, and spread of movement; usually associated with excess of 'background' movement *(synkinesia);* and often with impulsiveness, impetuosity, irritability, insomnia, etc. Hyperkinesias are the opposite of *akinesias,* whether the latter be Parkinsonian, catatonic, or neurotic in nature. Akinesia and hyperkinesia are interconvertible – often quite suddenly and explosively so: such sudden switches are seen not only in manic-depression, but in hysteria, Parkinsonism, and especially catatonia.

HYPERTONIA. Excessive muscular tone – due to spasticity, Parkinsonism, nervous tension, local irritation, etc. That of Parkinsonism tends to affect opposing muscles symmetrically, producing a plastic or 'lead-pipe' (or sometimes a *'cogwheel'*) rigidity. A striking effect of L-DOPA (even in non-Parkinsonians) is to render muscular tone less than normal – *hypotonic* – sometimes so much so that normal postures cannot be maintained. Thus the muscles and postures of Parkinsonians tend to be *hard,* whereas those of choreics and anti-Parkinsonians tend to be *soft* (so called *'chorea mollis'*).

HYPOKINESIA. Reduced force, impetus, or spread of movement – a diminution of movement short of complete *akinesia.*

HYPOMANIA. Elation which is pathological, but less than manic.

HYPOPHONIA. Reduced vocal force.

KINESIA PARADOXA. The sudden, total 'conversion' of Parkinsonism to normality, or to hyperkinesia.

MASK.   The characteristically expressionless face seen in Parkinson-ism.

MICROGRAPHIA.   Microscopic handwriting.

MYDRIASIS.   Pupillary dilatation.

MYOCLONUS.   Sudden violent jerks of a primitive and lowly organ-ised type, involving anything from fractions of muscle-groups (*myokymia,* myofibrillary twitchings) to the entire body-muscula-ture (lighting-spasms, *'blitzkrampf'*). Such movements may be ex-perienced by all of us, e.g. as we are falling asleep.

NARCOLEPSY.   One of the many sleep-disorders particularly com-mon in post-encephalitic patients. Narcolepsy is sudden, irresist-ible sleep, sometimes only a few seconds in length, and usually filled with vivid dreams; often associated with this are *cataplexy* (sudden loss of all muscle-tone, often brought on by excitement or laughter), *sleep-paralysis* (inability to move for several seconds or minutes after waking), *sleep-talking, sleep-walking,* nightmares, night-terrors, and excessive restlessness and movement during sleep (see also *sleep disorders*).

OCULOGYRIC CRISES.   Attacks of forced deviation of gaze, often associated with a surge of Parkinsonism, catatonia, tics, obsessive-ness, suggestibility, etc., etc.

OPHTHALMOPLEGIA.   Paralysis of gaze.

OPISTHOTONOS.   See *emprosthotonos.*

OREXIA.   Incontinent gluttony, voracity, greed. Its privative *(ano-rexia)* may be used to denote either simple loss of appetite, or positive refusal to eat, voracity-in-reverse. (All negative or priva-tive words here – *akinesia, aboulia,* etc. – may also be used to denote a simple lack, a contrariety, or both.)

PALILALIA, PALIPRAXIS.   See *echolalia.*

PARESIS.   Partial paralysis.

PERSEVERATION.   A tendency to indefinite continuation, or repeti-tion, of nervous processes – self-stimulating, self-reinforcing, self-maintaining, scarcely controllable: a basic pathological state, the antithesis of *'block'* (see *catalepsy, echolalia, rigidity,* etc., which are instances of such inertia).

PULSION.   Push, thrust – of an uncontrollable type. Thus one speaks of Parkinsonian propulsions, retropulsions, lateropulsions, etc. Variously qualified as *im*pulsions, *com*pulsions, *re*pulsions, etc., the term and concept necessarily pervade descriptions of experience and behaviour at *every* level.

RIGIDITY. A primary symptom in Parkinsonism, but also manifest at higher levels, as *gegenhalten* (paratonic rigidity), catatonic rigidity, hysterical rigidity, and neurotic rigidities and obstinacies. The transfixion of a limb (or the entire body, or all being) by the dynamic opposition of opposing innervations, producing a state of *clench,* or *spasm.* If the opposing impulses alternate, instead of coinciding, we see *tremor, flutter, hesitancy, vacillation,* etc. – also basic phenomena in Parkinsonism and neurosis.

SATYRIASIS. Excessive sexual appetency, urgency, or hunger: the venereal equivalent of *bulimia.*

SEBORRHOEA. Increased secretion of sebum, causing greasiness of the skin.

SIALORRHOEA. Increased salivation.

SLEEP DISORDERS. Unusual forms and transforms of sleep were particularly common in the early days of the sleeping-sickness, and have become familiar again as 'paradoxical' effects of L-DOPA. Such sleeps tend to be imperative, often sudden, profound, and usually resistant to interruption: they are of two basic types – swoon-like sleeps, wells of perseveration, into which patients may sink deeper and deeper (analogous to *catalepsy*), or inhibitions and obstructions of consciousness (analogous to *block*). If suddenly awoken from such pathological sleeps, patients may instantly fly into a rage or frenzy – a phenomenon analogous to 'kinesia paradoxa,' or to the notorious explosiveness of depressed or catatonic patients (see also *narcolepsy*).

TACHYCARDIA. Rapid heart-rate.

TACHYKINESIA. Excessive speed of movement – often associated with excessive force and abruptness; very characteristic of Parkinsonism (especially when activated by L-DOPA), of frenzies, manias, and tic-disorders; one speaks, similarly, of tachyphemia, tachyphrenia, etc.

TACHYPHRENIA. Accelerated thought.

TACHYPNOEA. Rapid breathing.

TIC. A sudden, complex, compulsive movement – more highly organised and constant in form than myoclonic jerks, jactitations, chorea, etc. A tendency to tic – seen in its most florid form in tic-disease (Gilles de la Tourette's syndrome) – is *also* common in neurotic and especially schizophrenic disorders, and in (active or activated) Parkinsonism. Tics of immobility, or tonic tics, resemble catalepsy, and indicate the functional similarity of such tics with catatonia. Higher-level tics tend to proliferate, to induce *counter-tics,* and to be built up into idiosyncratic mannerisms, affectations, impostures, etc.

TONUS.   Muscle tone (increased in hypertonia, decreased in hypotonia, bizarre in paratonia, or *'gegenhalten'*).

TORTICOLLIS. Maintained asymmetric spasm of neck-muscles, forcing the head to one side – a dystonic symptom which may be 'organic' (e.g. Parkinsonian) or 'functional' (e.g. hysterical) in nature. One speaks, similarly, of *tortipelvis.* The general term *torsion-spasm* denotes contorting spasms affecting the trunk and neck (compare *athetosis*). Similar writhing movements and contortions may, of course, affect being-as-a-whole: thus one may speak of a *moral athetosis,* and torturing states of *emotional torsion.*

BIBLIOGRAPHY

Anonymous. 1974. Editorial: 'Medical Literature,' *British Clinical Journal* 2:3.

Auden, G. A. 1922. 'Encephalitis Lethargica and Mental Deficiency,' *British Medical Journal* 1:165.

Briggs, John; and Peat, David F. 1989. *Turbulent Mirror.* New York: Harper & Row.

Bruner, Jerome. 1966. *Toward a Theory of Instruction.* Cambridge, Mass.: Harvard University Press.

Bruner, Jerome. 1986. *Actual Minds, Possible Worlds.* Cambridge, Mass.: Harvard University Press. (See especially Ch. 2, 'Two Modes of Thought.')

Calne, Donald. 1970. *Parkinsonism: Physiology, Pharmacology, and Treatment.* London: E. Arnold.

Calne, D. B.; and Lees, A. J. 1988. 'Late Progression of Post-Encephalitic Parkinson's Syndrome,' *Canadian Journal of Neurological Science* 15(2):135–138.

Calne, D. B.; Stern, G.; Laurence, D. R. M.; Sharkey, J.; and Armitage, J. 1969. 'L-DOPA in Post-Encephalitic Parkinsonism,' *Lancet* I:744.

Charcot, Jean-Marie. 1880. *De la Paralysie Agitante: Leçons sur les Maladies du Systeme Nerveux.* Paris: Adrien Delahaye, pp. 439–467.

Clough, C. G.; Plaitakis, A.; and Yahr, M. D. 1983. 'Oculogyric Crises and Parkinsonism: A Case of Recent Onset,' *Archives of Neurology* 40(1):36–37.

Cotzias, G. C.; Van Woert, M. H.; and Schiffer, L. M. 1967. 'Aromatic Amino Acids and Modication of Parkinsonism,' *New England Journal of Medicine* 276:374–379.

Crosby, Alfred W. 1990. *America's Forgotten Pandemic: The Influenza of 1918.* Cambridge: Cambridge University Press.

Cruchet, R. 1927. 'The Relation of Paralysis Agitans to the Parkinsonian Syndrome of Epidemic Encephalitis,' *Lancet* I:264.

Culliton, Barbara J. 1990. 'Emerging Viruses, Emerging Threat,' *Science,* 19 January, 279–280.

Dorros, Sidney. 1989. *Parkinson's: A Patient's View.* Cabin John, Md.: Seven Locks Press.

Duvoisin, Roger C. 1978. *Parkinson's Disease: A Guide for Patient and Family.* New York: Raven Press.

Edelman, Gerald. 1990. *The Remembered Present: A Biological Theory of Consciousness.* New York: Basic Books.

Fahn, S. 1974. ' "On-off" Phenomenon with Levodopa Therapy in Parkinsonism,' *Neurology* 24:431–441.

Fine, Edward J.; Soria, Emilio D.; and Paroski, Margaret W. 1990. 'Tremor Studies in 1886 through 1889.' *Archives of Neurology* vol. 47, no. 3:337–340.

Fuller, John G. 1969. *The Day of St. Anthony's Fire.* London: Hutchinson.

His Majesty's Stationery Office. 1918. 'Report of an Enquiry into an Obscure Disease, Encephalitis Lethargica.' London.

Gaubius, H. D. 1758. *Institutiones Pathologiae Medicinalis.* Leiden: S. N. J. Luchtmans.

Geertz, Clifford. 1973. *The Interpretation of Cultures.* New York: Basic Books.

Glass, Leon; and Mackey, Michael C. 1988. *From Chaos to Clocks: The Rhythms of Life.* Princeton: Princeton University Press.

Gleick, James. 1987. *Chaos.* New York: Viking.

Goffman, Erving. 1961. *Asylums.* Garden City, N.Y.: Anchor Books.

Gould, Stephen Jay. 1989. *Wonderful Life: The Burgess Shale and the Nature of History.* New York: W. W. Norton.

Gowers, W. R. 1893. *A Manual of Diseases of the Nervous System.* Philadelphia: Blakiston (2nd ed.). See esp. vol. II, pp. 636–657.

Greenough, A. and Davis, J. A. 1983. 'Encephalitis Lethargica: Mystery of the Past or Undiagnosed Disease of the Present?,' *Lancet* I(8330):922–923.

Hall, Arthur J. 1924. *Epidemic Encephalitis.* Bristol: Wright & Sons.

Hardie, R. J. 1984. 'On-off Fluctuations in Parkinson's Disease: A Clinical and Neuropharmacological Study.' M.D. Thesis, Cambridge University.

Hardie, Richard J. 1990. 'Levodopa-related Motor Fluctuations,' in *Parkinson's Disease,* edited by G. Stern. Baltimore: Johns Hopkins University Press.

Hardie, R. J.; Lees, A. J. and Stern, G. M. 1984. 'On-off Fluctuations in Parkinson's Disease: A Clinical and Neuropharmacological Study,' *Brain* 107:487–506.

Hess, Walter Rudolf. 1954. *Diencephalon.* New York: Grune & Stratton.

Howard, R. S. and Lees, A. J. 1987. 'Encephalitis Lethargica: A Report of Four Recent Cases,' *Brain* 110 (1):19–33.

Jelliffe, Smith Ely. 1927. *Post-Encephalitic Respiratory Disorders.* Washington, D.C.: Nervous and Mental Disease Publishing Co.

Jelliffe, Smith Ely. 1932. *Psychopathology of Forced Movements and the Oculogyric Crises of Lethargic Encephalitis.* Washington, D.C.: Nervous and Mental Disease Publishing Co.

Johnson, J. and Lucey, P. A. 1988. 'Late Progression of Post-Encephalitic Parkinson's Syndrome,' *Canadian Journal of Neurological Sciences* 15(2):135–138.

Kraus, P. H.; Bittner, H. R.; Klotz, P.; and Przuntek, H. 1987. 'Investigation of Agonistic/Antagonistic Movement in Parkinson's Disease from an Ergodic Point of View,' in *Temporal Disorders in Human Oscillatory Systems,* edited by L. Rensing et al. New York: Springer Verlag.

Langston, J. William. 1989. 'Current Theories on the Cause of Parkinson's Disease,' *Journal of Neurology, Neurosurgery and Psychiatry* special supplement:13–17.

Langston, J. William; and Irwin, Ian. 1986. 'MPTP: Current Concepts and Controversies,' *Clinical Neuropharmacology,* 9(6):485–507. New York: Raven Press.

Laplane, D.; Levasseur, M.; Pillon, B.; Dubois, B.; Baulac, M.; Mazoyer, B.; Tran Dinh, S.; Sette, G.; Danze, F.; and Baron, J. C. 1989. 'Obsessive-Compulsive and Other Behavioural Changes with Bilateral Basal Ganglia Lesions,' *Brain* 112:699–725.

Luria, A. R. [1932] 1976. *The Nature of Human Conflicts.* Reprint. New York: Liveright.

Luria, A. R. [1968] 1987. *The Mind of a Mnemonist.* Reprint. Cambridge, Mass.: Harvard University Press.

Luria, A. R. [1972] 1987. *The Man with a Shattered World.* Reprint. Cambridge, Mass.: Harvard University Press.

Luria, A. R. 1977. *The Making of Mind.* Cambridge, Mass.: Harvard University Press.

Mandelbrot, B. B. 1977. *Fractals: Form, Chance and Dimension.* San Francisco: W. H. Freeman.

Mandelbrot, B. B. 1982. *The Fractal Geometry of Nature.* San Francisco: W. H. Freeman.

Marsden, C. D. and Parkes, J. D. 1976. ' "On-off" Effects in Patients with Parkinson's Disease on Chronic Levodopa Therapy,' *Lancet* I:292–296.

Martin, James Purdon. 1967. *The Basal Ganglia and Posture.* London: Pitman Medical Publishing.

McKenzie, Ivy. 1927. 'Discussion on Epidemic Encephalitis,' *British Medical Journal* ii:632–634.

Meige, Henry; and Feindel, E. 1902. *Les Tics et Leur Traitement.* Paris: Masson.

Mitsuyama, Y.; Fukunaga, H.; and Takayama, S. 1983. 'Parkinson's Disease of Post-Encephalitic Type Following General Paresis – An Autopsied Case,' *Folia. Psychiatry and Neurology (Japan)* 37(1):85–93.

Nauta, W. J. H. 1989. 'Reciprocal Links of the Corpus Striatum with the Cerebral Cortex and Limbic System: A Common Substrate for Movement and Thoughts?' in *Neurology and Psychiatry: A Meeting of Minds,* edited by J. Mueller. Basel: Karger.

Onuaguluchi, Gilbert. 1964. *Parkinsonism.* London: Butterworth.

Parkes, C. M. 1972. *Bereavement.* London: Tavistock; and New York: International Universities Press.

Parkinson, James. 1817. *An Essay on the Shaking Palsy.* London: Sherwood, Neely & Jones. (The original is very rare, but a facsimile was published in 1959 by Dawson in London.)

Penfield, W. and Perot, P. 1963. 'The Brain's Record of Visual and Auditory Experience: A Final Summary and Discussion,' *Brain* 86:595–696.

Podvoll, Edward M. 1990. *The Seduction of Madness.* New York: HarperCollins.

Prigogine, Ilya. 1980. *From Being to Becoming.* San Francisco: W. H. Freeman.

Rail, D.; Scholtz, C.; and Swash, M. 1981. 'Post-encephalitic Parkinsonism: Current Experience,' *Journal of Neurology, Neurosurgery and Psychiatry* 44(8):670–676.

Sacks, O. 1969. 'L-DOPA for Progressive Supranuclear Palsy,' *Lancet* II: 591–592.

Sacks, Oliver W. 1970. *Migraine: Evolution of a Common Disorder.* Berkeley and Los Angeles: University of California Press.

Sacks, O. W.; and Kohl, M. 1970a. 'Incontinent Nostalgia Induced by L-DOPA,' *Lancet* I:1394–1395.

Sacks, O. W.; and Kohl, M. 1970b. 'L-DOPA and Oculogyric Crises,' *Lancet* II:215–216.

Sacks, O. W.; Kohl, M.; Schwartz, W.; and Messeloff, C. 1970a. 'Side-Effects of L-DOPA in Post-Encephalitic Parkinsonism,' *Lancet* I:1006.

Sacks, O. W.; Messeloff, C.; Schwartz, W.; Goldfarb, A.; and Kohl, M. 1970b. 'Effects of L-DOPA in Patients with Dementia,' *Lancet* I:1231–1232.

Sacks, O. W.; Messeloff, C. R.; and Schwartz, W. 1970c. 'Long-term Effects of Levodopa in Severely Disabled Patients,' *Journal of the American Medical Association* 213:2270.

Sacks, O. W.; Ross, S. J.; de Paola, D. P.; and Kohl, M. 1970d. 'Abnormal Mouth-Movements and Oral Damage Associated with L-DOPA Treatment,' *Annals of Dentistry* 29:130–144.

Sacks, O. W. 1971. 'Parkinsonism – A So-Called New Disease,' *British Medical Journal* 4:111–113.

Sacks, O. W. 1972. 'The Great Awakening,' *The Listener,* 26 October.

Sacks, O. W.; Kohl, M. S.; Messeloff, C. R.; and Schwartz, W. F. 1972. 'Effects of Levodopa in Parkinsonian Patients with Dementia,' *Neurology* 22:516–519.

Sacks, O. W. 1975. 'The Nature of Consciousness,' *Harper's,* December.

Sacks, O. W. and Carolan, P. C. 1979. 'EEG Findings in Post-Encephalitic and Tourettic Patients,' *Proceedings of Annual Meeting,* New York: Metropolitan EEG Society.

Sacks, O. W. 1981. 'Witty Ticcy Ray,' *London Review of Books,* 19 March. (Also reprinted in Sacks, 1985.)

Sacks, O. W. 1982a. 'Acquired Tourettism in Adult Life,' in *Gilles de la Tourette Syndrome,* edited by A. J. Friedhoff and T. N. Chase. New York: Raven Press.

Sacks, O. W. 1982b. '*Awakenings* Revisited,' in *Advanced Medicine 18,* edited by M. Sarner. London: Pitman Books.

Sacks, O. W. 1983. 'The Origin of *Awakenings,*' *British Medical Journal* 287:1968–1969.

Sacks, Oliver. 1985. *The Man Who Mistook His Wife for a Hat.* New York: Summit Books.

Sacks, Oliver. 1986. 'Clinical Tales,' in *Use and Abuse of Literary Concepts in Medicine,* Literature and Medicine 5, edited by J. T. Banks. Baltimore: Johns Hopkins University Press.

Sacks, Oliver. 1987. Foreword to A. R. Luria, *The Man with a Shattered World.* Cambridge, Mass.: Harvard University Press.

Sacks, Oliver. 1989. 'Neuropsychiatry and Tourette's.' in *Neurology and Psychiatry: A Meeting of Minds,* edited by J. Mueller. Basel: S. Karger.

Sacks, Oliver. 1990a. 'Luria and Romantic Science,' in *Contemporary Neuropsychology and the Legacy of Luria,* edited by E. Goldberg. Hillsdale, N.J.: Erlbaum.

Sacks, Oliver. 1990b. 'Post-Encephalitic Syndromes,' in *Parkinson's Disease,* edited by G. Stern. London: Chapman and Hall.

Shenker, Israel. 1969. 'Drug Brings Parkinson Victims Back into Life.' *New York Times,* August 26.

Spitz, R. A. 1946. 'Anaclitic Depression,' *Psychoanal. Study Child* 2:313–342.

Tilney, Frederick; and Howe, Hubert S. 1920. *Epidemic Encephalitis.* New York: Paul B. Hoeber.

Todes, Cecil. 1990. *The Shadow Over My Brain: My Struggle with Parkinson's Disease.* Gloucestershire: Windrush.

Trétiakoff, C. 1919. 'Contribution a l'étude de l'anatomie du locus niger,' Thèse de Paris. (1921) *Rev. Neurol.* 592.

Turner, W. A.; and Critchley, M. 1925. 'Respiratory Disorders in Epidemic Encephalitis,' *Brain* 48:72–104.

Turner, W. A.; and Critchley, M. 1928. 'The Prognosis and Late Results of Postencephalitic Respiratory Disorders,' *Journal of Neurology and Neuropathology* 8:191.

Vaughan, Ivan. 1986. *Ivan: Living with Parkinson's Disease.* London: Macmillan.

Vogt, C.; and Vogt, O. 1920. 'Lehre der Erkrangungen des striären Systems,' *Journal für Psychologie und Neurologie* 26s:43–57.

von Economo, C. 1918. *Die Encephalitis Lethargica.* Wien.

von Economo, Constantin. 1931. *Encephalitis Lethargica: Its Sequelae and Treatment* Oxford: Oxford University Press.

Wilson, S. A. K. 1940. 'Paralysis Agitans,' in *Neurology,* edited by Ninian Bruce. London: Arnold. See also Wilson's chapter on 'Epidemic Encephalitis' in the same book.

Wimmer, August. *Chronic Epidemic Encephalitis.* London: Heinemann.

Winfree, Arthur T. 1980. *The Geometry of Biological Time.* New York: Springer Verlag.

Woodcock, A. and Davis, M. 1978. *Catastrophe Theory.* London: Pelican.

Zeeman, E. C. 1976. 'Catastrophe Theory,' *Scientific American* 232: 65–83.

INDEX

Aaron E., 65n, 190–98, 250, 255, 269n, 304–5, 341–43
aboulia, 9
absence, pathological, 9, 14
acceleration of movements, 103n
acceptance, 266
accommodation, 62–63, 106–7, 253n, 265–75, 289, 291
activation, devices for, 346–47
addiction, 251n; to L-DOPA, 252–57
adjustment of dosage, 48, 251, 255n, 257–59, 351
admission psychosis, 161–62
adverse reactions to L-DOPA, 235n, 243–65. *See also* case histories
affective compulsions, 17
age-related deterioration, 315
agnosia, 343, 344
agrypnia (inability to sleep), 13–14n
akathisia, 6, 15, 120–21, 154–55
akinesia, 7–8, 15, 27n, 286, 363–64
akinetic amimia, 347
akinetic episodes, 258
alcohol, 31n, 253n; James and, 325
algorithms, 281, 348
amantadine, 34n, 58, 125, 167, 175, 200, 218, 300–301, 308–9; and brain activity, 329
amphetamines, 27n, 252n
anachronistic states, 113n
anticholinergic drugs, 27n, 91
anti-DOPA, 252n
anti-histamines, 58
apomorphine, 27n
apraxia, 343, 344
Aprill, Arnold, 373
arithmomania, 132n
arousal, excessive, 104–5, 120–23; with L-DOPA, 153–54
arrests, paroxysmal, 95–97, 112
arsephenamine, 31n
art, therapeutic, 281–85
Artane, 191, 199
asylums, xxvi–xxvii
athetosis, 6n, 16

attention defects, 63–64n, 166, 240–41
Auden, G. A., 17–18n
Auden, W. H., 18n
autochthonous thinking, 81–82n
auto-command, 270
automatism, 285
awakening, phenomena of, xxv–xxvi, 231n, 235–43, 247–48n, 262, 266n, 275, 327–32; *See also* case histories
Awakenings, Sacks, xxv–xxvi, xxxi, xxxvi–xxxvii; dramatic interpretations, 367–86; publishing history, xxi–xxiii, xxxiv–xxxvi, xxxviii
Awakenings, films, 373–86; documentary, 46n, 65n, 96n, 295–96, 309, 315, 368–69

Barbeau, A., 34
barbiturates, 58
Barnes, Peter, *Drummer,* 378–79n
basal-ganglia, and memory, 83–84n
behavior disorders, 110–11, 180–83; with L-DOPA, 159–60, 185–88
behavioral neurology, 14–15n
beneficial effects of L-DOPA, 202–3, 235–36n, 236–37, 278, 292–95, 298–99. *See also* case histories
Bernard, Claude, 21, 266, 330
Bert E., 243–44n
biological thinking, 273–74
bipolar L-DOPA reactions, 291–92, 296–98
block, 16, 18; with L-DOPA, 85–86, 215
Boswell, James, 264
bradykinesia, 8n
brain: and accommodation, 267; damage to, 21, 32–34; L-DOPA and, 251–52; studies, 237n
brain activity, 308–9; in awakenings, 327–32
brain cell transplants, 34n, 336

brainstem, 15n
breakdown, signs of, 250
bromocriptine, 34n
Browne, Sir Thomas, 71n, 224, 234,
     243, 261, 266, 269n, 365
Bruner, Jerome, 382
Buber, Martin, 227n
butyrophenones, 5, 58, 252n

cachexia, 93
Calne, D. B., 315n
care for patients, 234
care-taking accommodation, 271n
Carolan, P. C., 327
Cartesian physiology, 261n
case histories, xxxvii, 229–30;
     individual, 39–219, 289–311
catalepsy, 15, 240–41
catastrophe theory, 355n, 356
catatonia, 15–16, 18, 96–98, 363;
     hyperkinetic, 103n; L-DOPA and,
     236
Cecil M., 202–3, 278, 306, 314, 341
cell transplantation, 336
cerebral cortex, 267
chaos theory, 98n, 354–65
character, 17–18n, 229; L-DOPA and,
     293–94
Charcot, Jean-Marie, xxvi, 4, 6, 7, 9,
     11, 27n, 320
chemopallidectomy, 27n, 117
children, symptoms, 17
chorea, 16, 194–98
chronic hallucinations, 214–15n
chronic hospitals, xxvi–xxvii, xxix
clinical approach, 226n
cocaine, 252n; Freud and, 31, 323–24
coercive institutions, 25n
command negativism, 16
communication, doctor-patient, 225–34
community, post-encephalitic, 65–66n
compulsions, 16–17, 55, 102–3;
     counting, 131–33n; See also tics
Conrad, Joseph, 231n
consciousness, 239n; James and, 325
contactual reflexes, 281–82
Conti, Tom, 375, 378n
controlled hallucinosis, 214
Cooper, Irving, 192n
coping behaviors, 63n, 106–7, 114,
     270–75, 345–49
cortisone, 31
Cotzias, George, xxvii, 28, 34, 255n
crash, after treatment high, 254–57
crises, 18–20, 204; oculogyric, 17,
     40–42; periodicities, 360n; psychic
     causes, 47, 49, 53n; respiratory,
     39–40, 46–50; unusual, 188. See
     also case histories

Cruchet, R., 13n
Culliton, Barbara J., 321

Dali, Salvador, 284
Dallas, Duncan, 368
Darwin, Charles, 287
Davis, J. A., 321
deaths of patients, 125–28, 182–83,
     188, 189, 277, 290, 296, 298,
     303–5, 310, 313, 314; from grief,
     127n
delirium, 168–69, 183, 238n, 239n,
     301; Kantian, 286; kinematic, 113
dementias, 238n, 244n
Dench, Judy, 370–71
De Niro, Robert, 46n, 375–86
dependence on L-DOPA, 159. See also
     addiction
Deprenyl (selegiline), 337
depression, 9; with L-DOPA, 52–53;
     stimulants and, 252n
de Quincey, Thomas, 225–26n, 253n
diabetes, 363n
diagnosis, 226n
diencephalic syndromes, 65n
diencephalon, 15n
Dionysiac disease, 17–18n
discontinuation of L-DOPA, 353. See
     also case histories
discourse, types of, 225–27
disease, 237, 249, 250, 263, 268; and
     health, 238–39; metaphysical
     views, 223–34
DL-DOPA, 34n
documentary film of *Awakenings*, 46n,
     65n, 96n, 295–96, 309, 315,
     368–69
Donne, John, 22, 223–24, 225, 229n,
     246, 249–50, 263
dopamine, xxvii, 31; deficiency of, 34
dopamine agonists, 34n, 333
dosage: adjustment of, 48–49, 251,
     255n, 257–59, 351; correct, 248n
drama of *Awakenings*, 367–86
drawing style, L-DOPA and, 155n
dream alterations, 154–55n
drug-induced Parkinsonism, 5
Drummer, Barnes, 378–79n
dynamic vision, 206
dynamical diseases, 363
dystonia, 16, 77, 99, 171, 188

Easter psychosis, 171
echolalia, 16; with L-DOPA, 189
echopraxia, 16
Edelman, Gerald, 83–84n, 239n
Edith T., 60–61n
Ed M., 211n, 278, 282, 330
Ed W., 63n, 357–58, 360–61, 361n,

Ed W. *(cont'd)*
378, 381; record of symptoms,
363
Edward J., 192n
EEG (electro-encephalography),
308–9, 327–32; effects of music,
282
Eldepryl (selegiline), 337
electrical activity of brain, 308–9;
awakenings, 327–32
Eliot, T. S., 60n, 275
Ellis, Havelock, and mescal, 326
emotional response: increased with
L-DOPA, 70–73, 122; lacking,
67–69
emotions: stressful, and Parkinsonism,
191–93n; unstable, L-DOPA and,
54–57, 201n
encephalitis lethargica, xxv, 4–5, 12–23,
32, 319–21; hyperkinetic form,
39–40; individual cases, 67,
74–75, 88, 116, 129, 148, 180,
188, 202–3; new cases, 314;
respiratory crises, 46n;
sub-clinical, 161n
"enkieness," 27n, 380
environment, 65–66, 268, 295; and
accommodation, 270–75; and
post-encephalitic symptoms,
21–22, 25–27n
environmentally-caused Parkinsonism, 5
epidemics of sleeping sickness, xxv,
4–5, 12–14, 319–21
epilepsy, 249n, 358n; *petit mal,* 95–96;
seizures, 19n
ergot poisoning, 14n
existential medicine, 285–87
exorbitance, 250–51, 253, 254n;
opposite states, 256–57; tendency,
262n
explosive disorders, 15
explosive reactions to L-DOPA,
99–102, 146–47, 178, 186, 189
external command, 270, 345–49

Faraday, Michael, 230
Feindel, E., 229n
festination (hurry), 3, 6–7, 343–44. *See
also* case histories
films. *See Awakenings,* films
folk medicine, 28n
Forster, E. M., 283
Foster, Michael, 344n
fractals, 360n
Frances D., 39–67, 114, 201n, 231n,
248n, 260, 267, 270, 289–90,
293, 339, 340, 343, 345, 347

Frank G., 180–83
freezing, 43–44, 63–64n, 202, 339
Freud, Sigmund, 229, 231, 246, 264;
and cocaine, 31, 323–24; and
sleep, 269n
Fuller, John G., 14n

Gaubius, H. D., 285
Geertz, Clifford, xxxvii-n
George W., 190n, 198–201, 305–6,
352
Gertie C., 113n, 165–70, 235n, 277,
298–302, 307, 313
Glass, Leon, 360–62
Goethe, Johann Wolfgang von, 232
Gowers, W. R., 6, 8, 249n, 360n
grasp-reflexes, 123
Greenough, A., 321
Gregory, Richard, 343
grimaces, 89–92, 144
Gunn, Thom, 17n

hallucinations, 18, 138, 161, 301;
kinematic, 113; with L-DOPA,
167–70, 173–75, 189, 214–15
haloperidol, 123, 157, 252n
Hardie, Richard, 355n
hatred, 130
health, 224, 228, 233–34, 237–38,
268
Helen K., 8n
Hesse, Hermann, 275
Hester Y., 95–115, 162–63n, 206,
231n, 243n, 257, 262n, 273, 277,
278, 291–92, 302, 313, 347,
351–52, 369
hiccups, 138
higher faculties of post-encephalitic
patients, 20
Highlands Hospital, 10, 26–27n,
270n, 375; last survivors, 314–16
Hoffman, Dustin, 382n
holism, mystical, 31n
holistic neurology, 239–40
home, need for, 272
homeostasis, 266–67
Hornykiewicz, O., 34
horse-back riding, 348–49
hospitalization: deaths during strikes,
313; Parkinson's disease and,
305–6
hostility, 18
humming, 89–90, 98, 181, 182
hunger, with L-DOPA, 153, 155
Huntington's chorea, 195n
Hyman H., 161n
hyoscine, 91
hyoscyamine, 27n

hyperkinesia, 363
hyperkinetic states, 103n; *encephalitis lethargica,* 39–40
hypothalamus, 15n; disorders of, 129

Ida T., 176–79, 231n, 273, 304
identification, diagnostic, 226n
illness, 263; metaphysical view, 223–34
individuality of patient, 21–22, 228, 259–65, 268–73
industrial toxins, 335
inertia, Parkinsonian, 7, 9n, 345–46
inertia-less states, 111n
infinite sets, 249n
influenza epidemic, 13n
inner space, 256n, 257n
insomnia, 14n, 80, 153, 154
instability, emotional, L-DOPA and, 201n
institutions, 64–66, 272; coercive, 25n; and treatment response, 216–17n
intelligence of post-encephalitic patients, 20
involuntary movements, 16, 250. *See also* tics
Irmgard H., 155n

James, Henry, 239n
James, William, 7n, 31n, 266n, 324–25
Jelliffe, Smith Ely, 18, 19–20n, 21, 46n, 55n, 65n, 78n, 81–82n, 229n, 320
Joseph F., 315
Journal of the American Medical Association, Sacks letter, xxxi–xxxii
Joyce, James, 79, 98n
juvenile Parkinsonism, 320

Kant, Immanuel, 61n, 283, 286
Keynes, Maynard, xix
A Kind of Alaska, Pinter, xxxviii, 369–71
kinematic-mosaic vision, 206, 257n
kinematic states, 112–13
kinesia paradoxa, 10, 363–64, 379
Kohl, Marjorie, 52–53, 85n, 370

Langston, William, 333–35
Largactil (thorazine), 185
Lasker, Larry, 373
Lawrence, D. H., 241n, 242–43
L-DOPA, xxvii–xxviii, xxx–xxxi, 27n, 28, 34–35, 231–34, 279–80; accommodation to, 265–75; awakening experience, 235–43; and brain activity, 328; outpatient

treatment, 202–3; and Parkinson's disease, 190n, 193–98, 200–201; reactions to, xxxvii, 20, 22, 333, 351–65; tribulations of, 243–65. *See also* case histories
Lees, A. J., 315n
Leibniz, Gottfried Wilhelm, 227–29, 233, 261, 283, 286–87, 339
Leonard L., xxviii, 7, 203–19, 242, 247n, 248n, 250, 256, 257, 264, 273, 307–11, 367, 369; De Niro as, 380–86; EEG, 328–30; film story, 374–75
Lesch-Nyhan syndrome, 55n
liability to illness, 246–47
life changes, Parkinsonism and, 191–93n, 238n
Lillian T., 63n, 245n, 271n, 313, 315, 369; film of, 385–86
Lillian W., 18–19n, 78–79n, 231n
The Listener, article, xxxiii–xxxiv
lock-jaw, with L-DOPA treatment, 203
Lorenz, Konrad, 354n, 356–57, 359
love, 273; of patients, 288
lucid intervals, 238n
Lucy K., 140–47, 201n, 264, 297
Luria, A. R., xxxiv–xxxvi, 229n, 280, 287, 300, 348, 360; *The Nature of Human Conflict,* 114n, 271n

McKenzie, Ivy, xxviii
Mackey, Michael C., 362–63
macro-tics, 110
Magda B., 67–73, 244n, 260, 273
maintenance dosage, 248n
major tranquillizers, 5, 58
man, characterization of, 229
Mandelbrot, B. B., *The Fractal Geometry of Nature,* 364–65
manic behavior, with L-DOPA, 156
Mann, Thomas, 18n
mannerized tics, 110, 136
MAO (mono-amine oxidase) inhibitors, 335–36
Margaret A., 148–60, 201n, 295–96, 369
Maria G., 110, 183–88, 231n, 261–62, 262n
Mark, Margery, 314, 321
Marshall, Penny, 375–78
Martha N., xxxv-n, 113n, 170–76, 260, 261, 262n, 277, 300–303, 353, 362
Martin, James Purdon, 55n, 114n, 280–81, 284, 288
Mary T., 314
mask-like face, 42, 68, 89, 151, 204
mathematical compulsions, 131–33n

mathematics, 274n; chaos theory, 354–57
Maurice P., 10–11n, 211n
measures of scale, 346–48
mechanical medicine, 226n, 227–28, 273
medicine, xviii–xix, 285–87; and metaphysics, 28–32, 224–34; and philosophy, 279–80
megaphonia, 202, 341
Meige, Henry, 229n
memory, 19–20n; L-DOPA and, 260n; post-encephalitic, 82–83; updating, 83–84n
Mencken, H. L., 13n
mental state, Parkinsonian, 166–67
mescal, Ellis and, 326
metaphors for health, 241n
metaphysical approach: to medicine, 28–32, 224–34; to side effects of L-DOPA, 262–65
microambulation, 341
micro-crises, 151, 204
micro-tics, 110
migraine, 98n, 206n, 358n
Migraine, Sacks, xviii
Miller, Jonathan, 327, 384n
mimetic therapy, 347
minor tranquillizers, 58
miracle drugs, 28, 31–32, 323–26
Miriam H., 82n, 128–40, 260, 277, 278, 292–95, 304, 313, 347, 380
Miron V., 161–64, 211n, 265, 273, 296–98
moments, perception of, 113n, 260–61n
mood-swings, 88, 89, 150–51
mother, abnormal relationship with, 141–47, 208, 213, 216, 217n, 264
motor deterioration, age-related, 315
Mount Carmel hospital, xxv–xxx, 24–27, 210n, 270n, 277–78, 296–97, 313–14; administrative change, 53n, 64–65; L-DOPA use, 34–35
movement: disorders of, 6–9, 42–43, 59–60, 63–64n, 193; ease of, 270; and memory, 83–84n
MPP+, 335
MPTP (1-methyl-4-phenyl-1,2,3,6-tetra-hydropyridine), 334–36
music, therapeutic, 60, 60–62n, 117, 125, 160, 270, 281–84, 295–96, 348; EEGs, 330
mystagogic drugs, 31–32n
mysticism, 30–31n; medicine and, 228

narcoleptic patients, 252n
Nathan G., 71n
Nature, 274; therapeutic effect, 160
Nauta, Walle, 237n
needs: for illness, 246–47, 263–64; unfulfilled by L-DOPA, 251
negative disorders, 9, 14, 72n
nervous system, disorders, xxviii
neuroanatomy, 237n
neurochemistry, 33–34
neurodynamical disorders, 362
neurology, xxvi, 288; behavioral, 14–15n; case histories, 229–30; language of, 233; schools of, 239–40
neuroses, 17–18, 25n, 231, 241n, 252n
neurotic symptoms, 39–40
Newton, Isaac, 201n, 339
Nietzsche, F. W., 279, 289
nightmares, 74–75; with L-DOPA, 154
nitrous oxide, James and, 324–25
nonlinearity, 98n, 356–61
nothingness, 381; thinking of, 75–76n

obsessions, 18
obstructive disorders, 15
oculogyric crises, 17, 19n; in patients, 40–184 passim
Onuaguluchi, Gilbert, 331–32
oral mania, 121
orphans, 127n, 128–29
Orwell, Sonia, 371
oscillations of response, 107, 124, 215–16
outpatients, 305–6

pacing, 270
palilalia, 16; in patients, 59–214 passim
paralysis agitans, 5, 33
paranoia, 104–5, 161
Parkes, Walter, 373
Parkinson, James, 3, 32
Parkinsonian patients, xxvii–xxviii, 259, 284–86; weight-loss, 93n
Parkinsonism, 4–11, 17n, 25n, 32–34, 40, 63–64n, 165, 190–91, 231–34, 319; infinite quality, 97–98n; and L-DOPA, 235–43; periodicities, 360n; post-encephalitic, 15–23; psychic causes, 53n; space-time perceptions, 339–49; sudden-onset, 333–37; treatments, 27n, 333–37
Parkinson's disease, 3–11, 14–15, 190–201, 278–79, 291, 335, 363; accommodation, 267, 271;

Parkinson's disease *(cont'd)*
   L-DOPA and, xxxvii, 20, 236,
      244n, 250, 255, 278–79, 304–6
paroxysmal symptoms, 95–97, 112,
      148–49, 158–59
passivity of Parkinsonism, 7, 345–46
Pasteur, Louis, 228
patients, individuality of, xxviii–xxix,
      7–8n, 259–65, 268–73,
Pavlov, I. P., 254n, 256n, 285
Penfield, W., 19n
perceptual inertia, 9n
pergolide, 34n
periodicities, 360n
Perot, P., 19n
perseveration, 8, 9
persona, 239n
personality: changes, 54n; disorders,
      159–62; L-DOPA and, 50, 159–60,
      293–94
personal space and time, 340–49
PET scanning, 334–36
phenothiazides, 5, 58, 252n
philosophy, medicine and, 279–80
physicians, 287–88
Pinter, Harold, 369–71, 381; *A Kind
   of Alaska,* xxxviii
plants, medicines from, 28n
Podvoll, Edward M., 358n
Poincaré, Henri, 355–56
positive disorders, 14–15, 72n
post-DOPA states, 52–57, 59n, 92–94
post-encephalitic patients, xxv–xxvi,
      xxvii–xxxi, 10–11n, 25–27, 35,
      93n, 271, 277–79, 288–89; case
      histories, 39–189, 202–19,
      289–306, 313–16, 375–77, 385;
      EEGs, 327–32; and L-DOPA,
      65–66n, 235n, 236–43, 244n,
      250, 255–57; MAO inhibitors
      and, 335n; symptoms, 14–20,
      361–62n; unhospitalized, 202n,
      306
post-encephalitic syndrome, 5, 6, 8,
      20–23, 148–49; and age, 314–15;
      incubation period, 161n; L-DOPA
      and, 304
posture, 284–85; disorders of, 42,
      90, 181, 184; Parkinsonian,
      193
predictability of science, 353
prehuman behaviors, 55–56n, 231–32n
presence, pathological, 9–11, 14
Prigogine, Ilya, 353, 354–56, 365
Proust, Marcel, 260–61n
pseudo-Parkinsonism, 235n
psychically caused symptoms, 49, 53n
psychic influences, 65n

psychoses, 17–18, 161, 252n; reactions
      to L-DOPA, 72–73
pulsion (push), 6–7, 43
punishment, illness seen as, 183, 207

Rachel I., 188–89, 244n, 257, 267
radical medicine, 280
radio adaptation of *Awakenings,*
      371–73
rages, 142, 180, 184; with L-DOPA,
      185–86
rationalization of tics, 136
reactions to L-DOPA, 248n, 254n,
      351–65; individuality of, 228,
      259–62
Reeves, John, 371–72
reflexive states, 249n
relationships, 26; dependent, 213n;
      therapeutic, 66, 115, 126–27,
      160, 178–79, 226n, 272, 281–82,
      292
retarded motions, 162n
rigidity, 5–6, 15, 27n; of Parkinson's
      disease, 193, 199. *See also* case
      histories
Robert O., 88–94, 296
Rolando P., 116–28, 303
romantic science, 287
Rosalie B., 330
Rose R., 16, 72n, 74–87, 201n, 206,
      260, 264, 290, 327–28, 369,
      370–71
Ross, Carmel, 372n, 378n

Sachs, Bernard, 13n
sailing, 349
Sam G., 82–83n
Samuels, Jackie, 373, 380
scale: disparities of, 340–44; measures
      of, 346–48
schism, tendency to, 262n
schizophrenia, 15–16, 214–15n;
      L-DOPA and, 243–44n, 261–62;
      misdiagnosis, 278n;
Schopenhauer, Arthur, 247
science, predictability of, 353
scientific medicine, 285–87
scintillating tics, 110n
selegiline (Deprenyl or Eldepryl), 336
sensitivity to L-DOPA, 107, 196–97,
      218, 236, 248n, 307–8, 352
severity of disease: and
      accommodation, 267; and L-DOPA
      effect, 236, 244
sexual arousal, with L-DOPA, 119–21,
      122, 210–12, 214, 216
Seymour L., 235n, 343–44
Shaw, Richard, 321

side-effects of L-DOPA, xxxvii, 48, 250, 262, 245–46. *See also* adverse reactions to L-DOPA
Siegel, Ralph, 357
skin disorders, 134
sleep: adequate, 268–69; disorders of, 13–14n, 88, 129, 149–50
sleeping sickness. *See encephalitis lethargica*
sodium amytal, 58
somatic compliance, 18, 65n
space, Parkinsonian perceptions, 339–49
spasticity, 6n
Spitz, R. A., 127n
sporadic cases of *encephalitis lethargica*, 321
sports abilities, 24n
stage version of *Awakenings*, 373
stationary states, 111–12
Stern, Gerald, 10n
stimulants, addictive, 252n, 326
stimulation, response to, 254n
strengths, personal, 266–75
stress: and Parkinsonism, 191–93n; L-DOPA and, 269–70
striatal dopamine, 336
subcortical function, studies, 15n
substantia nigra, 15n, 32–33; damage to, 334–36
sudden-onset Parkinsonism, 333–37
suggestion, 270
supreme moment, addiction and, 253n
surgical treatments, 27n, 32n, 117
swimming, therapeutic effect, 6n, 125
Sylvester, James Joseph, 274n
Symmetrel, 58
synkinesis, 250
synthetic opiate, brain damage from, 334
syphilitic Parkinsonism, 235n
systems, chaotic, 355n

technological medicine, 226n
thalamotomy, 27n, 192n
therapy, 268
thirst, excessive, 148, 149, 153, 155
thorazine (Largactil), 105, 157, 185
thought, speed of, 8–9n, 136
tics, 16–17, 18, 73n, periodicities, 360n; phases, 364; response to L-DOPA, 253n. *See also* case histories
Tighe, Lillian, 377–78
time-lapse, reactions to, 72n, 82–83, 87, 100–101n
tissue transplants, 34n
titration, 248n, 251
topism, mystical, 30–31n

Topist neurology, 240
torticollis, 6n, 16, 171
Total Institution, 64–66
touch, therapeutic, 60–61n, 281–82, 349
Tourette's syndrome, 24n, 55n, 103n, 110n, 122n, 132n, 293, 380; drawings, 155n; treatment, 252n
toxic Parkinsonism, 235n
trance-like states, 75–77; EEGs, 327–28
tranquillizers, 5, 58, 252n
transfinite cardinals, 249n
tremor, 3, 5–6, 15, 27n, 360; of Parkinson's disease, 193, 199
Trétiakoff, C., 32
tribulation, 243–65, 266n, 328–29
trismus, with L-DOPA, 203
turbulence, 354

understanding: diagnostic, 226n; of Parkinsonism, 7–8
unease, 250
unpredictability of response, xxxv–xxxvi-n, xxxvii, 353–54

The Varieties of Religious Experience, James, 324–25
Vaughan, Ivan, 64n
viral diseases, 321
Vogt, C. and O., 32
von Economo, Constantin, 12, 13n, 14, 32, 319, 320–21
voracity, 121, 155, 156, 177, 187, 210–12

water, therapeutic effect, 6n, 125
weather, 354
weight-loss, progressive, 93–94
Wells, H. G., "The New Accelerator," 103n
Weschler, Lawrence, 166n
Whose Life Is It, Anyway?, 378n
Wilbur F., 24n
will: absence of, 9; perversions of, 7n
Williams, Robin, 375–86
Wilson, Kinnier, 13n, 33, 252
Winfree, Arthur T., 360
Wings (play), 378n
Wittgenstein, Ludwig, xviii, 227n, 232
work, therapeutic, 164
writing: compulsive, 104–6; therapeutic, with L-DOPA, 212–13

youthful appearance of post-encephalitic patients, 77, 87, 143, 204, 309

Zaillian, Steve, 274, 285